Chris Carmichael's
Food for Fitness

Chris Carmichael's

Food for

Eat Right
to Train Right

Fitness

CHRIS CARMICHAEL

with **JIM RUTBERG** *and* **KATHY ZAWADZKI**

Foreword by LANCE ARMSTRONG

G. P. PUTNAM'S SONS

NEW YORK

ıllP

G. P. Putnam's Sons
Publishers Since 1838
a member of
Penguin Group (USA) Inc.
375 Hudson Street
New York, NY 10014

Library of Congress Cataloging-in-Publication Data
Carmichael, Chris, date.
  [Food for fitness]
  Chris Carmichael's food for fitness : eat right to train right / Chris Carmichael with Jim Rutberg and Kathy Zawadzki; foreword by Lance Armstrong.
      p.   cm.
  ISBN 0-399-15194-X (alk. paper)
  1. Athletes—Nutrition.   I. Rutberg, Jim.   II. Zawadzki, Kathy.   III. Title.
  TX361.A8C37   2004
  613.2'02'4796—dc22   2004044623

Printed in the United States of America
10   9   8   7   6   5   4   3   2   1

This book is printed on acid-free paper. ♾

BOOK DESIGN BY TANYA MAIBORODA

To Mom and Dad:
You guys were my first coaches and my best. I love you.

CONTENTS

Part ③   Sports Nutrition from All Angles

FOREWORD
Lance Armstrong

AS ATHLETES, WE CAN ALL RELATE TO ONE ANOTHER BECAUSE
we share a common starting point. We all began as novices in our re-
spective sports, and no matter how skilled we became, we all remember
those first training rides. We learned the skills, we sought guidance from
those who came before us, and we improved.

When Chris told me he was writing a book on sports nutrition, I immediately lent my support to the project because I've seen firsthand the
effects that food can have on performance. Like many new athletes, I
paid little attention to what I ate when I started out, and for a while I was
successful in spite of the food I was eating.

Perhaps the biggest lesson I've learned about sports nutrition is that
paying attention to it can make your dreams come true, and neglecting
it can be your undoing. During the Tour de France, my teammates and I
are eating machines; we eat and drink constantly from the time we get up

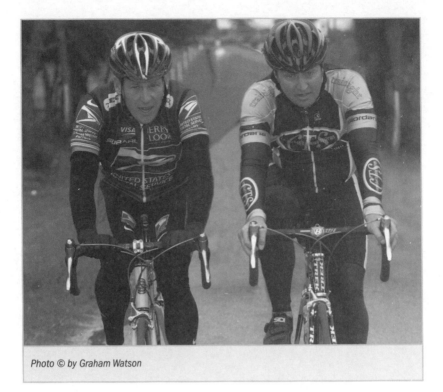

Photo © by Graham Watson

until we go to bed, and yet there have been times when I've felt that unpleasant feeling that comes when you know you're running out of gas. And in the end, all of the training and determination in the world can be undone by something as simple as eating or drinking too little.

Your goals may not include winning the Tour de France, but you should pursue them with the commitment and passion they deserve. I believe knowledge is a powerful tool, and the information and advice in this book will help you achieve your goals, just as it helped me achieve mine.

Chris Carmichael's
Food for Fitness

INTRODUCTION

"GO OUTSIDE" WAS PROBABLY THE BEST THING MY MOTHER ever told me to do, and she told me it all the time when I was growing up in Miami, Florida. Riding a bicycle was a fun way to get from here to there, so out I went, and in the heat of a southern-Florida afternoon, I could move fast enough to create a breeze. Even though there were several sports or games going on in the neighborhood on any given afternoon, I was much more interested in riding my bike. On a bike, I could get away. I could explore more territory, and even though I rarely rode any farther than the three miles to Biscayne Bay, I felt much more "worldly" than my friends who never ventured more than a block from home.

Competition didn't really interest me until I entered my first bike race when I was nine years old. The race couldn't have been more than two miles, but by the time I crossed the finish line in third place, I was hooked. I started riding more, but the concept of training never occurred to me.

As much as I loved cycling, I was really a pinball fanatic. There was an arcade on my way home from school, and on most afternoons, my bike was locked up outside as I honed my skills. One day, when I was twelve years old, I locked my bike up as usual and came out a few hours later to find it had been stolen. I walked straight into the bike shop that was next-door to the arcade and asked the owner for a job. I knew I was going to have to go home and tell my father I had lost my bike, but I wanted to be able to tell him I had a way to earn money to replace it. The owner of the shop gave me a job sweeping the floors, but he had a few conditions. I wasn't supposed to talk very much, and if he found out my grades were dropping, he would fire me.

The Dade Cycle Shop was a racers' store. There were racing bikes hanging in the windows, and it wasn't really the place folks took their children to get their first bicycles. The mechanics were all bike racers, and it was one of the only places in town where you could buy magazines that covered professional racing in Europe. When my work was done, I read everything I could get my hands on and listened to the mechanics telling bike-racing stories.

Working at Dade Cycle Shop was when I learned about the concept of training for the first time. Up to that point, I had entered a few races and done pretty well, but my "training" had merely consisted of riding my bike to and from school and Biscayne Bay. The racers who worked in the shop let me tag along on their training rides, even though I was several years younger than they were. Keeping up was difficult in the beginning, but they helped me learn about staying out of the wind and pacing myself. Within a few months, I was able to hold my own.

Though the racers from the shop taught me a great deal, there were several lessons I had to learn on my own. They were the same lessons all active people learn at some point: exercising in the afternoon after skipping lunch leaves you lightheaded and delirious, chili dogs should not be eaten right before hard workouts, and in a pinch a candy bar and a Coke will get you home.

Getting Serious

As I started going on longer and harder training rides, my mom noticed I was always hungry. Even though I was younger and smaller than either my brother or sister, I was soon eating much more food than they were. Meals at our house were almost always healthy; Mom cooked meat, chicken, fish, or pasta, and there was always some form of a vegetable and a salad. I didn't eat anything different than what everyone else in the family was eating; I just ate *more* of it. When I was living at home, I never had a problem getting enough food to fuel my exercise habits.

After I finished high school, I started traveling more to compete in higher-level races, and that was when I realized there was a connection between what I ate and how I performed on the bike. With my food budget largely dependent on the amount of money I was earning through race winnings, and with my sporadic ability to win any money at all, there was no way I could afford to buy or prepare meals like the ones I had eaten at home.

As a natural consequence, I started eating less, even though my activity level was higher than ever. My weight started to fall, and though many people would have seen that as a positive thing, I didn't have any excess weight to lose. My body was searching for energy, and it found what it needed in my muscle tissue. I started losing muscle mass, and with it, the ability to train and race effectively.

Lack of food was affecting my ability to achieve my goals, and I quickly realized I was setting myself up for a vicious cycle. Being successful in races was my only means of earning the money I needed in order to eat more. But I couldn't be successful in races unless I could train effectively, which I couldn't do unless I had more to eat. The dilemma forced me to change my view of food.

Fueling the Fire

I started to look at food solely as fuel. My goal was to get as many calories and as much energy as I could for as little money as possible. Grocery shopping took on a whole new meaning. The grocery store was like a fantasy world, with aisle upon aisle of wonderful, tasty, nutritious foods I couldn't afford. Every week I would walk up and down the aisles for up to two hours, looking at all the things I wanted to eat. But by the time I reached the checkout line, I had the same old assortment of rice, pasta, canned foods, potatoes, and mystery meat. I saw fresh fruit and vegetables as luxury items I could only buy when they were on sale, and even then I still went for the cheapest stuff: bananas, oranges, or apples. Salads were almost completely out of the question: Although I could buy the lettuce, it was too expensive to buy all the rest of the ingredients that go into a salad. More important, I could buy several meals' worth of pasta or potatoes for what it would have cost me for one good salad.

To add even more complication to my food situation, I was traveling up and down the East Coast with a friend, living out of a van. We had a cooler we could fill with ice, but nothing we could use to cook anything. We found places to stay in the houses of friends and strangers, and we cooked as well as we could in their kitchens. Perishable items like fruits, vegetables, meat, and dairy products didn't travel very well in those conditions, so they usually had to be purchased and eaten in the same day.

For aspiring athletes in any competitive sport, life is often feast or famine. When you win prize money, you eat well and splurge on things like good cuts of meat and chicken, spaghetti sauce from a bottle instead of a can, and fresh vegetables like broccoli, squash, spinach, and avocados. If you do really well, bring on the ice cream. When times are lean and you barely have the gas money to get to your next event, it's back to pinto beans, potatoes, canned tuna, and peanut butter.

Professional Bliss

I spent the early '80s racing as an elite amateur in the U.S. and Europe, and I was selected to the 1984 U.S. Olympic cycling team. Not long after the Olympics in Los Angeles, I signed a contract to race for 7-Eleven, the newly formed American professional cycling team. The team was going to split time between racing in the U.S. and in Europe, but the big goal was to get into the Tour de France.

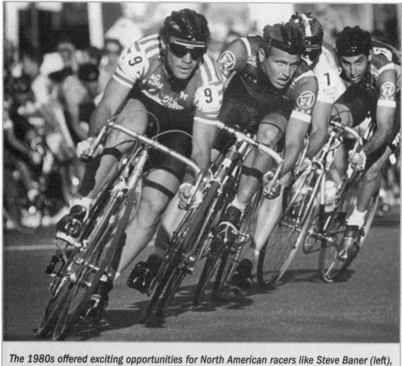

The 1980s offered exciting opportunities for North American racers like Steve Baner (left), me, and Doug Shapiro (far right). Photo © Chris Carmichael

Cycling was a European sport, as it still is, and in the early '80s, Americans, Kiwis, Aussies, and Canadians all started to infiltrate the European peloton. We were all outsiders, invaders of a sort, and we had to prove our right to stay. The racing and lifestyle were difficult, but I think we all felt a pioneer's pride that sustained us through the worst of it. I wanted to conquer the world, and every racer and director who cursed my presence strengthened my resolve to stay and succeed. Along the way, there were a lot of cultural and language barriers to overcome, and by 1986, when the 7-Eleven team became the first American team to enter the Tour de France, I think we all understood obscenities in six or seven languages.

As a professional cyclist with a paycheck and a share of the team's haul of prize money, I was finally able to increase the quality and variety of my diet. Of course, that was only true when I had any control over what I was eating. We traveled and lived together for weeks at a time, and the team usually ate together in the hotels where the race organizers had booked us. Dinner and breakfast were whatever the hotel chef had available and knew how to make. Lunch was usually eaten on the bike if you were racing, or in a roadside café if you were training.

In the end, at least nutritionally, I wasn't much better off than when I had been traveling around the U.S. as an amateur. Every hotel chef in France seemed to cook off the same menu, and since the hotel was trying to feed the whole racing team (and sometimes two or three teams), as well as all the support staff, they shopped the same way I had back home: buy the most food for the least amount of money. We just couldn't seem to get away from pasta, potatoes, and mystery meat.

When I was in Italy between races, I could take advantage of the great local markets that exist in every European town. There were farm-fresh vegetables, dark breads, and wonderful cuts of meat. Although I was still viewing food primarily as fuel, I had grown to appreciate how it tasted as well. I took the time to learn to cook and looked forward to the times between racing trips to experiment with new recipes.

During the same period in the United States, the fast-food industry was exploding. Every time I traveled back to the U.S., the number of McDonaldses, Burger Kings, and Kentucky Fried Chickens I saw amazed me. I started seeing a growing disparity between the diets that Europeans and Americans consumed, but I didn't give it much thought. As an athlete, I was very self-focused, and as long as I could eat the foods that would allow me to perform at my best, it didn't really matter to me what other people were eating.

Trading Places

After suffering a broken femur in a cross-country skiing accident and three subsequent knee surgeries, I decided that 1989 would be my last year as a professional cyclist. I had spent more than ten years completely immersed in cycling, and I wasn't really sure what I was going to do afterward. While I was recovering from surgeries and making repeated returns to professional cycling, I had learned a great deal about exercise science and physiology. One of my primary teachers in that department was Dr. Edmund Burke, the physiologist for the U.S. Olympic cycling team and the author of several of the most respected texts on endurance training. He encouraged me to consider coaching as a career, and when Jiri Mainus contacted me to coach some junior development camps for USA Cycling, I decided to give it a try.

I quickly realized I enjoyed coaching and had an aptitude for it. One of Ed Burke's greatest gifts was his ability to explain complicated physiological principles in a way that anyone could understand, and it was one of the most important traits I learned from him. I found I was able to bridge the gap between sports science and the practical challenges facing the athletes I was working with, and I was proud to help develop some of the young, talented riders in the National Team program, including Lance Armstrong and George Hincapie.

After working as the Men's Road Coach for the 1992 U.S. Olympic cycling team, I was promoted to the position of National Coaching Director for USA Cycling and put in charge of delivering the most technically, psychologically, and physically prepared athletes to the Atlanta Olympic Games. After the Games, I wanted to try something different. One of the things I had trouble with at USA Cycling was that we had developed a tremendous amount of information and knowledge, but it was only available to elite athletes in the National Team program. I wanted to find a way to work with a broader scope of athletes and make quality coaching available to everyone.

The next few years consisted of standing by Lance during his fight against cancer, consulting for various companies within the cycling and fitness industries, and picking up individual coaching clients. The combination was critical because Lance's comeback from cancer challenged me as a coach, the consulting work exposed me to many types of business models, and my individual clients helped me become more customer-oriented.

The business model for Carmichael Training Systems began to crystallize in the spring of 1999. With the help of my wife, Paige, and Simon Essl, Carmichael Training Systems was launched that September.

Working with Lance Armstrong through his comeback from cancer to the top step of the Tour de France podium completely changed the way I approached coaching. After several surgeries and rounds of chemotherapy, Lance was a shell of his former self. His genetic gifts were still there, but the aerobic engine that had previously propelled him to a World Championship and two Tour de France stage victories had nearly vanished. Psychologically, he was a different man as well. Where he had been extremely self-confident in his abilities as an athlete, the experience of fighting cancer into remission had left him uncertain about his future and his goals. Throwing him back into the type of hard training he had previously endured was out of the question.

As a coach, I went back to the basics. The aerobic system is the limiting factor in endurance athletic performance, so we set about rebuilding Lance's aerobic engine. The major shift in my coaching methodology occurred a few months after Lance started training again. The old school of thought was to push an athlete very hard to fatigue him, then let him rest for a short while so he could repeat hard efforts again. In Lance's case, pushing him that hard led to such intense fatigue that he had to take one or two days off before he could perform again. The cycle was too hard on him physically and emotionally, and most important, we weren't seeing the results we wanted.

To solve the problem, I eased up on the training load by adjusting the intensity down a notch. Using heart-rate monitors and powermeters, I found the point at which his body switched from providing energy primarily from his aerobic system to providing it from his anaerobic system. When I kept primarily using his aerobic system, he could exercise longer, recover more quickly, and maintain his motivation better. The really phenomenal result was that his fitness started improving by leaps and bounds.

I also applied a similar idea to Lance's nutrition program. At the same time I was focusing his training, I focused his diet as well. I knew that in order for him to progress, he had to match the fuel he was taking in with the work he was putting out. And as the months passed and his training changed, so did his nutrition program. During portions of the year when the nature of his workouts meant burning more carbohydrate or relying more on fat, he consciously modified his diet. This concept of periodizing eating in much the same way as you periodize training is a central idea in this book and will be discussed in more detail in later chapters. I've successfully applied these concepts to beginner through world-class athletes with strikingly similar results:

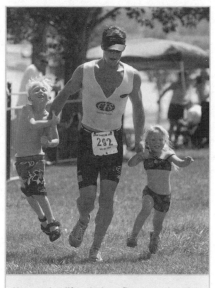

Your active lifestyle benefits more than just you; share the fun with the people around you. Photo © by Cliff Grassmick

more energy, better performance, faster progress, and optimal body weight.

Less Pain, More Gain

The concept of training with less pain for more gain was born, and by the end of July 1999, we had proven that this new training methodology could prepare an athlete to win the most grueling athletic event in the world, the Tour de France.

Since 1999, Carmichael Training Systems coaches have applied the same coaching methods I use with Lance Armstrong to help thousands of amateur and recreational athletes achieve their goals.

In the beginning, the majority of the athletes that worked with CTS coaches were cyclists, but as the business grew, I started noticing that people were signing up to achieve a wide variety of goals. Some people were looking to improve performance, some hoped to lose a little extra weight, and still others were seeking the motivation and direction a coach could provide. When I took a step back to consider the bigger picture, I realized that the group of athletes my company was working with represents a distinct and growing population in the United States: active people.

You're Your Own Breed

You might be an accountant with two kids and a passion for cycling on the weekends, or you could be a mother of three trying to balance the needs of your children and your need to run to maintain sanity, or you might have a secret desire to enter the triathlon being offered in your city next spring. Regardless of your profile, you are already an active person who has made the commitment to exercise for health, fitness, well-being—maybe all three.

But what does an active person like you need to eat in order for you to achieve your health and training goals? As you read, I'm going to give you a blueprint to help you match your eating to your activity level. You'll also learn some of CTS's revolutionary training methods, which have been proven effective over and over in the professional and amateur athletic arenas. Mostly, I want to provide you with the information that pertains directly to you, but has been missing from previous nutrition and diet books.

As you approach this book, take a look at the four sections we've created. First, we'll cover some circumstances that make athletes a unique segment of the population. Next, we'll delve into the nutrients your body needs, the best ways to get them, and ways you can tailor your diet to fuel your activity level. Third, we'll cover sports nutrition for specific groups, from adolescent nutrition (parents: a must-read!) to nutrition for Masters athletes. Lastly, our fourth section provides great performance and recovery recipes, sample meal plans, and suggestions to put all of this information to practical use.

The New Training and Nutrition Revolution

My hope is that by the time you finish this book you will think of food in a new way: as the fuel that enables you to achieve your dreams and goals.

In this context, each and every nutrient plays an integral role, and each will enhance the type of activity you are pursuing. As many books as I've read, written, and collaborated on, I will be the first person to tell you that a relationship with a coach will help you progress faster and farther than any book can. The concepts, principles, and ideas in this book have to be applied to your unique situation and personality in order for them to work, and that can be difficult to do without the help of a coach. That's why we're offering a free month of CTS Nutrition Coaching to everyone who purchases this book. (You can find more details on how to take advantage of this offer on page 415.) Working with a coach for fitness and nutrition is new to many people, but I believe it can be of real benefit. By utilizing the methods that have worked for thousands of athletes and active people, both amateur and professional, you will learn to make food your ultimate fuel for optimal performance.

Chris Carmichael, January 2004

PART

What It Means
to Be an Athlete

1

FOOD FOR FITNESS

Welcome to the Privileged Minority

For too long, active people in the United States have been a marginalized segment of the population. You are a minority group living in a society struggling to cope with serious health issues. Most of the books and health-related information available out there are targeted at the majority, making it difficult for you—an active person—to discern what information applies to your specific needs.

I'm sure the people who wrote many of the most popular diet books had the best of intentions. They wanted to help people lose weight and lead healthier lives, but they approached the subject almost entirely as a problem with the foods people eat. Many nutritional approaches focus on treating a problem, pitting nutrient against nutrient in a battle over what (if anything!) can be consumed. The assumption is that some food

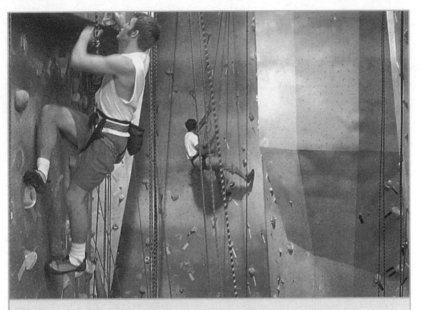

Exercise is an integral part of an active person's lifestyle, and a means to achieve personal, health, and fitness goals. Photo © by Craig Watter Photography

has to go; but instead of eating less of everything, they eliminate a whole category of nutrients. Overweight people lose weight, but active people lose energy. Rather than focus on food first, I focus on exercise as the key to achieving weight loss and fitness goals. And when you focus on exercise first, you immediately realize that all foods have their place in an active person's life. To fuel your workouts and reach your goals, you have to eat a balance of carbohydrate, protein, and fat. The foods you stopped eating after reading popular diet or nutrition books could be the very ones that, as an active person, you need to achieve your athletic goals.

Watching the National Waistline

It's not difficult to see that the health status of the American population has been declining for decades. In the past forty years, rates for overweight and obesity have reached epidemic proportions, and now we also lead the world in the incidence of cardiovascular disease. According to data from the most recent National Health and Nutritional Examination Survey (NHANES 1999–2000), nearly two-thirds of adults in the U.S. are overweight (Body Mass Index [BMI] > 25), and over 30% of adults are obese BMI = 30 or more). The incidence of overweight and obesity has increased for all racial and ethnic groups, both genders, and all age groups. One of the most striking examples is the prevalence of overweight and obesity among children, which increased threefold between 1980 and 2000. Excessive bodyweight has been shown to be a contributing factor in the development of heart disease, stroke, certain types of cancer, Type 2 diabetes, arthritis, respiratory problems, and some psychological disorders, including depression. While genetics play a role in the development of many diseases, lifestyle-related factors including nutritional choices, smoking, substance abuse, and exercise significantly influence your chances of staying healthy.

The government and medical professionals initiated three major responses to America's growing waistlines and diminishing health: diets, medical interventions, and exercise. As you might have noticed, over the past few decades, diets and medical interventions have been the more popular choices by far, but have yet to lead to lasting results for many people. Those people who proactively increased their activity levels by participating in exercise programs, however, have significantly improved their health and quality of life.

Why are diets and medical interventions more popular than exercise for controlling body weight? Because they don't interfere with your schedule. Let's face it: It's easier to pop a pill or simply eliminate certain foods from your diet; your work schedule stays the same, and you can still spend time with your family. On the other hand, making time for exercise can be difficult. Believe me, as the husband of a (great and wonderful) wife, the father of two incredible kids, and the owner of a growing company, I don't find training time easy to come by. My kids and my family come first, but I do my best to fit exercise into my schedule at least four times a week because I know it's the best way to stay healthy.

The health of the American population will *not* be dramatically improved by only changing the foods we eat or discovering a new wonder drug, because neither the foods nor the medicines address the whole problem. The results so many people have been looking for can really be achieved by combining exercise with a varied and complete diet. Active people have already figured this out, and your moderate-to-high level of fitness has improved your quality of life and reduced your risk of developing several diseases.

Dinner Outgrew Its Plate

For a long time, the standard round dinner plate bought by restaurants was 10 inches in diameter. When portion sizes grew to the point at which the food no longer fit on the plate, restaurants began ordering 12-inch plates, which is the new standard. Larger portions appeal to our sense of value, a fact not lost on marketers and restaurateurs. Everyone likes to get more for their money, and some studies have shown that larger portion size is one of the factors consumers consider when choosing restaurants. The increasing popularity of buffet-style restaurants illustrates the extreme end of this trend.

Increasing portion sizes aren't difficult to find; just visit any sit-down restaurant or fast-food joint. Consider the option to increase the size of your French fries and drink at fast food restaurants (McDonald's had "Supersizing," Wendy's has "Great Biggie," and Burger King has "King Size"), or the advent of the 64-ounce "Double Gulp" from 7-Eleven. Even movie-theater popcorn has increased in size, to the point that a typical large popcorn with butter contains over 1,500 calories and more than 120 grams of fat. There's even evidence that portion sizes have increased more rapidly in the United States than in other countries. Identically named fast food products (large fries, large soda) weigh more in the U.S. than they do in the United Kingdom and Italy.

Over the past few decades, the activity level of the average American adult has also decreased. The technological advancements that have made our lives more efficient and comfortable have also led us to become more sedentary than ever before. Our reliance on automobiles, even for the shortest of trips, as well as our utilization of computers, dishwashers, washing machines, and ridable lawn mowers have reduced the amount of energy we expend on normal daily activities. Here's the scary part: As the amount of energy we expend each day has decreased, the amount of food we consumed has increased. Comparing dietary-intake surveys from the late '70s to similar surveys today, you can see a per-capita increase of about 200 kilocalories per day. Similar research shows that the food supply in the United States (total food produced, plus imports, less exports) now supplies about 500 kilocalories per person per day more than it did in the 1970s.

High Fat vs. Low Fat

Over the past twenty years, there has been a big movement to reduce the amount of fat in the typical American diet. Even the U.S. government got involved because the health benefits of a low-fat diet were so influential. They led to changes in government policy, affecting nutrition programs in schools, hospitals, and the military. The American Dietetic Association replaced the Four Basic Food Groups with the Food Pyramid in an effort to reduce fat intake and improve the health of Americans. After a lot of time, money, and effort, the eating habits of Americans shifted and we started eating less fat. During the same period of time, however, the incidence of overweight, obesity, and cardiovascular disease continued to rise. What happened? Were the researchers wrong about fat?

No, they were right to recommend that Americans reduce their fat intake, but we misinterpreted what we were told. We heard the part about a reduced fat intake leading to a reduced risk of disease, and figured that meant we were free to eat anything we wanted as long as it was low in fat. The food companies helped out by pumping out hundreds of new, low-fat versions of our favorite snacks. But instead of eating a few low-fat cookies, we ate the whole bag. We switched from consuming high-fat foods to consuming an overabundance of low-fat carbohydrate foods. In another twist of misinterpretation, carbs got blamed for the resulting weight gain, even though the increase in calories and our continued lack of physical activity were the real culprits.

Eat Right to Train Right

The American College of Sports Medicine's recommendation for getting adequate exercise is to walk 30 minutes, at least three days per week. This recommendation was not designed with you in mind; they wrote it for people who can't stand the idea of exercising. Your fitness level has already progressed way beyond the point at which ninety minutes of walking each week would have a positive effect.

Making Exercise a Priority

You are the people who get up early to train before work, take your workout clothes with you so you can exercise at lunch, and find ways to involve your children in your training program. Climbing stairs or walking to the far end of the parking lot doesn't leave you winded, and you secretly enjoy the way it feels when you first start to sweat. You are an active person, and the majority of the health and nutritional information currently available is not targeted toward you. You have already conquered the most serious problems afflicting the majority of Americans. Exercising regularly has already reduced your risk for cardiovascular disease, hypertension, diabetes, and the host of other disorders associated with being inactive and overweight. In contrast, the average American population is so sedentary that *any* activity would be a move in the right direction. In fact, during undergraduate and graduate-level classes on exercise prescription, students are taught that the number-one goal is to make an American *move*.

Active Eating for Active Living

In the context of an active, athletic lifestyle, food has to be thought of in a new way. We have to move beyond thinking about food as the primary determinant of body weight, and see it as the fuel that enables us to achieve our goals. I can't stand the old adage that you are what you eat. You're *not* what you eat, you're a combination of the things you eat, do, think, believe, and feel. When I'm working with Lance Armstrong to prepare him for the Tour de France, I am involved in every aspect of his

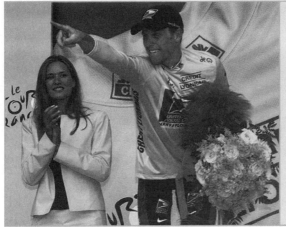

Lance Armstrong's ability to win the Tour de France comes from maximizing his potential in everything he does. Photo © by Graham Watson

life, from his training to his nutrition, his goals to his personal life. Achieving your goals and living a successful, enjoyable life is a matter of maximizing your potential in *every* aspect of what you do. A great training program integrated into a misguided life won't work, but when everything works together, you can achieve any goal you set your sights on.

My interest in sports nutrition stems from my years as an athlete and a coach, which means that I'm approaching the subject from the sports side rather than the nutrition side. While the clinical nutritionists, doctors, and researchers focus strictly on the foods, I'm focused on helping people achieve their fitness, weight, and performance goals. As a result, I see sports nutrition as just one component of an active person's overall performance plan. Omitting training from a sports-nutrition book is like giving you all the parts to a Ferrari engine without showing you how to put them together. By including extensive information on training combined with nutrition, I hope to help you fire up that engine.

Straight Talk About Calories

Nutrition and activity levels are inexorably linked, whether you're talking about performance or weight loss. It's misleading to promote the idea that what you eat doesn't matter as long as you only consume as many calories as you burn. The truth is, some foods provide better fuel than others, meaning more of their calories are clean-burning energy. Glucose (one form of carbohydrate) can burn hot and fast; foods readily broken down to glucose can efficiently provide clean-burning fuel. In contrast, burning lactose, a carbohydrate found in dairy products, is like trying to burn damp logs. It'll burn if the flame is hot enough, but it's troublesome and not your best first choice.

Not All Calories Are Created Equal

In terms of performance and health, it's also misleading to say that a calorie is a calorie, regardless of where it comes from. That's only the case after food is broken down to its simplest units, at the moment it is ready to be thrown into the metabolic fire—*then* a calorie is a calorie. In the process of getting from the grocery store to your cells, however, not all foods are equal. Some foods bring additional positive benefits along with their calories, while others bring either nothing or else ingredients that pollute your body and contribute to the onset of disease. Wholesome, unprocessed, or minimally processed foods bring vitamins, phytochemicals, minerals, and trace elements into your diet—nutrients that you need and benefit from but that you'd miss out on by eating only bleached white rice, refined sugar, and imitation cheese spread (also available in an aerosol can).

The quality of a given kind of food you consume directly influences the balance of nutrients versus pollutants that it provides. Peanut butter, for instance, can be a great source of protein, unsaturated fat, phytochemicals, and even vitamins. But low-quality peanut butter can instead be a source of a lot of unnecessary refined sugar and harmful trans-fat (partially hydrogenated oils). While we'd all like to eat only the highest-quality foods available, we often have to make choices based on price. It's not necessary for you to spend all of your money buying organic and unprocessed foods; many medium-priced options offer a good compromise between optimal health and performance benefits and the realities of living on a budget.

Straight Talk About Exercise

The Amount and Type of Exercise You Do Does Matter

It's about time we took care of some misleading statements about exercise. Dr. George Sheehan wrote many monthly columns for *Runners' World* magazine over a 25-year period, and in his last essay on running, published ten years after his death in the November 2003 edition, Dr. Sheehan provided one of the best explanations as to why athletes continue training. He wrote:

> We know that the effects of training are temporary. I cannot put fitness in the bank. If inactive, I will detrain faster than it took me to get in shape. And since my entire persona is influenced by my running program, I must remain constantly in training. Otherwise, the sedentary life will inexorably reduce my mental and emotional well-being.
>
> So, I run each day to preserve the self I attained the day before. And coupled with this is the desire to secure the self yet to be. There can be no letup. If I do not run, I will eventually lose all I have gained—and my future with it.

You May Never Regain the Fitness or Body You Had at Twenty-Two

Your fitness goals need to realistically take your lifestyle and priorities into account. It might be great to win races against guys half your age or fit into the jeans you wore in high school, but what would you have to give up to get there: the time you spend with your wife or kids, your next raise or promotion, the chance to go on a real vacation, or great food you've worked so hard to be able to afford? Life is a balance, and it's all right for training and competition to decrease in priority as you get older, so long as you remain committed to training at some level.

Training Doesn't Cancel Out Bad Decisions

The positive health effects of training should not be seen as a counterbalance to behaviors that increase your risk of disease. Abusing alcohol or tobacco products is hazardous to your health, no matter how fit you may be. Saturated fat and increased levels of LDL cholesterol increase athletes' risks of developing coronary artery disease the same way they do for sedentary people. Your fitness may reduce your risk, but it is not a license to eat irresponsibly or to expect few or no consequences.

There's No Perfect Training Program

If there was, it would have been published long ago and everyone would be using it to achieve the best performances. We are all different, and what works for you may not help your best friend at all. The perfect training program is the one that is built around *your* unique physiology and goals, and that works to improve *your* fitness.

There's No Shortcut to Success

Don't look to a supplement to make you stronger or a sports drink to give you the edge over the competition. They have their place in sports, but they cannot replace hard work. People start looking for shortcuts

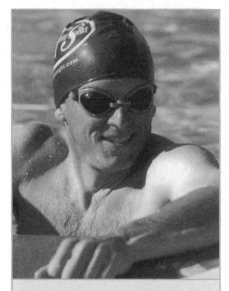

Mike Pigg, seen here coaching at a CTS Multisport Camp, earned his legendary status in triathlon by working hard and never seeking a shortcut to success. Photo © by @Porter Foto

when they lose respect for their goals. If you don't care enough about the goal to do the work to achieve it, you should find a goal that you're more passionate about.

Training Changes Throughout the Year

If you're doing the same workouts now that you did more than four weeks ago, you need to revise your training program. Not only does training have to progress in order to continue being effective, it has to be organized to develop your energy systems optimally and in the right order. It also has to have variety so you stay motivated and headed in the right direction.

Understanding Caloric Intake

Your body doesn't have a counter that resets at midnight, and there is no penalty for eating a little more one day and a little less the next. The difficulty with publishing recommendations for nutrition is that some people take them to extremes. If you recommend 3,000 calories per day, that's what they'll consume; no more, no less. Likewise, when I tell people they should slightly reduce their caloric intake during rest days and regeneration weeks, they nearly stop eating altogether. Eating a little less on days when you're not training as much doesn't mean cutting your caloric intake in half or skipping meals. It means pouring a little less cereal in the morning, putting a little less meat or cheese in your sandwich for lunch, and letting someone else have "the big piece of chicken" at dinner.

I don't want you to eat calories today to specifically balance out the energy you expended today. Your nutrition program has to supply the fuel for a machine that never stops running and that operates for varying amounts of time at every level from idling to full throttle. When you focus too intently on today's calories, you're trying to apply a static, immobile number to the dynamic, mobile environment in your body. That's too narrow an approach to nutrition. Instead, look at caloric intake over a rolling three-day window of time instead of looking at each day in isolation.

2

PERIODIZATION: THE ROAD MAP TO OPTIMAL PERFORMANCE

The Concept of Periodization

Long-term and dream goals can seem unrealistic and unachievable because the chasm between here and there seems too massive. You might be saying, *How am I going to run a marathon if I can't run a mile without stopping?* Or, *The last time I did yoga I was sore for days; how am I going to survive three classes a week, plus aerobic training?* I hear you. The best way to make goals less intimidating is to break them into smaller, more readily achievable pieces. Periodization is the process of breaking the year into segments so you progress through a planned series of steps. Sounds restrictive and highly regimented, doesn't it? In truth, periodization is just the opposite: it provides a road map to your goals and gives you the confidence and flexibility to make changes or deal with setbacks and still get where you want to go.

I've been using periodization with Lance Armstrong and all of my athletes for years. One of the reasons my coaching methods have been more successful than other periodized programs is that I extend the concept into the athletes' nutrition programs. Different training periods require different fuel mixtures, and when the fuel matches your demands, you reap huge rewards. Think of it in terms of a race car: When I was coaching Indy-Car driver Eliseo Salazar, he came to drive a race at the Pikes Peak International Raceway. We sat down to talk about his training and nutrition program, and he said, "You know, it's like in the car. When we come here, to high altitude, we have to run a different fuel because the air is so thin. The car won't run fast here with the fuel from sea level." Likewise, the food you eat to power your aerobic workouts in the winter isn't the right fuel mixture to achieve the speed and power you want in the summer.

How Periodization Works

I break the year into four big segments or mesocycles, known as the Foundation, Preparation, Specialization, and Transition periods. Each period is then broken down into four-week blocks, also referred to as macrocycles. Macrocycles are broken down into microcycles, which are typically seven days long to correspond with a calendar week. In summary, microcycles combine to form macrocycles, which combine to

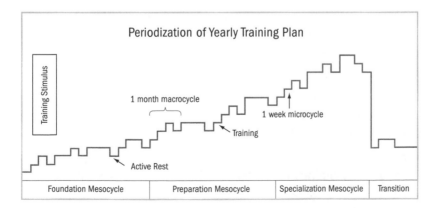

form mesocycles, and mesocycles work together to form a periodized training program that leads you to success.

The primary role of periodization is to arrange workouts and nutrition so that you reach your goals. Each period has a broad training goal, and each month in the period is focused on training that contributes to achieving it. The benefit of periodization is that by training the components of fitness individually, you can make greater gains in each component, and subsequently make huge gains in overall performance.

What Does Periodization Have to Do with Nutrition?

The amount of energy you burn changes as you go through weeks, months, and a full year of training. If you're eating the same basic number of calories all year, there is most likely a portion of the year when you're eating more food than you need. Likewise, there's almost certainly a portion of the year when your training burns more calories and demands more nutrients than you're consuming. As your training addresses different goals in different months of the year, you need to make sure you're eating enough food—and the right kind of it—to support your workouts.

Beyond the number of calories you're eating, your training also influences the *kind* of food you eat. As exercise intensity increases, so does the amount of carbohydrate you burn. When you're training harder and are more active than your nutrition program can support, you hinder your ability to make training progress and perform at your best.

You have to give yourself the fuel and recovery time to support your training load. During your peak activity season, it's great that you're out there burning energy—that's what you spent all that time training for— but don't waste all your hard work by shortchanging your performance with poor nutrition. The food you eat has to supply clean-burning energy for activity as well as nutrient-rich fuel to refill your tanks between exercise bouts, maintain the integrity of your immune system, and keep your muscles and other tissues healthy. To accomplish these tasks, you need to replenish the carbohydrates you burned so you can start your next workout with muscles full of glycogen. You also need to consume enough protein to produce the enzymes your aerobic system uses to burn carbohydrate and fat in the aerobic system.

Carbohydrate is the most versatile energy-producing fuel you have. It can be stored in a variety of forms, redistributed around the body as needed for energy or storage, generated from protein via gluconeogenesis (literally "making new glucose"), and utilized to produce energy rapidly for powerful activities and slowly for endurance activities. You can store far more fat energy than carbohydrate, but you can't do nearly as much with it.

Applying Periodization to Your Nutrition Program

The first step in applying the concept of periodization to your nutrition program is figuring out how much you are already eating. A three-day dietary record is the most effective way to do this, and you can enter the results into a nutrition software program to determine where your calories are coming from. This is the type of dietary record that CTS nutrition coaches use when they work with members. Don't bother with a five-day dietary record unless you really enjoy tracking everything you eat. The results you get after three days are very similar to the ones you'll get after five.

A dietary record is a good way to take a snapshot of your normal diet and examine it for its nutrient composition. You want to record everything you eat and drink for a full three-day period, keeping track of the portion sizes as well. Make sure the three days you choose for your record represent normal eating habits. For instance, your dietary recall shouldn't include Thanksgiving dinner, your child's birthday party, or your attempt to eat the 72-ounce steak at Billy Bob's Chowline just so you can get it for free.

When you view the analysis of your dietary record, realize that you most likely ate more calories than you said you did. I don't doubt your honesty; it's just that studies show that people consistently underreport nutrient intakes. The problem isn't so much from underestimating portion size (although that is a problem too), as it is from forgetting snacks, ingredients in combination foods (e.g., mayonnaise on a sandwich), or a side-dish from a meal.

The primary information you're looking for on your dietary-record report includes your total daily caloric intake and the percentages of that intake from carbohydrate, protein, and fat. You should also be able to find the grams of each macronutrient (carbohydrate, protein, fat). Some software will calculate your grams per pound for macronutrients, but many do not. To determine this number, divide the number of carbohydrate grams you consumed by your weight in pounds.

Make Changes Gradually

Making major changes to your nutrition program, like eliminating foods, altering the balance of nutrients, or changing your daily caloric intake by more than 500 calories, can be significant shocks to your body. Your body is used to the way you've been eating and training, and it has all the enzymes, hormones, and other substances that it needs to handle the load. When you make major changes, your body has to rapidly reestablish homeostasis (balance). In the process, you may experience gastrointestinal distress or fluctuations in energy as your body figures out how to process a new fuel mixture to meet new demands. If you make changes more gradually, the transition to burning new fuels for new demands proceeds much more smoothly. You also have a better chance of sticking to those changes long-term.

People drop out of exercise programs because they fail to integrate training into their already-busy schedules, or because their training doesn't match their goals or fitness level. If you're always struggling to fit exercise into your schedule, then it's time to carve a little permanent time out of your day that is reserved for exercise. For some of you, that might mean training before the day really gets going; for others, it might mean arranging your work schedule so you can take a longer lunch break or leave a little early a few times a week.

See It Through

Compliance, or lack thereof, is the number-one reason diets and exercise programs fail for many people. It doesn't matter if you're on the best nutrition-and-training program in the world; if you don't stick with it, it can't work for you. When you make small changes to your nutrition or training program, rather than large sweeping ones, you are more likely to make those changes a permanent part of your normal routine. For instance, if you're trying to change the composition of your nutrition program, focus on modifying your breakfast this week, stick with that change for an additional week, and then make changes to your lunch. Sure, you could make all the necessary changes in one day, but doing so significantly reduces the chances that any of those modifications will last more than a month.

Seek Advice

Arranging a training and nutrition schedule can seem overwhelming, and there are plenty of resources available to help you design the best plan for your needs. I encourage you to take advantage of the special nutrition coaching offer located on the last page of this book. Working directly with a coach is your best option, because studies have shown that people are most likely to stick with an exercise and nutrition plan when they are working one-on-one with a coach.

For those of you who don't want to work with a personal coach on an ongoing basis or feel you can't afford one, I'd suggest scheduling a few visits with a fitness-and-nutrition professional. During these visits, your goal should be creating the framework of a fitness-and-nutrition plan that you can live with. Make sure to keep a diary as you progress along this plan so you can show it to your fitness-and-nutrition professional in the future, especially when you want or need to make changes in your program.

Required Reading Before Applying Periodization to Your Nutrition Program

Understanding What You're Burning and When You're Burning It

It's important to realize that you burn carbohydrate, protein, and fat simultaneously whenever you exercise, regardless of the intensity of the workout. There is no such thing as an exercise that only burns fat, and there is never a condition where you can exercise effectively when you are totally depleted of carbohydrate, protein, or fat. Burning any one of these nutrients for energy requires the presence of the others.

Likewise, every time you exercise, you utilize all three of your primary energy systems: the immediate energy system, the anaerobic system, and the aerobic system. As the intensity of your workout changes, the percentage of your energy being delivered from each of these systems

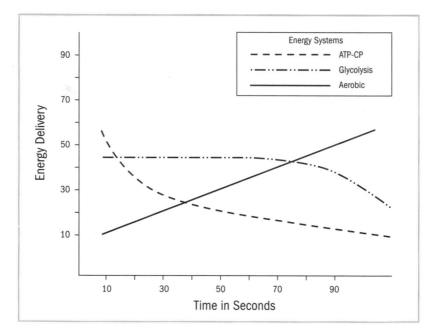

Adapted from Energy Yielding Macronutrients and Energy Metabolism in Sports Nutrition, *edited by Judy A. Driskell and Ira Wolinsky (Boca Raton, Florida: CRC Press, 2000), page 15.*

shifts; and with those shifts, there are changes in the amount of carbo-hydrate, protein, and fat being broken down for energy.

Several factors determine how cleanly your body operates. The foods you eat influence the availability of clean-burning fuels, and your fitness level influences the choices your body makes regarding which fuel to burn at what time. The cleanest way to burn fuel is with oxygen, using the aero-bic system. The immediate energy system is pretty clean too, but it's not a major energy supplier. In fact, it can only supply energy for about 8 to 15 seconds of work. The anaerobic system is the real troublemaker, though. It's absolutely necessary, and the energy it supplies gives you the power to accelerate, sprint, and lift weights; but it's also a dirty, inefficient, smoke-belching, self-limiting system. That's why your training and nutritional choices should favor the development and use of your aerobic system: the clean, efficient, high-energy, unlimited energy system.

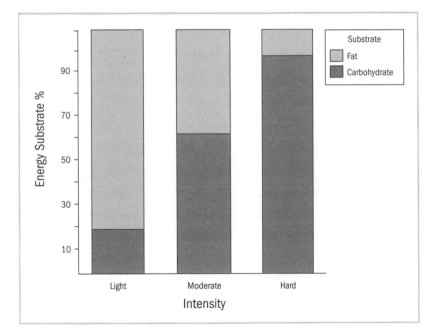

Adapted from Energy Yielding Macronutrients and Energy Metabolism in Sports Nu-trition, *edited by Judy A. Driskell and Ira Wolinsky (Boca Raton, Florida: CRC Press, 2000), page 22.*

At low intensity levels (20 to 25 percent of maximal effort), most of your energy is derived from fat. You utilize fat from food and that has been mobilized from adipose (fat) tissues, transported through the blood, and delivered to muscle cells. It's important to note, however, that in order for your muscles to burn fat in the aerobic system, carbohydrate has to be present. In conditions where your body is depleted of carbohydrate, the rate at which you burn fat decreases, and your capacity for high-intensity exercise disappears.

As the intensity of exercise increases to 40 to 50 percent of maximal effort, you're burning about a 50/50-percent mixture of fat and carbohydrate, and almost all of that fuel is being burned by the aerobic system. The carbohydrate you're burning is coming primarily from blood glucose and glycogen. The percentage of energy derived from carbohydrate increases as intensity increases, in part because you need energy more quickly than it can be liberated from fat. Interestingly, if it were possible to only burn fat for energy, you would be limited to exercise under 60 percent of your maximum effort. There is also some contribution from the anaerobic system, but at this level of intensity, it is very low.

The shift from deriving energy from a balanced mixture of fuels to burning much more carbohydrate occurs when you increase the amount of energy coming from the anaerobic system. Fat can only be oxidized through aerobic metabolism, but carbohydrate is burned aerobically *and* anaerobically, so when the aerobic system's relative contribution to energy production diminishes, the percentage of energy coming from fat decreases. However, the percentage of energy derived from carbohydrate steadily increases as exercise intensity increases.

The relative contribution of fat to energy production steadily decreases as exercise intensity moves from about 50 percent to 85 percent of maximal effort. This is the range where the aerobic system is still providing a large portion of your energy but can't completely keep up with the demand. The anaerobic system is providing some of your energy also, which increases the total percentage of energy coming from carbohydrate. As your exercise intensity increases above 85 percent of maximum effort, the percentage of your energy coming from fat

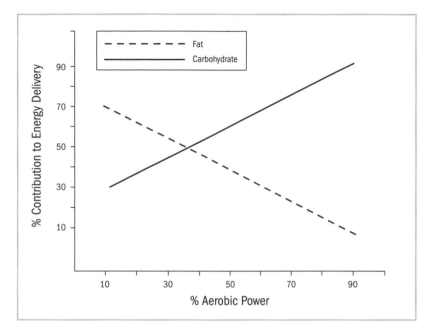

Adapted from Energy Yielding Macronutrients and Energy Metabolism in Sports Nutrition, *edited by Judy A. Driskell and Ira Wolinsky (Boca Raton, Florida: CRC Press, 2000), page 19.*

decreases even more, even though you're still burning a lot of fat. It represents a lower percentage because you're burning so much more carbohydrate.

I know this might be a little technical, but stay with me a bit longer. Training increases the work you can do at a given intensity or means you can do the same amount of work at a lower intensity than before. Some people with strong aerobic engines can operate at over 85 percent of maximum effort and still burn a balanced fuel mixture by continuing to rely primarily on aerobic metabolism. Other athletes may experience the shift to increased anaerobic metabolism at low intensity levels, like 70 percent of maximum effort. The goal of endurance training is to increase the work your aerobic engine can do, thereby increasing your ability to continue burning a mixture of fuels as exercise intensity increases.

What Does All This Mean for You?

People use this information in two ways: to determine the nutrients they need in order to perform in training or competition, or to determine the type of exercise they need to do in order to burn a maximum amount of a given nutrient. Dieters often focus on the latter of the two, and structure their exercise programs around burning fat. They advocate low-intensity exercise because it is primarily powered by energy derived from fat. It seems logical—you want to burn fat, so you exercise at a level that burns primarily fat—but it's not a very effective means of reaching your goals.

You may derive the highest percentage of your energy from fat when you exercise at low aerobic intensities, but when you increase your intensity to 45 to 65 percent of maximal effort, you burn more total calories *and* more fat. The *percentage* of energy produced from fat decreases, but the absolute amount of fat burned increases. Low-intensity aerobic exercise is also less likely to induce enough of a training load to improve fitness, especially for active people like you who have been exercising for a while. Since the intensity is so low, it would take hours of continuous work to overload the aerobic system and cause positive training adaptations.

Busy people like you want to use their time effectively. Most of the active people we coach at CTS have 60 to 90 minutes to exercise during weekdays. When their goals are reducing fat mass and improving body composition, increasing their workout intensity ups the total calories burned and amount of fat burned, as well as increases the training load applied to the aerobic system. My first goal is to improve their aerobic engine, because a stronger aerobic engine has the ability to burn more fat for fuel.

As an athlete seeking to improve your performance, you need to look at the type of training you are doing, then determine the nutrients you need in order to optimize the effects of that training. For instance, when you're training for endurance and your workouts are long but not very intense, you know you're going to be burning a balanced mixture of fuels for the vast majority of the workout. Your diet, therefore, should provide energy from carbohydrate, protein, and fat.

Improve Your Fitness with Heart-Rate Training

Your heart rate can give you a good indication of which energy system you are currently using, and the availability of accurate and affordable heart-rate monitors such as the Nike Triax models have made this valuable information increasingly useful. At CTS, our coaches use heart-rate intensities to prescribe training for athletes in a wide variety of sports, including running, cycling, walking, rowing, hockey, motorsports, and basketball. We use the CTS Field Test™ to determine the heart-rate

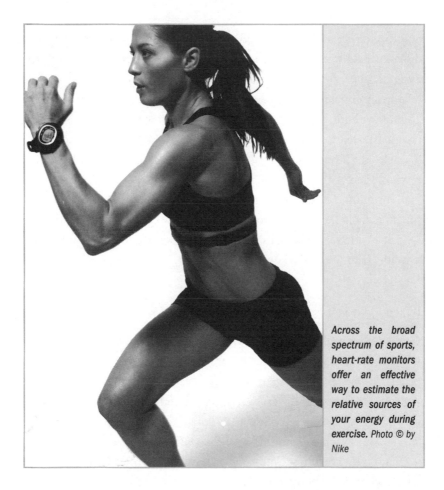

Across the broad spectrum of sports, heart-rate monitors offer an effective way to estimate the relative sources of your energy during exercise. Photo © by Nike

intensities that correspond to training different energy systems. This test is the cornerstone of the training programs we design for our members, so much so that we encourage new members to complete the CTS Field Test before we build programs for them.

Lance Armstrong has access to the most sophisticated laboratory equipment in the world, and yet I still primarily rely on field tests to evaluate his training progress. Lance doesn't compete in a lab, so I need to know how his training is affecting his ability to ride a standard bicycle, on regular roads, and in normal conditions.

The CTS Field Test

Since we coach athletes in a wide variety of sports, we have developed different field tests to determine members' fitness levels accurately and establish appropriate heart-rate intensities for training. If you were to take a running field test and apply the heart rates calculated from it to a cycling workout, your actual training intensity would be higher than it should be. Heart rates seen while running are higher than during cycling because you have to support more of your body weight, and thus use more oxygen. This can significantly change the effect a workout has on your training, because instead of stressing your aerobic engine, you might actually be stressing your anaerobic system. While we coach athletes in a wide variety of sports, the two primary exercise tests we use are a cycling field test and a running field test.

Which Field Test Is Right for You?

Generally, we look at the nature of your training activities to determine whether the CTS Cycling Field Test or CTS Running Field Test is more appropriate for you. If your sport is weight-bearing, meaning you are carrying your body weight on your feet, or significantly involves both upper and lower body muscles, you should complete the running field test. Such sports would include running, soccer, rowing, and cross-country skiing.

The cycling field test is more appropriate for athletes participating in sports where your body weight is largely supported by a machine. These

Are Motorsports Really Athletic Events?

Many people have inquired about the efficacy of aerobic training for motorsports, as the perception is that the machine is doing all the work. When I put a Nike Triax Elite heart-rate monitor on a race-car driver or a motocross rider, however, I quickly realize they maintain high heart rates all the way through their competitions, indicating that their aerobic engines are working hard. They are using a lot of muscle to counteract G-forces and maintain control of the machines. During competitions, Motocross Champion Tim Ferry has to race in several heats to earn his way into the finals. By improving the strength of his aerobic engine, Tim reduces his reliance on his anaerobic system during the early heats. This preserves his glycogen stores, allowing him to line up for the finals with more carbohydrate energy than his competitors. This gives Tim more fuel to power his muscles and his brain during the final, enabling him to make the split-second decisions that make the difference between winning and losing. We have noticed the same effects in our work with AMA Superbike champion Miguel Duhamel and Indy Car driver Eliseo Salazar.

sports include cycling and motorsports. I have also found that cycling is more effective than running for improving the aerobic conditioning of hockey and basketball players. These sports are more sprint- and power-oriented, and endurance running hinders players' performances in sport-specific practices. These athletes should utilize the cycling field test and integrate cycling training into their programs.

Interpreting Field-Test Data

While I will provide instructions on calculating specific heart-rate intensities for workouts in the appendix, the more important issue right now is to explain how heart-rate intensities correlate with fuel use. In the scientific literature, exercise intensities are usually described as a percentage of VO_{2max}, which can be defined as the maximal rate of oxygen uptake, delivery, and consumption by the body during maximal exertion. The trouble is, it takes sophisticated lab equipment to determine a person's VO_{2max}, making it an impractical measure of intensity for most of us.

I have found over the years that using average heart rates from the CTS Field Test, as opposed to VO_{2max} tests or maximum-heart-rate tests, yields better responses from athletes at all ability levels and minimizes any risk of over-training. I also prefer using average heart rates because they are indicative of an athlete's true response to the entire duration of the effort.

Lactate threshold is the exercise intensity at which you start to produce lactic acid, a byproduct of anaerobic metabolism, faster than you can process and clear it. As a result, the acid accumulates, which decreases your muscles' ability to generate power. You're creating lactic acid right now as you sit in a chair reading this book, but only a little bit, and your body can easily process it, so it doesn't accumulate. When lactic-acid levels in the blood rise dramatically, you have crossed over your lactate threshold and are generating a lot of your energy from your anaerobic system. Since this point correlates with a specific heart rate for a given activity (like running or cycling), we can say that your lactate-threshold heart rate determines the point where you go from primarily using your aerobic system for energy to primarily using your anaerobic system for energy.

The average heart rate you see from a CTS Field Test is usually slightly above your lactate threshold. While we know this from experience with thousands of athletes, we also know there is no way to confirm absolutely that this is true for you without lab testing. During an eight- to ten-minute all-out effort, most athletes are able to maintain an intensity above their lactate thresholds; if the test is longer, say 20 to 30 minutes, the average heart rate usually corresponds very closely with a person's lab-tested lactate-threshold heart rate.

Not only have I found that the CTS Field Tests accurately determine real-world training intensities for athletes of all ability levels in a variety of sports, but I have also found that they provide an easily understandable way to explain the way fuel usage changes as exercise intensity increases. More important, it helps you, as an athlete, apply this information directly to your own training and nutrition programs.

Sports scientists keep repeating their mantra that unless you know your lactate threshold and VO_{2max} as the results of a laboratory test, there's no way to absolutely know how your training intensities compare to these values. I agree with them, but I also believe that most people don't need exact numbers for lactate threshold and/or VO_{2max} to see improvement in their training. We've proven as much with the thousands of athletes who have been coached by CTS coaches. Less than 10 percent of our members have been tested in a lab, but they've all been on training programs designed with training intensities derived from their CTS Field Tests. These athletes continue to achieve their goals, from gaining fitness to losing weight, and from finishing their first 10k run to winning the Tour de France.

As a coach who works in the real world, I realize that active people need a good way to estimate the way their training intensities compare to physiological performance markers. The numbers presented below are approximate values and ranges based on what I have seen in more than 15 years of coaching athletes.

Percent of CTS Field Test Average Heart Rate	Heart Rate Range (based on 185 bpm* average from CTS Field Test)	Energy System(s) Providing Most of the Energy	Approximate Balance of Fuel Use (Carbohydrate-Fat) (excludes small contribution from protein)	Approximate Percentage of VO_{2max}
<65%	<120	Aerobic	30-70	20-35
65-85%	120-153	Aerobic	50-50	35-50
85-88%	153-163	Mostly Aerobic & Little Anaerobic	60-40	50-65
88-95%	163-176	Aerobic & Anaerobic	70-30	65-80
95-100%	176-185	Mostly Anaerobic & Little Aerobic	80-20	80-85
>100%	>185	Anaerobic	>90-<10	85-100

*beats per minute

For those of you who are familiar with heart-rate intensities for specific workouts, like those found in *The Ultimate Ride, The Lance Armstrong Performance Plan,* or a variety of magazine and website articles published over the past several years, you may notice that these calculations don't always correspond to the heart-rate values for CTS workouts. This is because heart-rate intensity is only one of several variables that determine the efficacy of a workout. The percentages in the preceding table are meant to illustrate the relative contributions of energy from carbohydrate and fat as exercise intensity increases. Heart-rate intensities for individual workouts will be described with the field test information in the appendix.

Reading the Ranges

In the next couple of chapters, I'm going to recommend ranges for carbohydrate, protein, and fat consumption in each of the four periods. One of the questions I am asked most frequently about this information is, *Well, how do I know if I should eat at the low end of the ranges or the high end?*

The answer to this question lies in your training load. As you'll read shortly, the recommendation for carbohydrate during the Foundation Period is 2.5 to 3 grams per pound. If you're training fewer than eight hours each week, shoot for the low end of the gram/pound ranges. Your goal would therefore be 2.5 grams of carbohydrate per pound. Athletes training between eight and twelve hours per week should shoot for the middle of the ranges, in this case 2.75 grams of carbohydrate per pound. If you're training more than 12 hours per week, you should be eating at the high end of the range. The table below illustrates the nutrient requirements for the Foundation Period, as correlated with weekly training hours.

Weekly Training Hours	< 8	8–12	>12
Carbohydrate (g/lb)	2.5	2.75	3.0
Protein (g/lb)	.50	.55	.60
Total Calories for a 165-lb athlete	2,750	3,025	3,300

For those athletes performing at a level that requires training more than 16 hours per week, your energy requirements may be even higher than those covered in the ranges given, and your nutrition program may be more complicated. If you're training that much, you're obviously very committed to performing at a high level, and you should invest some time and money to sit down with a nutrition coach to make sure you're getting the nutrients you need to perform at your best.

3

THE CARMICHAEL
NUTRITION PROGRAM

ALTHOUGH RUNNERS, CYCLISTS, CROSS-COUNTRY SKIERS, and soccer players use very different workouts in their training programs, they all benefit from training on a program that progresses through the four main periods of the year. The exact workouts a triathlete performs in the Specialization Period are completely different than those a cross-country skier performs, but the goals and the characteristics of the period are the same. Likewise, the nutritional characteristics of the Specialization Period would be very similar for athletes in these two sports, even though the exact food choices may be different.

Nutrition and Training Across the Four Periods

Across all sports, I've seen the positive results athletes achieve when they pattern their nutrition programs after their training. The concept is simple: When what you're burning for fuel and what you need for opti-

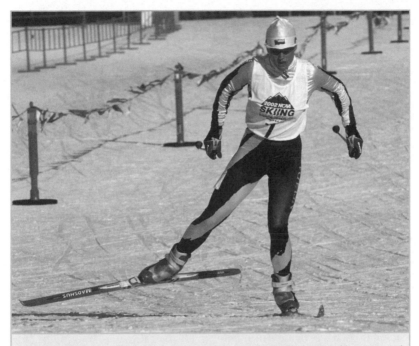

Katerina Hanusova, an Olympic cross-country skier, professional mountain-bike racer, and CTS member, uses sport-specific training and nutrition to maximize her performance.
Photo © by David Prediger/NCAA Photos

mal performance change, you need to change your nutrition program accordingly. Over the years, I've found that applying the simple concept of periodizing nutrition provides my athletes with everything they need to train and compete at their best.

I focus on ensuring that an athlete gets enough carbohydrate and protein to meet his or her needs by relating the characteristics of the training period to the person's body weight. I end up with a prescription for a certain number of carbohydrate grams per pound of body weight along with a certain number of protein grams per pound of body weight. I then use these numbers, in relation to the four periods of the training year, to estimate their goal for total daily caloric intake. Fat ends up being the remainder of their calories after calculating carbohydrate and protein. I've made sure the amount of fat in this program is relatively low, but not so low that people have to consciously spend time avoiding fat.

The key here, however, is that the human body doesn't care about mathematics. Any number you calculate that is supposed to predict or quantify what's happening inside your body or what it needs can only be regarded as an estimate. The numbers I calculate for my athletes, and the numbers you will undoubtedly calculate for yourself soon, are merely starting points. They may need to be adjusted up or down based on the details of your training program as well as your fitness and body-weight goals. However, for many of the athletes I work with, especially active fitness enthusiasts and amateur athletes, adjustments aren't necessary.

Determine Your Current Training Period

If you have not been training consistently and are just starting a training program, begin with the Foundation Period. Noncompetitive athletes, fitness enthusiasts, and active people sometimes have a little more trouble placing themselves in a training period. Historically, your training has remained the same all year, and it most closely resembles Preparation Period Training. There is an aerobic component and an anaerobic component to your training, but neither receives enough attention to lead to significant progress. Essentially, you have a choice, and your decision may be largely influenced by the time you have left before your goal. If you have several months before your goal event or active season, it would best for you to start with the Foundation Period so you can maximize the strength of your aerobic engine. If, however, your goal event is only a few months away, you should place yourself in the beginning of the Preparation Period.

I rarely recommend that anyone start a structured program in the Specialization Period. If you're in your most active season already, changing your training isn't going to do you much good. The modifications you can benefit from are to get more rest and make sure you're supplying your body with the nutrients it needs for success. Once your most active season is over, go straight into the Transition Period and progress from there.

If you're uncertain, this is one of the times when it is best to be conservative. Attempting to accelerate your progress can be risky and hard on your body. I'd rather see you arrive at your goal event healthy, fresh, and with a little less power than you could have had. The alternative is uglier: You're at increased risk of suffering an illness or injury that keeps you from participating in your goal event at all, or hinders your performance to a greater extent than being a little undertrained.

Periodization and Nutrition at a Glance

It is nearly impossible for anyone to doggedly adhere to fixed macronutrient intakes and percentages. It's not practical, or necessary, to weigh your food or pre-plan every meal so that it has just the right amounts of carbohydrate, protein, and fat. What's more, doing so would be to miss the bigger picture. There's nothing magical about eating 2.5 grams of carbohydrate per pound or making protein 14 percent of your total calories. These things need to be viewed as details of a much more far-reaching concept.

Here are my nutritional guidelines for average daily intake during training days. Intake on rest and recovery days should be reduced about 10 to 15 percent.

110-lb Athlete:

Period	Total Calories	Carbohydrate		Protein		Fat	
		%	Grams	%	Grams	%	Grams
Foundation	1,700–2,000	65	275–330	13	55–65	22	40–50
Preparation	2,000–2,400	65	330–385	13	65–80	22	50–60
Specialization	2,500–2,800	70	440–500	14	90–100	16	65–75
Transition	1,500–1,800	60	220–275	18	65–80	22	35–50

120-lb Athlete:

Period	Total Calories	Carbohydrate		Protein		Fat	
		%	Grams	%	Grams	%	Grams
Foundation	1,800–2,200	65	300–360	13	60–75	22	45–55
Preparation	2,200–2,600	65	360–420	13	75–85	22	50–60
Specialization	2,700–3,100	70	480–540	14	95–110	16	50–55
Transition	1,600–2,000	60	240–300	18	75–85	22	40–50

135-lb Athlete:

Period	Total Calories	Carbohydrate		Protein		Fat	
		%	Grams	%	Grams	%	Grams
Foundation	2,100–2,500	65	340–400	13	65–80	22	50–60
Preparation	2,500–2,900	65	400–475	13	80–95	22	60–70
Specialization	3,100–3,500	70	540–610	14	110–120	16	55–60
Transition	1,800–2,200	60	270–340	18	80–95	22	45–60

150-lb Athlete:

Period	Total Calories	Carbohydrate		Protein		Fat	
		%	Grams	%	Grams	%	Grams
Foundation	2,300–2,800	65	375–450	13	75–90	22	55–65
Preparation	2,800–3,200	65	450–525	13	90–105	22	70–80
Specialization	3,400–3,900	70	600–675	14	120–135	16	60–70
Transition	2,000–2,500	60	300–375	18	90–105	22	50–60

165-lb Athlete:

Period	Total Calories	Carbohydrate		Protein		Fat	
		%	Grams	%	Grams	%	Grams
Foundation	2,500–3,000	65	410–500	13	80–100	22	60–75
Preparation	3,000–3,500	65	500–575	13	100–115	22	70–85
Specialization	3,700–4,200	70	660–740	14	130–150	16	65–75
Transition	2,200–2,700	60	330–410	18	100–115	22	55–70

180-lb Athlete:

Period	Total Calories	Carbohydrate		Protein		Fat	
		%	Grams	%	Grams	%	Grams
Foundation	2,800–3,300	65	450–540	13	90–110	22	65–80
Preparation	3,300–3,900	65	540–630	13	110–125	22	80–95
Specialization	4,100–4,600	70	720–810	14	140–160	16	70–80
Transition	2,400–3,000	60	360–450	18	110–125	22	60–75

195-lb Athlete:

Period	Total Calories	Carbohydrate		Protein		Fat	
		%	Grams	%	Grams	%	Grams
Foundation	3,000–3,600	65	490–585	13	100–120	22	70–85
Preparation	3,600–4,200	65	585–680	13	120–140	22	85–100
Specialization	4,400–5,000	70	780–875	14	155–175	16	80–90
Transition	2,600–3,200	60	390–485	18	120–140	22	65–80

Seeing the Bigger Picture

Look at the year as whole, starting with the Foundation Period, and you should see trends develop. For instance, your caloric intake follows the same trend as your training. Caloric intake increases as training volume and intensity increase during the Foundation, Preparation, and Specialization periods. It then falls during the Transition Period so you can restart the cycle. Following this general trend is more important than strictly increasing your carbohydrate intake from 2.5 to 3 grams per pound. While changes in carbohydrate and protein intakes track together, fat intake rises through the Foundation and Preparation periods, then stays constant or falls during the Specialization Period. It can be a challenge to reduce fat intake while increasing overall calorie consumption, which is part of the reason the Specialization Period is relatively short. And in this case, the more important trend is the increased percentage of carbohydrate calories, as opposed to the reduction in fat calories. You can't be overly clinical when you think about nutrition, because that's not how you live your life.

Body Weight Across the Year

Following a periodized nutrition program, you will most likely notice that your body weight will stay nearly constant, if not decrease, from the beginning of Foundation through the end of Transition. Your fitness will improve, your performances will be better than ever before, and even though your caloric intake will increase for most of the year, your weight will stay roughly the same.

By patterning your nutrition program to match your training, you eliminate periods of the year where your caloric intake and energy expenditure are vastly mismatched. People who consume a low-calorie, low-fat diet all year out of fear of gaining any weight tend to eat as if they are in the Transition or Foundation Period all year. They usually encounter a more active period of the year when their caloric intake is far too low to meet their energy demands. They tend to lose weight during this time, which they view as progress, but their athletic performance suffers in the short term, and their training progress stagnates in the long term.

At the other end of the spectrum sits the athlete who eats like the Specialization Period lasts all year. He has no trouble meeting his energy demands during the most intense portion of his season, but he quickly gains weight through the Transition Period and spends most of the Foundation and Preparation periods struggling to lose it again. When your eating correlates to your training load, you naturally maintain a more constant body weight throughout the year without having to deprive yourself of food or force yourself to exercise longer just to burn off excess weight.

Nutrition and Training During the Foundation Period

Building Your Power and Strength from the Ground Up

The Foundation Period sets the tone for your entire training year because it is your opportunity to lay the groundwork for everything you want to accomplish in the Preparation and Specialization periods. I view training as the process of building the CTS Pyramid of Success™. While the details of all the Pyramid's levels are outside the scope of this book, I mention it because it is a great illustration of the importance of the Foundation Period. Located in the third level of the Pyramid, the Foundation Period is the first part of physical training and must support the weight of everything above it. The size and strength of this foundation determines how high you can build your Pyramid of Success. If you rush the Foundation Period and move on to Preparation too soon, you're limiting the heights

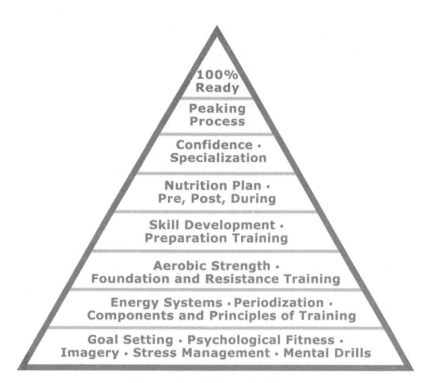

Figure 2: The CTS Pyramid of Success

to which you can aspire within this training year, and risking that the entire structure may collapse under the pressure applied later in the year.

The training during the Foundation Period focuses on aerobic development and strength training. Improving the power and capacity of the aerobic engine requires workouts that overload the aerobic system for prolonged periods of time. This means doing endurance workouts that are longer and of moderate intensity. You might exercise at a level you can sustain for an hour or several hours with minimal interruptions. The key is to maximize the amount of energy you are deriving aerobically while minimizing the energy contribution from your anaerobic system.

The Foundation Period lasts about four months, or four to five four-week training blocks. For people living in the Northern Hemisphere and participating primarily in summer sports, this period usually occupies the late fall and winter months (November to February, give or take a month or two). For folks who want to be in the best shape for winter sports, the Foundation Period would occupy the spring and early sum-mer months (May to August, give or take a month or two).

How to Get What You Need in the Foundation Period

Carbohydrate: 2.5–3 g/lb

The high volume and low-to-moderate intensity of the endurance train-ing in the Foundation Period mean you will rely on a balanced mixture of carbohydrate and fat for the majority of your fuel for those workouts. The longer the workouts, the higher the reliance on fat for energy, since your glycogen stores only last 90 minutes (2 to 3 hours if you eat/drink carbo-hydrates while exercising). During exercise lasting more than 90 minutes at intensities above 65 percent of maximal effort, fatigue sets in just as you deplete your muscle-glycogen stores. You have limited stores in your muscles and liver, and it makes sense that you're forced to slow down as your fuel tank nears empty. As you run out of high-octane fuel, your body must rely more heavily on fat for fuel. Although you have virtually un-limited supplies of fat, it doesn't supply energy as quickly. As a result, you can continue to exercise, but the intensity level you can sustain decreases.

Strength-training workouts will also place a high demand on carbo-hydrate stores, because strength-training activities like weight lifting and some styles of yoga and Pilates involve powerful movements. To rapidly get enough energy for these activities, you use your anaerobic system, which is almost entirely powered by carbohydrate. As a result, you burn through carbohydrate stores as well during these activities.

In order to ensure that you are ingesting enough carbohydrate to re-plenish your glycogen stores before your next endurance or strength workout, you should ingest 2.5 to 3 grams of carbohydrate per pound of body weight every day during the Foundation Period. For a 165-pound (75 kilogram) person, this would equate to about 410 to 500 grams of carbohydrate. As a total number, it might seem like a huge amount of food, especially considering it contains between 1,640 and 2,000 calories. However, when you spread those grams out over four or five meals and intermittent snacks, it is very easy to consume 100 to 125 grams of car-bohydrate in a meal or snack.

Protein: 0.5–0.6 g/lb

The Recommended Daily Allowance for protein is 0.8 grams per kilogram of body weight (approximately 0.35 grams per pound), and the average American diet provides close to twice that amount. For a long time, athletes have been gulping down massive portions of protein in the form of shakes, powders, raw eggs, tuna fish, and lots of meat. They figured they needed it for energy and for the amino-acid building blocks their bodies required for muscle growth and repair as well as immune-system maintenance. The problem is, science has shown that consuming above .9 grams of protein per pound per day (2 grams per kilogram per day) has no additional benefits. You can convert some of the excess to glycogen in the liver, and much of the rest is converted to fat for storage. Oversupplementation with protein is a waste of money.

As an athlete, you do need more protein than the RDA calls for, but the increase is small, and most people don't need heavy supplementation to meet it. Instead of 0.35 grams per pound per day, athletes in the Foundation Period should consume 0.5 to 0.6 grams of protein per pound of body weight. This means the same 165-pound athlete mentioned above would need 80 to 100 grams of protein to meet his or her needs. As I mentioned, this is not much of a challenge for most people because they are usually eating at least this much already. More often than not, I've reduced athletes' protein intakes as a means of controlling their caloric intake, because they've been consuming much more protein than they need or can use.

During the Foundation Period, the protein you consume is essential in providing the amino-acid building blocks of enzymes and structures that your aerobic system needs to improve its capacity to cleanly burn carbohydrate and fat for energy. Without these enzymes and structures, along with cellular powerhouses (mitochondria) that are made of amino acids, you wouldn't have the machinery and tools to break down the carbohydrate that you're consuming.

Total Energy and Fat

After determining the absolute amounts of carbohydrate and protein you should consume, it's time to figure out how much fat you need to consume. And no, it's not a typo; I really meant to say "how much fat you *need* to consume." As we'll cover in later chapters, there are different kinds of fat, and they perform many crucial roles in your body. From an energy perspective, research suggests that the only way to restore your intramuscular stores of fat is through ingesting fat. The fat in your love handles can be burned for energy, and it can be moved from storage in adipose (fat) tissue to storage in muscles. This is an important consideration because intramuscular fats may play an important role in fat's contribution to energy expenditure during aerobic exercise, especially prolonged aerobic exercise like that found in the Foundation Period.

Consuming too much fat, on the other hand, has well-proven and serious disadvantages. Excess fat is quickly and efficiently stored in adipose tissue, leading to increased fat mass. It can contribute to increased blood triglyceride levels and increased blood pressure, as well as to the development of cardiac disease and diabetes. Generally, as an athlete, you should keep your fat intake between 12 and 30 percent of your caloric intake, and further limit your intake of saturated fat to between 6 and 10 percent of your caloric intake.

Up to this point, I haven't mentioned carbohydrate or protein consumption in terms of percentages of total caloric intake, only grams per kilogram of body weight. However, after making a recommendation for fat intake based on a percentage of total caloric consumption, the natural question is: fat intake should be 12 to 30 percent of *what*?

Total Energy

I use the grams-per-pound value for carbohydrate as the basis for determining a starting point for total caloric intake and composition. Given the characteristics of the Foundation Period, you need to derive 65 percent of your total caloric intake from carbohydrates in order to support your training. Going back to our 165-pound athlete, consuming 2.5 to 3 grams of carbohydrate per pound of body weight yields a carbohydrate requirement of approximately 410 to 500 grams, or 1,640 to 2,000 calories. If this represents 65 percent of his or her daily energy needs, then total caloric intake needs to be approximately 2,500 to 3,000 calories.

Rather than determine a percentage for protein and then figure out how many grams per pound it would take to get that percentage, I determine the best absolute amount of protein an athlete needs and let the percentage work itself out. Keeping to the recommendation of 0.5 to 0.6 grams per pound, protein would contribute 80 to 100 (320 to 400 calories) for our 165-pound athlete and represent 13 percent of total caloric intake. Compared to nutritional trends that dominated the literature in the 1990s, 13 percent may seem very low; many popular nutritional programs advise 25 to 30 percent of calories from protein. I advise a lower protein percentage because I am basing it on the optimal number of grams per pound of body weight that your body can absorb, process, and actually use to balance your energy, recovery, and developmental needs. The fact that the percentage is lower is irrelevant because the important thing is to get the absolute amount your body needs.

Basing your protein intake on grams per pound is best because it gives you a much better idea of how much protein you need to consume. Since carbohydrate represents the largest portion of your total calories, and meeting those requirements can mean several meals or meals with relatively large portions, it is very easy for you to overeat protein. On your plate, the meal looks well-rounded because the high-protein food looks like it's in proper proportion to the larger carbohydrate portion. However, carbohydrate-rich foods like pasta, rice, potatoes, and vegetables tend to be less dense than protein-rich foods, meaning that a 100-gram pile of pasta takes up much more room than a 100-gram piece of chicken. Athletes, and all people, tend to dish food onto plates in ways that are appealing to the eye or look "normal," like they saw when they were kids or see when they go to restaurants. Oftentimes, when athletes serve themselves an appropriate amount of carbohydrate-rich food, they compliment it with an oversized serving of protein-rich food.

Fat

After the carbohydrate and protein intakes have been determined, the remainder of the calories in your nutrition program come from fat. During the Foundation Period, fat represents 22 percent of total caloric intake. The important caveat, however, is that the fat should come from healthy sources. You should be looking to meet this caloric requirement with monounsaturated and polyunsaturated fats, since they are less detrimental to your cardiovascular health than saturated fats and hydrogenated oils (trans-fats). Fats from vegetable sources, like avocados and nuts, contain none of the cholesterol found in fats from animal sources. And fats found in fish, both omega-3 and omega-6 fatty acids, have been shown to decrease the risk of developing some forms of cardiovascular disease. More details on fats, their sources, and their actions will be explained in Chapter 8.

Continuing to follow our example of the 165-pound athlete, 22 percent of 2,500 total calories works out to be 550 calories. Since there are nine calories in every gram of fat, 550 calories is the equivalent of about 61 grams of fat.

As I mentioned earlier, any numbers that are calculated to predict or explain what's happening in your body are merely starting points. For instance, it is unrealistic for anyone to maintain their caloric intake in exact proportions. Rather, the goal of presenting gram-per-pound values and macronutrient percentages is to help you understand the relative proportions of your energy that should come from carbohydrate, protein, and fat.

I have noticed that this is a very realistic approach for athletes. Before, when I recommended that an athlete consume 60 to 65 percent carbohydrate and 20 percent protein, their actual caloric intake soared well above what was recommended. The foods they were eating to reach their carbohydrate and protein requirements had enough obvious and hidden fat that they really struggled to keep the fat intake, and hence total caloric intake, down. In the end, the goal of eating more protein was leading to drastically increased caloric and fat intakes. Now, when I base protein intake on grams per pound and am less concerned with the percentage it works out to be, my athletes can more easily stay within their recommended caloric intakes; intakes that provide them with the energy they need to perform at their best, without the extra, unintended calories that lead to weight gain.

Foundation Period

Carbohydrate-Protein-Fat Percentages: 65-13-22				
Body Weight (pounds)	Total Calories	Carbohydrate (g)	Protein (g)	Fat (g)
110	1,700–2,000	275–330	55–65	40–50
120	1,800–2,200	300–360	60–75	45–55
135	2,100–2,500	340–400	65–80	50–60
150	2,300–2,800	375–450	75–90	55–65
165	2,500–3,000	410–500	80–100	60–75
180	2,800–3,300	450–540	90–110	65–80
195	3,000–3,600	490–585	100–120	70–85

Nutrition and Training During the Preparation Period

The Preparation Period follows the Foundation Period and builds upon the gains you've made in aerobic conditioning and strength. During this period, the intensity of your workouts will increase, and you will make the transition from gaining strength and power in the gym to becoming more powerful in your sport. The aerobic and strength work from the Foundation Period should have been specific to the demands of your primary sport, but your primary goals were to improve your aerobic engine's capacity and the amount of total work you could do. The Preparation Period is the portion of the year when you more directly apply your increased capacity to your specific sport or activity. As the higher-intensity workouts lead to their desired adaptations, you will feel faster, stronger, and more powerful than you did at the same time last year.

You don't just *feel* better; you are in fact stronger and more powerful because your aerobic engine can deliver more power than it could last year. This is very influential because it means that you can sustain a higher pace or power output before your anaerobic system has to kick in. And when your anaerobic system does start to contribute energy, it's starting from a higher level and can propel your performance to a higher total workload than ever before. The development of your anaerobic power is absolutely dependent on the strength of your aerobic engine.

Speed, Power, and Technique

For athletes in power sports, this is the portion of the year when a speed component should be added to your movements. The Foundation Period training increased your ability to generate force and repeat that action over and over with less fatigue. During the Preparation Period, your training should focus on performing the components of your sport or activity more quickly and with less recovery. For instance, football players may change their weight-lifting regimen to incorporate speed into their lifts. Instead of just squatting a given weight and focusing solely on the mass being moved, we're looking for the athlete to perform the lift faster and to accelerate the mass more quickly.

The Preparation Period typically lasts two to three months, or three to four macrocycles. For people living in the Northern Hemisphere and primarily participating in summer sports, this period usually occupies the late winter and spring (March to May, give or take a month or two). For folks who want to be in the best shape for winter sports, the Preparation Period would occupy summer and early fall months (September to November, give or take a month or two). This is the portion of the year where you start to develop the sport-specific speed, power, and technique that will be key to achieving your fitness or competition goals.

Since the volume of training is still pretty high and your intensity of training continues to build on the Foundation Period, your total energy requirement also increases as you enter the Preparation Period. The higher intensity causes an increase in carbohydrate usage, especially since your harder workouts call for a higher energy contribution from the anaerobic energy system. Your protein requirement also increases, since harder workouts cause more stress to muscles and your immune system.

How to Get What You Need

During the Preparation Period, you are still consuming 65 percent carbohydrate, 13 percent protein, and 22 percent fat, but the increased intensity of your training necessitates about a 15-percent rise in your daily caloric intake.

In order to meet your energy needs during the Preparation Period, you need to eat 3 to 3.5 grams of carbohydrate per pound and 0.6 to 0.7 grams of protein per pound. The amount of fat in your diet naturally increases along with the increases in carbohydrate and protein. The relative proportions of carbohydrate, protein, and fat are the same as they were during the Foundation Period; the only thing that changes is the amount of food you're eating.

Recommending an increase in grams of macronutrients per pound is more effective than asking athletes to increase their caloric intake by about 15 percent. When described as a percentage increase, 15 percent is perceived as a license to heap more food on your plate, but in reality it only has small effects on portion sizes. For most people, increasing carbohydrate intake from the Foundation Period to the Preparation Period is only an addition of 60 to 90 grams per day. Spread across four to five meals and other snacks, this represents small increases (15 to 20 grams— less than one ounce) during each meal or snack.

Children aren't the only ones who take a mile whenever you give them an inch. As a coach, I've found that recommending that an athlete increase caloric intake by 15 percent results in increases twice that high. All of a sudden, athletes who are working out longer and harder than they were two months ago start gaining weight. A few years ago, I was working with a very busy executive who wanted to lose some weight and throttle his cycling buddies on the weekend group rides. As a connoisseur of great food and wine, he was thrilled that increasing the intensity of his training meant he could eat more, but like so many people, he went overboard. Rather than increase his 1½-cup serving of pasta by half a cup, he doubled it to three cups; and that was just the beginning. Overall, he had nearly doubled the portion sizes of everything he ate.

Preparation Period

Carbohydrate-Protein-Fat Percentages: 65-13-22				
Body Weight (pounds)	Total Calories	Carbohydrate (g)	Protein (g)	Fat (g)
110	2,000–2,400	330–385	65–80	50–60
120	2,200–2,600	360–420	75–85	50–60
135	2,500–2,900	400–475	80–95	60–70
150	2,800–3,200	450–525	90–105	70–80
165	3,000–3,500	500–575	100–115	70–85
180	3,300–3,900	540–630	110–125	80–95
195	3,600–4,200	585–680	120–140	85–100

I'm rarely concerned with a few pounds here or there throughout the year, but for an athlete who has been working hard to maintain or lose fat mass and improve body composition, gaining weight in the Preparation Period can be a blow to self-confidence and self-esteem. By achieving the increase in calories through small increases in grams per pound, athletes are less likely to overinflate their daily caloric consumption.

Nutrition and Training During the Specialization Period

Faster Than a Speeding Bullet

You spend the entire year getting ready for the Specialization Period. This is the time of year when you are your strongest, fastest, and most prepared for optimal performance. If you love outdoor sports in the summer, you might want to plan your Specialization Period for June to August or July to September. If winter sports are your favorites, you might want the months of December to February or January to March to encompass your Specialization Period.

Competitive athletes build their periodization plans around being optimally prepared for one event or a series of events. In Lance Armstrong's case, the Tour de France falls right in the middle of his Specialization Period. The period begins about six weeks prior to the beginning of July, the month when the three-week race is held. In these final weeks building up to the Tour, Lance's training is very intense, but the volume decreases. He spends fewer hours on the bike than during the Preparation Period, but his workouts are harder than at any other time of the year.

The training intensity in your Specialization Period needs to be very high, because this is the time of year when you are working on systems that supply energy for maximal efforts. To overload the aerobic system in the Foundation Period, you worked out longer and at an aerobic intensity. When you wanted to apply a training stress to your anaerobic system, you worked out near your lactate threshold during the Preparation Period. Now that you want to improve your ability to deliver maximum power with both your aerobic and anaerobic systems, your workouts have to be at their most intense.

The positive side of increased intensity is that the workouts are shorter and your overall training volume decreases. The harder you work, the more recovery you need; and in the Specialization Period, you're either working at full-throttle or you're resting. Failing to get enough rest during the Specialization Period will undermine your performance more than any other factor can. With insufficient recovery, you won't be able to give your best efforts in training, and you may jeopardize your chances of reaching your goals. Even if you have no desire to compete, there is most likely a portion of the year when you would like to be in your best shape. Some active people don't necessarily train for specific events, but rather aim to be in top condition to participate in a variety of activities in a given season. The summer-sport enthusiast, for instance, strives to be in good shape as the summer begins because outdoor

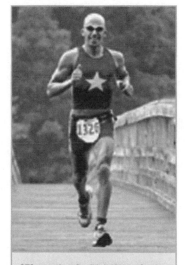

CTS member Dr. Rick Kattouf enjoying the fitness he works to develop for the Specialization Period. Photo © by Brightroom Photo

activities are more fun when you're physically prepared for them. Down-hill skiers and snowboarders aim to be in top shape when the snow starts falling because the ski season only lasts for a few months. They don't want to waste half the season skiing half-days and feeling tired before they get in shape. Being in optimal shape for your favorite season of the year gives you the opportunity to make the most of that season while it lasts.

How to Get What You Need in the Specialization Period

Nutrition plays a major role in the success of your Specialization Period. High intensity training and participation in goal events requires a lot of carbohydrate for fuel, and the workouts during this period will burn through your glycogen stores faster than during any other portion of the year. The stress induced by these workouts increases the importance of protein in your nutrition program, and there is a lot of muscle repair going on in the Specialization Period. The immune system takes a beating during this period as well. Ironically, as you get closer to performing at your absolute best, your risk of getting sick increases. After working so hard to be in top shape, you don't want to let yourself be undermined by poor recovery and nutritional choices.

For instance, the Specialization Period is not the time to actively try to lose weight. Your increased exercise intensity and competitions may naturally cause you to lose a few pounds, but you should not purposely restrict your caloric intake during this part of the year in an effort to drop weight. Many people decide they have to be a certain weight in order to compete or perform at their best. But what ends up happening, a lot of times, is that the caloric restriction needed to achieve that body weight conflicts with the increased caloric intake they need to support their activity level. As a result, workout quality diminishes, recovery suffers, and fitness erodes. CTS coach Brad Huff learned the hard way during his racing career. During the course of one racing season, he restricted his diet to the point that he lost 25 pounds, going from 165 pounds to 140 at 5 foot 10 inches tall. Instead of getting faster, he started suffering from small, nagging injuries and losing power. Guys he used to ride away from on hills now left him behind, and his racing results were erratic and disappointing. Brad's season ended abruptly with a career-threatening Achilles tendon injury. Two years later and at 180 pounds, Brad returned to racing and had his most successful season to date. He was able to handle the day-to-day intensity of training, his ability to recover improved, and even his ability to climb hills improved (despite his increased weight). The best times of the year to actively pursue weight loss are during the Foundation and Preparation periods. During the Specialization Period, full energy tanks will improve your performance more than dropping a few pounds will.

To meet the extreme demands of training, participation, and/or competition, your energy intake reaches its peak during the Specialization Period. Carbohydrate intake can reach 4 to 4.5 grams per pound of body weight, and endurance athletes like marathon runners, road cyclists, mountain bikers, and Ironman triathletes may need to further increase this to 5 grams per pound. Studies of Tour de France cyclists reveal that their carbohydrate intake often reaches 5.5 grams per pound (12 grams per kilogram) during the three-week event.

With the absolute amount of carbohydrate so high during this period of the year, it needs to represent more than 70 percent of total calories. I increase the percentage of calories from carbohydrate from 65 percent to 70 percent during the Specialization Period in order to keep an athlete's total caloric intake from soaring too high. At 4.5 grams of carbohydrate per pound, a 165-pound athlete would consume 740 grams of carbohydrate each day. This is a whopping 2,960 calories, nearly as many as the total daily caloric intake during the Foundation Period! If 2,960 calories were to represent only 60 percent of total calories, this athlete would be eating nearly 5,000 calories. In some cases, this would be appropriate, but for most athletes, 5,000 calories a day is several hundred too many, even during the Specialization Period. Instead, carbohydrates should represent 70 percent of your total daily caloric intake during the Specialization Period. For the 165-pound athlete consuming 4.5 grams per pound, this keeps total daily calories at about 4,200—enough for energy, recovery, and optimal performance.

As total caloric intake reaches its peak during the Specialization Period, so does your protein intake. You should aim to eat 0.8 to 0.9 grams

Specialization Period

Carbohydrate-Protein-Fat Percentages: 70-14-16				
Body Weight (pounds)	Total Calories	Carbohydrate (g)	Protein (g)	Fat (g)
110	2,500-2,800	440-500	90-100	65-75
120	2,700-3,100	480-540	95-110	50-55
135	3,100-3,500	540-610	110-120	55-60
150	3,400-3,900	600-675	120-135	60-70
165	3,700-4,200	660-740	130-150	65-75
180	4,100-4,600	720-810	140-160	70-80
195	4,400-5,000	780-875	155-175	80-90

of protein per pound of body weight to maintain your immune system and lean-muscle mass. This amount will also provide enough calories to account for protein's 5- to 15-percent contribution to total exercise energy expenditure. With carbohydrate representing a higher proportion of total calories and ranging from 4 to 4.5 grams per pound, protein's percentage contribution increases to about 14 percent during the Specialization Period.

Fat represents around 16 percent of your total daily caloric intake during the Specialization Period. This is lower than during either of the two previous periods of the year. Essentially, the 5-percent increase in calories from carbohydrate is made possible by reducing your fat intake. In terms of fat grams, you're eating about as many in the Specialization Period as you were in the Foundation Period.

The Specialization Period is the only time of the year when you should pay a little more attention to your fat intake. You need a lot of energy during this period, and the fuel you're looking for is clean-burning carbohydrate. You also need an elevated protein intake for your muscles and immune system. When you're consuming so much food, it's easy to believe that any food you can get your hands on is all right to eat. Many athletes can meet their carbohydrate and protein needs, but they inadvertently pile on mountains of excess fat calories in the process.

Nutrition and Training During the Transition Period

Regeneration, Yes; Vegetation, No

It's important that your Specialization Period doesn't exceed a maximum of about 12 weeks. Lance's season is essentially over after the Tour de France, and he takes some time to relax, reflect on the season, and physically and mentally recuperate. The Transition Period should be an important part of everyone's training program, but it's often overlooked. Many highly motivated people don't readily see the benefit of taking it easy for several weeks, preferring to continue training in pursuit of new goals. They fail to see that recuperation is an essential part of pursuing their next goal.

Many months of focused training takes a toll on your body and mind. The Transition Period functions as a recovery period on an annual scale. You recovered between intervals so you could better perform your workout. You also took recovery days and regeneration weeks during the Foundation, Preparation, and Specialization periods. Now it's time to apply the concept of overload and recovery to your entire training year by taking one or two months of active recovery.

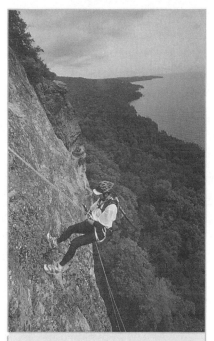

You shouldn't mistake the Transition Period for a prolonged vacation from training. If you were to stop exercising completely for a month, it would take you another two months just to regain the fitness you lost. That means that after three months, you would only be as fit as you

The Transition Period is a perfect time to expand your horizons and try something new.
Photo © by Craig Watter Photography

were the last day of your season. It is difficult to make significant progress from one year to the next when you spend three months losing and regaining fitness.

The goal of training in the Transition Period is to maintain your aerobic conditioning. Since you've spent so much time building your aerobic engine, it would be a shame to let that fitness disappear. Fortunately, it doesn't take a huge amount of training to prevent the aerobic system from detraining. Your weekly training hours can be about 25 percent less than what they were during the Foundation Period, and you'll still get through the Transition Period with the majority of your aerobic capacity intact. Instead of sitting on the couch for weeks, reduce your training volume and intensity and take the regimen out of training. If you normally train five days each week, add another rest day. Spend time participating in different sports than you normally would.

How to Get What You Need

Since the volume and intensity of the Transition Period are lower than during any other portion of the year, your calorie intake needs to decrease. You're not burning as much energy on a daily basis, and if you continue eating as if you are, you will quickly gain weight. Gaining a few pounds is normal, even recommended, but aim to keep this weight gain to about a 5 percent increase (i.e., for a 100-pound person: about 5 pounds gained; for a 150-pound-person: about 8 pounds gained; for a 200-pound person: about 10 pounds gained).

Both the quantity and compostion of your nutritional program changes during the Transition Period. The greatest reduction in energy intake comes from carbohydrate. Instead of 65 to 70 percent of your caloric intake, carbohydrate should represent only 60 percent of your calories during the Transition Period. To achieve this, you should eat 2 to 2.5 grams of carbohydrate per pound of body weight.

Your protein intake should decrease to 0.6 to 0.7 grams per pound as a result of your decreased training volume and intensity. While this is a reduction compared to the Specialization Period, your protein intake during the Transition Period is the same as it was in the Preparation Period and higher than it was during the Foundation Period. Protein will represent about 18 percent of your calories during the Transition Period. Protein is important during this time of year because your body is busy repairing muscles and connective tissues, as well as performing other functions that were neglected while you were training hard. This is the reason that your protein intake during the Transition Period is the same as it was during the Preparation Period. Instead of committing most of its resources to struggling to recover before your next hard workout, your body relishes this opportunity to slow down and recuperate fully.

During the Transition Period, fat will comprise about 22 percent of your caloric intake. While this is an increase in percentage from the Specialization Period, the actual amount of fat you're consuming during the Transition Period is less than during any other part of the year. Fat represents a higher percentage of your calories because your total energy intake is reduced. As we've done before, let's apply these numbers to a 165-pound athlete. At 2 grams per pound, you'd be eating 330 grams or 1,320 calories of carbohydrate. If this represents 60 percent of your total caloric intake, you'd be shooting for a daily intake of 2,200 calories. Consuming 0.6 grams of protein per pound would add another 400 calories

Transition Period

Carbohydrate-Protein-Fat Percentages: 60-18-22				
Body Weight (pounds)	Total Calories	Carbohydrate (g)	Protein (g)	Fat (g)
110	1,500–1,800	220–275	65–80	35–50
120	1,600–2,000	240–300	75–85	40–50
135	1,800–2,200	270–340	80–95	45–60
150	2,000–2,500	300–375	90–105	50–60
165	2,200–2,700	330–410	100–115	55–70
180	2,400–3,000	360–450	110–125	60–75
195	2,600–3,200	390–485	120–140	65–80

(100 grams), leaving fat to contribute the last 480 calories. Fifty-three grams of fat contain about 480 calories, which represents about 22 percent of your total calories.

How Food Affects Your Training

Foundation Period

Since the aerobic system is the primary focus of the Foundation Period, this is a good time to explain the ways carbohydrate and fat work together to power your Foundation Period workouts. Generally speaking, you have to use moderate-intensity workouts to develop your aerobic engine. You see, if the intensity gets too high, you're demanding energy faster than your aerobic system can deliver it, so you call upon the anaerobic system to bail you out (you remember—the inefficient, smoke-belching, self-limiting system). When your goal is to train the aerobic system, you can't push so hard that your other energy systems come in to bail it out; rather, you have to train at an intensity that your aerobic system can sustain without asking for help.

Your body burns a fairly even mixture of fat and carbohydrate during workouts that develop your aerobic engine, and your body has some interesting ways of keeping the mixture just right. You have essentially unlimited stores of fat, but very limited stores of carbohydrate, meaning you can run out of carbohydrate after as little as 90 minutes of exercise.

Since blood glucose (sugar) is the preferred fuel that your brain and central nervous system uses, your body acts defensively when it senses you are running low on carbohydrates. Your body has elaborate and redundant mechanisms for maintaining blood-glucose levels at 90 to 100 milligrams per deciliter of blood (mg/dl). Your body doesn't have redundant controls on blood glucose so you can perform better as an athlete; it has them so it can supply the brain with a constant supply of fuel. Optimal athletic performance is a beneficial side effect.

When blood-glucose levels fall, either as a result of rapid absorption into muscle cells or the lack of ingested carbohydrates, the pancreas secretes a hormone called glucagon. This hormone stimulates the breakdown of glycogen in the liver, which has the effect of raising blood glucose levels. Glucagon also stimulates gluconeogenesis, which is the process by which glucose can be created from amino acids (protein), lactate, and glycerol in the liver. Interestingly, your liver can produce a maximum of about 100 grams of glucose per day this way, which is just about how much your central nervous system requires.

Preparation Period

As I have previously explained, you burn more carbohydrate for energy as your exercise intensity increases. During many of your workouts, you will be burning about 70 percent carbohydrate and 30 percent fat. The Preparation Period is characterized by training that stresses the upper reaches of your aerobic system yet also calls upon your anaerobic system. You're burning energy in a hotter fire, which means it burns faster, and hence you deplete your carbohydrate stores more quickly.

In endurance events like 10-kilometer runs, marathons, triathlons, and mountain bike races, the best performers are the ones who can sustain their highest pace the longest; in other words, the ones who slow down the least in the last third of the event. This affects non-competitive athletes as well, and is often associated with feeling great for the first two-thirds of a hike, century ride, or charity walk, followed by a gradual descent into misery by the finish. During the first long ride in a CTS training camp in Buellton, California, one of the camp guests kept pushing the pace on every hill early in the ride. The other CTS coaches and I suggested the person take it a bit easier, considering we were less than an hour into a four-hour ride. Sure enough, two hours later, I had my hand on the back of his jersey, pushing him up a hill because he was out of fuel and out of power. Fortunately, one experience like that was all he needed to learn his lesson, and according to the coach he's been working with ever since that camp, he's now the guy with fuel and power to spare on long rides.

In order to set a new personal record in your next 10k run, you don't need to run faster over the first five kilometers; you have to avoid slowing down as you approach the finish line.

Duration is the key to workouts that improve your ability to sustain a high pace. While short intervals are good for developing strength and maximum power, the only way to increase sustainable power is to complete longer, sustained intervals. These workouts burn a lot of fuel, which is why the food you eat is critical to supporting the workouts in the Preparation Period.

Specialization Period

During the portion of the year when you want to perform at your absolute best, you need to provide your body with a lot of clean-burning fuel in the form of carbohydrate. At the same time, you need to stock up on enough protein to keep your muscles and immune system healthy so you can recover in time to participate in your next workout or competition. And while you need fat in your nutrition program, the slight reductions in fat intake often lead athletes to shed a few pounds in the weeks leading up to their goal events. For some, this weight loss can lead to the perception that they are in even better condition. Athletes yearn to be lean, to be at "fighting weight" before a goal event. In many sports, a few pounds up or down have no effect on performance, so this weight loss has more of a psychological impact than a physiological one.

There are a few sports, however, where body weight has a significant impact on performance. In endurance sports that involve climbing hills or mountains, like distance-running, some triathlons, and some cycling events, losing a few pounds means having a little less weight to lift against gravity. It has been shown that reducing the weight of a bicycle or its rider leads to increased speed on climbs, even though the rider is performing the same, or even less, work.

During his final preparations for the Tour de France, Lance takes this theory to an extreme. We restrict his caloric intake to a level where he is in an energy deficit, even though he is still training heavily. It is a tricky balance to maintain, but then again, the Tour de France is both tricky and extreme. During this period of his training, Lance and I communicate via telephone and computer three to four times each day, constantly

monitoring and adjusting his training, eating, and resting with the
goal of delivering him to the start
of the Tour de France 100-percent
ready to rip his bike and the competition to pieces.

We walk a tightrope with Lance's
body weight. The goal is to reduce
his body weight without reducing
the amount of power he can produce on the bike. Unfortunately,
there is a point at which an athlete,
and this applies to every athlete,
starts losing power along with body
weight. All too often, when an athlete pushes past this point, it is difficult to quickly regain either the
weight or the power.

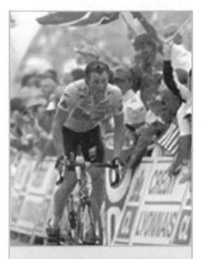

Lance Armstrong, minutes after his dra-
matic fall on Luz Ardiden, reestablishing
his lead as he approaches the finish line
of Stage 15 in the 2003 Tour de France.
Photo © by Graham Watson

Lance's nutrition and training program during the Specialization Period has garnered a great deal of attention because people are fascinated
by the fact that he weighs his food and arrives at the Tour both remark-
ably lean and amazingly powerful. It's crucial that everyone understands
something: Lance's nutrition program is designed to prepare him to win
one of the most extreme sporting events in the world. It's not a healthy
nutrition program that you should attempt to emulate. What no one
sees is that Lance gains six to ten pounds in the weeks following the Tour
de France. Maintaining his Tour weight or body composition would
make him ill if the race were much longer.

The Specialization Period is the fun part of the year, since it is the
time when you are able to perform at your best. With careful attention
paid to your nutrition program during these crucial months, you drastically increase your chances of reaching your goals and having the fitness
to fully enjoy all of your activities.

P A R T

The Best Fuels for the Job

2

4

MAKING THE RIGHT CHOICES

SO NOW COMES THE REALITY OF PUTTING THE CARMICHAEL
Nutritional Program together. When walking up and down the aisles at
the grocery store or looking at the many choices from a restaurant menu,
how do you know what's going to supply your body with the best fuel?
Your goal is as simple as it is complex: to choose foods with as high a nutritional value as possible. What do I mean by that? I mean choosing
foods that are nutrient-dense; that deliver fuel as well as beneficial vitamins and minerals.

With all of the advances in today's modern world, it's sometimes easy
to forget that the simplest things are the best. Recently, when I was
speaking to a group of junior cyclists and triathletes, I asked them for
examples of foods that contain carbohydrates. Their immediate responses
were "soda," "candy," and "Gatorade." It took them a while to get around
to fruits and vegetables. They were really surprised to learn that vege-

tables were a good source of carbohydrates! Likewise, it seems that many *adults* have forsaken natural foods for packaged and convenience foods. Eating natural foods allows our bodies to better absorb many of the nutrients we need as active adults. For example, eating *fresh* food helps ensure that you're getting plenty of fiber along with the vitamins and minerals; it also helps to keep your intake of salt and other additives down.

In addition to choosing whole foods, it is important to select a variety of foods. Our sports nutritionist at CTS sees dietary records with the same foods entered day after day. Once, she contacted a runner to ask him to repeat his dietary record because it appeared as if there was an error in the report—she had received two identical days of food records. After talking with the athlete, she realized that he ate the exact same thing (and not just cereal for breakfast, a sandwich for lunch, but the exact same cereal and the exact same sandwich) for days. The best way to ensure that your body receives the best fuel for training and recovery is to eat a wide *variety* of foods. Each food can offer its own special nutrients, and by eating a variety of foods throughout the day and from day to day, you can ensure that your body will be receiving all the necessary nutrients. If cereal is a favorite breakfast option, change the type of cereal from day to day, or mix two or more together. If a turkey sandwich is a favorite lunchtime meal, change the type of bread and type of lean meat, cheese, and vegetables from day to day.

The Carrier Method

I look at foods as vessels carrying supplies for the body. This is helpful because it illustrates that nutrients are not eaten in isolation. You may choose a food because you're after the carbohydrates it contains, but you're not just eating the carbohydrate portion. When you eat the entire food, you get everything else (the good and the bad) that it's carrying. I prefer to group foods into three categories: quality carriers, empty carriers, and pollutant carriers.

Quality carriers are the nutritional equivalent of the motor yacht:

powerful, impressive, and stocked with amenities. Empty carriers are more like your standard rowboat: a no-frills, unrewarding, and inefficient way to get where you're going. Finally, the pollutant carrier is essentially a garbage barge: a vessel whose cargo does you more harm than good. The table below shows some examples of foods that fit into these three categories.

Carrier	Quality Carriers "Motor Yacht"	Empty Carriers "Rowboat"	Pollutant Carriers "Garbage Barge"
Additional Cargo*	Vitamins, Minerals, Phytochemicals, Antioxidants, Fiber	Minimal amounts of beneficial nutrients	High amounts of harmful pollutants, including saturated fat, trans-fat, and excessive sodium
Food Examples	Spinach	Cola	Pork Rinds
	Whole-grain cereal and bread	Low-Fat Candy (i.e. Pixy Stix)	High-Fat Candy (i.e. Chunky bar)
	Salmon	Kool Aid®	Doughnuts
	Sweet Potatoes	Pretzels	Lard
	Kiwi Fruit	Low-Fat Cookies	French Fries
	Chicken Breasts	Iceberg Lettuce	Fried Chicken
	Brown Rice	White Rice	High-fat meats (e.g. pork ribs)
	Soy Milk		

*Each individually listed food may not contain all of these additional nutrients.

The next big question, however, is: How do you tell what category your food choices fit into?

Nutrient Density

A nutrient-dense food supplies many beneficial components per calorie, allowing that food to have the greatest positive impact on your health and performance. Foods that are less nutrient-dense aren't necessarily bad for you, but they're definitely less beneficial. A food's nutrient density can make the difference between its classification as a quality or empty carrier. Generally speaking, most fresh, natural foods are quality carriers. This includes fresh fruits, vegetables, nuts, grains, and lean cuts of meat, chicken, and fish. Within these groups, however, some foods are more nutrient-dense than others. In the next few chapters, I'll show you which specific foods provide the biggest nutrition bang for your buck.

Natural foods lose some of their quality and start heading toward the pollutant-carrier category as they are processed into convenience-oriented, pre-packaged foods. For instance, a fresh peach is a quality carrier because it supplies a lot of nutrients for the total calories it contains. In the process of being cooked, peeled, and canned in heavy, sweetened syrup, it becomes an empty-carrier food because the number of calories drastically increases and the nutrient concentration decreases, thereby reducing the food's ratio of nutrients to calories.

Many quality carriers are doomed to the pollutant-carrier category by the ways they are cooked. A lean cut of red meat, like an eye-of-round steak, is a quality carrier because it is a great source of protein, zinc, and iron. Grilled, it remains a quality carrier, but breaded and fried on the way to making southern-fried steak, it quickly becomes a pollutant-carrier food. The same is true of chicken when it is served as fried chicken, and potatoes, onions, and other vegetables that are commonly deep-fried.

Food Labels

While I will give you lists and tables of quality-carrier foods in the coming chapters, you should also know how to determine a food's quality on your own. The Nutrition Facts label on a food provides a lot of important information for athletes. The label lists the food's carbohydrate, protein, and fat content by telling you each nutrient's grams per serving. As I'll discuss shortly, serving size plays an important role in sports nutrition. It is up to you to use the information on the Nutrition Facts label to decide if a food is a quality, empty, or pollutant carrier.

You can do that by looking at the section of the food label that identifies the good stuff—the amenities you want to accompany your food choices. Fiber, vitamins A and C, the B-vitamins, calcium, and iron are required for optimal nutrition. Eating enough of these nutrients can improve your exercise training, recovery, and health, and can also help reduce the risk of some diseases and harmful conditions. The Nutrition Facts label displays the percentage of the recommended daily value (%DV) of these nutrients in one serving of the food. However, it's important to note that the %DVs are based on a 2,000-calorie-a-day diet, which is considerably lower than most athletes' daily caloric intakes. As we see in the periodization tables, caloric intake can range from 2,500 during Foundation to 4,200 in Specialization for a 165-pound athlete.

My advice is to use the %DV as a frame of reference for vitamin and mineral content. If the food has a negligible amount of vitamins (low %DV), it's probably not your best choice; go with something that has higher %DV numbers.

Even if a food has a lot of nutrients in it, you still have to look at its fat content to see if it can still retain its place as a quality carrier. You're looking for fat (of any kind) to comprise less than 30 percent of the food's total calories. You should also aim to further limit its content of saturated fat, trans-fat, and cholesterol, as these can contribute to the onset of several diseases. Trans-fat is not individually identified on most packaged foods,

Nutrition Facts

Serving Size 1 cup (228g)
Serving Per Container 2

Amount Per Serving

Calories 250	Calories from Fat 110

	% **Daily Value***
Total Fat 12g	**18%**
Saturated Fat 3g	**15%**
Trans Fat 1.5g	
Cholesterol 30mg	**10%**
Sodium 470mg	**20%**
Total Carbohydrate 31g	**10%**
Dietary Fiber 0g	**0%**
Sugars 5g	
Protein 5g	

Vitamin A	4%
Vitamin C	2%
Calcium	20%
Iron	4%

*Percent Daily Values are based on a 2,000 calorie diet. Your Daily Values may be higher or lower depending on your calorie needs.

	Calories:	2,000	2,500
Total Fat	Less than	65g	80g
Sat Fat	Less than	20g	25g
Cholesterol	Less than	300mg	300mg
Sodium	Less than	2,400mg	2,400mg
Total Carbohydrate		300g	375g
Dietary Fiber		25g	30g

Food label from the FDA's Center for Food Safety and Applied Nutrition (CFSAN)

and such labeling is not required until 2006, but if the words "partially-hydrogenated oil" or "hydrogenated oil" are in the list of ingredients, the food contains trans-fat.

In addition to the actual food label, there is an overwhelming amount of information to be found on food packaging. You must be aware of what this means, as food manufacturers use some terms to make you think a product is a quality carrier, when in fact it could be an empty or even a pollutant carrier. Here is a partial list of the FDA guidelines about the claims and descriptions manufacturers may use in food labeling to promote their products.

Claim	Requirements that must be met before using the claim in food labeling
Fat-Free	Less than 0.5 grams of fat per serving, with no added fat or oil
Low fat	3 grams or less of fat per serving
Less fat	25 percent or less fat than the comparison food
Saturated fat–free	Less than 0.5 grams of saturated fat and 0.5 grams of trans-fat per serving
Cholesterol–free	Less than 2 milligrams of cholesterol per serving, and 2 grams or less of saturated fat per serving
Low cholesterol	20 milligrams or less of cholesterol per serving, and 2 grams or less saturated fat per serving
Low calorie	40 calories or less per serving
Light (fat)	50 percent or less fat than in the comparison food (example: "Fifty percent less fat than our regular cheese.")
Light (calories)	$1/3$ fewer calories than the comparison food
High-fiber	5 grams or more fiber per serving
Low sodium	140 milligrams or less of sodium per serving
Very low sodium	35 milligrams or less of sodium per serving
"Good source of," "More," or "Added"	Provides 10 percent more of the Daily Value for a given nutrient than the comparison food

Source: U.S. Food and Drug Administration Center for Food Safety and Applied Nutrition. *A Food Labeling Guide* (September 1994). (Editorial revisions, June 1999).

Choosing Your Servings

In today's culture, where portion sizes have continued to increase, the technical definition of a serving size is actually quite small. The USDA Food Guide Pyramid recommends two to three servings per day from the food group containing meat, poultry, dry beans, eggs, and nuts. Well, the USDA is defining a single serving of meat as two to three ounces, and I can't remember the last time I saw a three-ounce piece of meat, chicken, or fish on a menu, or cooked such a small portion at home. More common actual serving sizes for athletes are in the four-to-six-ounce range for meats—double the USDA recommendations.

In Chapter 3, you read my recommendations for the number of grams of carbohydrate, protein, and fat your nutrition program should supply during each of the four periods of the year. Before I go on to recommend the best sources of these nutrients, you need to have an idea of appropriate portion sizes for athletes. Since many athletes eat one and a half times as many calories per day as sedentary people do, it makes sense that you're going to be putting larger portions onto your plate. However, this larger portion size is not a license to blindly heap the food on. The table on page 70 provides some reference points to help athletes determine appropriate portion sizes.

Other visual cues for determining portion sizes:

- One teaspoon is about the same size as the end of your thumb.
- There are three teaspoons in one tablespoon, or three thumb-portions.
- One cup of lettuce is often about four large leaves.
- A one-pint take-out Chinese food container holds two cups.
- A medium-sized baked potato is about the size of a computer mouse.
- One ounce of cheese is about the size of your entire thumb.
- A standard serving size for a pancake is about the size of a compact disk.

Food	USDA Serving Size	Looks like...	Normal Athlete's Portion	Looks like...
Cooked oatmeal, rice, pasta	1/2 cup	Ice-cream scoop	1–1.5 cups	Adult man's fist
Dry cereal	1 cup	1 large handful	1–1.5 cups	Two medium handfuls
Breads	1/2 bagel 1 slice of bread 1/2 pita pocket	n/a	1 bagel 2 slices of bread 1 pita pocket	n/a
Beans and legumes (peas, lentils, black beans, pinto beans, etc.)	1/2 cup	Ice-cream scoop; light bulb	1–1.5 cups	Adult man's fist
Nuts	1/3 cup	One handful	2/3 cup	Two handfuls
Meats	3 ounces	Deck of cards; palm of your hand	4–8 ounces	Checkbook; palm plus half of fingers
Fruit	1 medium-sized fruit; 1 cup cut fruit	Baseball; clenched fist	1 large fruit; two medium fruits; 1 cup cut fruit	Hand clasped around baseball
Peanut butter and similar foods	2 tablespoons	Golf or Ping-Pong ball	2–3 tablespoons	Racquetball

The Keys to Making the Best Choices

As you read the following chapters on carbohydrate, protein, fat, and vitamin choices, keep the following in mind.

There is no magic food.
You are going to perform at your best by eating a wide variety of foods, and the inclusion of one specific item will not magically boost your performance.

There are no evil foods.

No food should be considered completely off-limits. If you have a han-kering for deep-fried onion rings, eat a few. Just realize that onion rings and other pollutant-carrier foods should be consumed sparingly.

Keep an open mind.

Expand your horizons when considering foods that you'll include in your nutrition program. If you've never tried starfruit or mangoes, you're not sure you'd like barley, or the concept of eating cottage cheese makes you wince, I urge you to take some chances. Each week when you go to the grocery store, try to purchase one new, unusual-looking fruit or vegetable. You might just bump into a new favorite.

5

AN ATHLETE'S GUIDE
TO CARBOHYDRATES

Basic Facts About Carbohydrates

Carbohydrate forms the backbone of an athlete's nutrition program because it is the most versatile, energy-yielding nutrient you can consume. You can burn carbohydrate in either the aerobic or anaerobic energy system, store it in muscles and the liver as glycogen (preferred), or transform it into fat (last resort). Your liver can even make carbohydrate from protein to meet your needs for this clean-burning and efficient source of energy. Carbohydrate, in the form of glucose, is also the fuel your brain and central nervous system depend on for energy. As an athlete, the choices you make around the carbohydrates you eat play a large role in how effectively they contribute to your performance.

In recent years, the subject of carbohydrates has become much more complicated than it needs to be. People have been comparing the digestion rates of one food against another and the amount of insulin released after eating one food versus another, seeking to divide carbohydrates into "good" and "bad" categories. Some people skip the step of dividing them into two groups and simply banished them altogether. Improving athletic performance was not the motive behind these recommendations, and the people who made them were not talking to athletes. They were talking to sedentary individuals who consume too many calories and to diabetics who have trouble controlling blood sugar. The advice was given with good intentions—the goal was to improve people's health— but it came without enough information, especially for athletes.

While there are different types of carbohydrates in food, there is no such thing as a "bad" carbohydrate for an athlete. Simple carbohydrates (monosaccharides and disaccharides) are easy to digest and provide a lot of energy very quickly. Complex carbohydrates (polysaccharides, starch) provide a longer-lasting source of clean-burning energy that can keep you going for hours. Both are necessary parts of a high-performance nutrition program.

Simple Carbohydrates

When people talk about simple carbohydrates, they're talking about monosaccharides and disaccharides. Monosaccharides, the smallest units of sugar, include glucose, fructose, and galactose. Glucose is the sugar your body uses to fuel muscles, and it is the only fuel your brain and central nervous system can use for energy. Both fructose and galactose must be converted to glucose in the liver before they can be used for energy. Disaccharides are combinations of monosaccharides and are the common forms of sugar found in foods.

Sugars lose their sweetness as they increase in size, which has very important implications in food production. Dextrins are an intermediate form of sugar, caught somewhere between simple and complex carbohydrates. Carbohydrates can be provided with less associated sweetness by using slightly larger dextrins, like maltodextrin, in place of sucrose or dextrose. Conversely, when food processors need to make a normally bland or bitter carbohydrate sweeter, they sometimes add enzymes that

Simple Sugars	Type	Source	Sweetness
Fructose	Monosaccharide	Primarily fruit	Sweetest monosaccharide
Glucose	Monosaccharide	Fruits, vegetables, grains	Medium-sweetness monosaccharide
Galactose	Monosaccharide	Milk	Least-sweet monosaccharide
Sucrose	Disaccharide (fructose + glucose)	Sugar cane, table sugar	Sweetest disaccharide
Lactose	Disaccharide (glucose + galactose)	Dairy products	Medium-sweetness disaccharide
Maltose, dextrose	Disaccharide (glucose + glucose)	Germinating seeds, commercial foods	Least-sweet disaccharide
Maltodextrin	Dextrin (glucose polymer)	Sports drinks, commercial foods	Less sweet than either mono- or disaccharides

break some of the food's complex carbohydrates (starch) down into sweeter dextrins.

Simple carbohydrates have been given a bad reputation by non-athletes because they are found in junk food and candy, but the mistake is looking at the sugar by itself instead of looking at the entire food. Candy and junk food are a problem because their nutrient density is low; they're packed with calories but don't provide many beneficial nutrients. That's a characteristic of the candy bar as a whole, not the sugar itself. There's nothing wrong with simple sugars themselves, but they have been found guilty by association because they're in sweets.

Simple sugars are beneficial for athletes, especially during and after exercise. Eating or drinking carbohydrates during exercise spares stores of liver glycogen, meaning you can work out longer before your stores of carbohydrate energy are depleted. Since you're burning energy rapidly during sustained exercise, sometimes in excess of 12 calories per minute (during hard efforts in the Tour de France, Lance Armstrong and his competitors may burn more than 20 calories per minute), simple carbo-hydrates are beneficial because they provide usable energy quickly. Complex carbohydrates also play an integral role in providing energy during exercise, as I'll discuss shortly.

Immediately following exercise, eating or drinking carbohydrate improves recovery by rapidly replenishing depleted glycogen stores. Studies have shown that glycogen stores reach the same level whether people consume simple, complex, or a mixture of the two carbohydrate types. There is even some evidence that ingesting simple carbohydrates might increase the rate of glycogen replenishment.

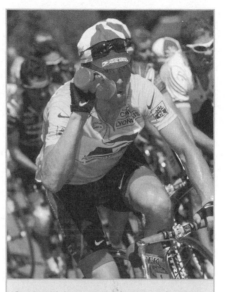

Sports drinks are good sources of carbohydrates, primarily from simple sugars like glucose and fructose, as well as from dextrins like maltodextrin. Photo © by Graham Watson

Complex Carbohydrates

These densely packed sources of carbohydrate energy are some of an athlete's best assets. The most important complex carbohydrates are starch and fiber. Foods high in polysaccharides, such as potatoes, pasta, brown

The best simple sugars for athletes are...	Because...
1. Dextrose, maltose	Its two glucose molecules can be absorbed and put to immediate use in muscles. The brain and central nervous system can pull them from the blood to burn for energy.
2. Sucrose	Its glucose can be used immediately, but the fructose must be converted to glucose in the liver before the body can use it.
3. Lactose	Its glucose can be used immediately. The galactose must be converted to glucose in the liver. Note: Many people have trouble breaking lactose down due to a deficiency of lactase, the enzyme necessary for lactose digestion.

rice, corn, and barley play a large role in an athlete's nutrition program because of their high carbohydrate concentration: Almost every calorie they provide comes from carbohydrate. In addition to providing lasting energy, grains and starches can help protect against muscular fatigue and help to enhance weight loss because they are mostly pure energy with no excess calories.

Fiber is a form of complex carbohydrate that your body does not break down. It is the indigestible part of food that gives whole grains, fruits, and vegetables their snap, crunch, and crispiness. Because it absorbs water in your stomach and expands, fiber also helps you feel full. And since your body can't digest it, fiber passes through you without adding calories. There are two kinds of fiber—soluble and insoluble—and you should aim to consume 25 to 35 grams of fiber every day. Soluble fiber is credited with lowering cholesterol levels, improving blood sugar control in diabetics, and delaying stomach emptying. Insoluble fiber helps remove carcinogens (potentially cancer-causing substances found in food) from your body.

Your body both produces and breaks down complex carbohydrates, depending on whether it needs to burn or store energy. Glycogen is the storage form of glucose in muscles and the liver. Under normal aerobic circumstances, when your muscles need energy, they break these massive, complex structures of polysaccharide back down to their most basic units. Glucose is then metabolized to carbon dioxide, water, and energy in the aerobic system. It is interesting to note that carbohydrates consumed as polysaccharides are broken down to individual simple sugars in the process of being digested, absorbed, and transported around the body. If they happen to come to rest as glycogen, it is only because your body has reassembled them back into a complex carbohydrate.

Your liver serves as the primary fuel tank for your brain and central nervous system. Muscles can absorb glucose and store it as glycogen, but they can't release glucose back into the blood. As a result, the liver is responsible for the majority of the brain's carbohydrate fuel. Glucose can also be transported from the liver to muscles during exercise when blood-sugar (glucose) levels are low. Liver glycogen is used overnight when you are sleeping, and by morning, most of this store is depleted.

That's why a high-carbohydrate breakfast is an important meal for athletes because it increases blood sugar for morning workouts, or it allows you to start an afternoon workout with fuller glycogen stores.

What happens if you already have full glycogen stores? The carbohydrates you ingest are broken down and absorbed into the bloodstream. Glucose can be immediately used for energy or stored as glycogen. If neither of these functions is needed (as in the case of a sedentary person with full glycogen stores), glucose can be converted to fatty acids in the liver. Interestingly, however, storing glucose as fat is one of the last things your body does with glucose. Your body will try to use glucose for several other purposes before it relegates it to storage in adipose tissue.

Spotting Quality-Carrier Carbohydrates

Fruits and Vegetables

Fruits and vegetables have always been considered a great source of carbohydrates, but some are better carriers than others. Generally speaking, the more vibrant and intense the color, the higher a fruit or vegetable's content of vitamins, minerals, antioxidants, and carotenoids. Carotenoids include beta-carotene, lutein, and lycopene, and evidence suggests these compounds found in colorful vegetables may help prevent degenerative eye diseases and some forms of cancer. (These micronutrients will be covered in more detail in Chapter 9.)

Vegetables

Dark green varieties of lettuce, like romaine or mignonette; red and yellow peppers, spinach, broccoli, and sweet potatoes are all high-quality carriers. In contrast, vegetables that lack color often contain fewer beneficial components. Since they still contain some vitamins, minerals, antioxidants, and phytochemicals, they are still considered quality carriers, but they shouldn't be your first choice at the vegetable stand. Iceberg lettuce, cucumbers, celery, and white mushrooms are good additions to many recipes, but athletes don't look to them as major sources of nutrition.

The table below lists a variety of vegetables, based on a nutrition score. The Center for Science in the Public Interest (CSPI) devised the scoring system by looking at vegetables' effectiveness in delivering seven nutrients: carotenoids, vitamins C and K, folate, potassium, iron, and fiber. While you should consume more of the high-scoring vegetables, low-scoring vegetables aren't bad for you; they just don't provide as many nutrients. If you're preparing mixed vegetables or a salad, make

Vegetable	Nutrient Score*	Nutrient Highlights	
		High in... (20–100+%DV)	Moderate (10–19%DV) or Adequate (5–9%DV) source of...
Sweet potato (baked, with skin)	424	Carotenoids, vitamin C	Potassium, fiber, folate
Spinach (raw)	287	Carotenoids, vitamin K	Folate, vitamin C
Red pepper	261	Carotenoids, very high in vitamin C	n/a
Butternut squash	176	Carotenoids, vitamin C	Fiber
Romaine lettuce	174	Carotenoids, vitamins C and K	Folate, potassium
Asparagus	163	Vitamin K, Folate	Vitamin C, carotenoids, fiber
Baked potato (with skin)	139	Vitamin C, iron, potassium, fiber	Folate
Green pepper	109	Vitamin C	Vitamin K
Frozen peas	104	Carotenoids, vitamin K	Fiber, vitamin C, folate, iron
Baked potato (without skin)	69	Vitamin C	Potassium, fiber
Corn	67	Carotenoids	Vitamin C, folate, potassium, fiber
Iceberg lettuce	45	Vitamin K	Carotenoids, folate
Onions	31	n/a	Vitamin C, fiber
Cucumber	14	n/a	n/a
Mushrooms (raw)	11	n/a	n/a

*Copyright 2002, CSPI. Adapted from *Nutrition Action Newsletter* (1875 Connecticut Ave., N.W., Suite 300, Washington, D.C. 20009-5728) July/Aug. 29(6), pages 13-15.

sure you have a few high-scoring vegetables in there, and then throw in any other vegetables you like.

While all vegetables supply beneficial nutrients, not all of them are good sources of carbohydrate fuel. For instance, spinach is packed with nutrients that support your health and performance, but a cup of it supplies less than six grams of carbohydrate, four of which are fiber. This certainly doesn't mean you shouldn't eat spinach, but you have to realize that it would take an enormous amount of spinach to fulfill a large portion of your daily carbohydrate energy needs. The same is true of the varieties of peppers and lettuces: great nutritional value, but low on fuel. The table below shows some of best vegetable choices for nutrient density as well as energy.

Vegetable	Grams of carbohydrate per cup
Baked potato (with skin)	51
Sweet potato (baked, with skin)	48
Garbanzo beans	45
White or yellow corn (boiled)	41
Butternut squash	21
Green Peas (boiled)	25

Fruits

Fruit has always been an essential part of an athlete's nutrition program. It functions both as an enjoyable treat in place of high-fat desserts, and as a quality carrier of carbohydrate, vitamin C, potassium, carotenoids, and fiber. When choosing fruit, there's really no way to go wrong, and even though some are more nutrient-dense than others, your favorite fruits should definitely be part of your sports nutrition program.

As they did with vegetables, the CSPI put together a scoring system for fruit. By using the parameters, the scoring system allows you to compare the nutrient densities of fruits and vegetables. The table on page 80 lists a variety of commonly available fruits. How do your favorites stack up?

Fruit	Nutrient Score*	Nutrient Highlights	
		High in...(20-100+%DV)	Moderate (10-19%DV) or Adequate (5-9%DV) source of...
Guava (1)	421	Carotenoids, very high in vitamin C	Potassium, fiber, folate
Watermelon (2 cups)	310	Carotenoids, vitamin C	Potassium, fiber
Grapefruit (1/2 pink or red)	263	Carotenoids, vitamin C	Potassium, fiber, folate
Kiwifruit (1)	233	Vitamin C	Potassium, fiber, folate, carotenoids
Cantaloupe (1/4)	200	Carotenoids, vitamin C	Folate, potassium
Orange (1)	186	Vitamin C, folate	Potassium, fiber, folate, carotenoids
Strawberries (8)	173	Vitamin C	Potassium, fiber, folate
Apricots (4)	156	Vitamin C	Potassium, fiber, carotenoids
Raspberries (1 cup)	106	Vitamin C, fiber	Potassium, folate
Blueberries (1 cup)	56	Vitamin C	Fiber
Banana (1)	54	n/a	Vitamin C, folate, potassium, fiber
Grapes (1.5 cups)	46	Vitamin C	Potassium, fiber
Avocado (1/2)	44	n/a	Vitamin C, folate, potassium, fiber
Apple (1)	43	n/a	Vitamin C, potassium, fiber
Raisins (1/4 cup)	24	n/a	Potassium, fiber

*Copyright 1998, CSPI. Adapted from *Nutrition Action Health Letter* (1875 Connecticut Ave., N.W., Suite 300, Washington, D.C. 20009-5728), *www.cspinet.org/nah/fanfruit.htm*.

A fruit's score only gives an indication of its nutrient density; it doesn't tell you which ones provide large amounts of carbohydrate for fuel. For instance, eating half a pink grapefruit is a great way to get carotenoids and vitamin C, but it's also a lot of work for only 50 calories. On the other hand, just one banana has a lower nutrient density but provides about 30 grams of carbohydrate and about 120 calories. The table below shows the amount of carbohydrate you get from select fruits.

Fruit	Grams of carbohydrate serving
Raisins (1/4 cup, packed)	33
Banana (1 large)	30
Pear (1 medium)	25
Grapes (1.5 cups)	24
Watermelon (2 cups)	22
Blueberries (1 cup)	21

Grains, Pasta, and Cereals

Most grains, including wheat, rice, rye, and barley, have to be processed to some extent before they are edible. This often means cracking, splitting, or removing the hulls that protected the grain while it was still attached to the plant. During this process, the bran and germ are often removed, and with them go much of the fiber, minerals, and antioxidants. Look for foods containing whole grains, even if they have been ground into flour. Look for "100-percent whole-wheat" breads that have one or more of the following close to the top of the ingredient list: whole-wheat flour, cracked wheat, rolled oats, barley, and rye. And you don't have to go to specialty bakeries to find decent bread; there are plenty in the grocery-store aisles. Look for multigrain breads, especially those that also contain seeds, like sunflower, sesame, and flaxseed.

Beyond breads, grains are used to produce foods that are staples in the diets of many cultures. Basic pasta, in any shape or size, is made from flour, water, and salt. The flour can be made from several grains, and you can find whole-grain varieties of pasta in most grocery stores. But as an athlete, you should look beyond pasta and brown rice for variety and more quality carbohydrates. Other than the obvious 100-percent

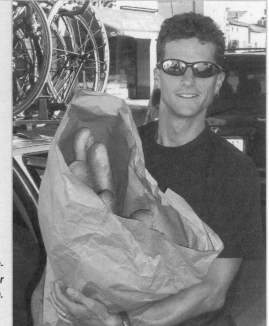

CTS Coach Jim Lehman carrying one day's worth of bread for the CTS Tour de France Camp.
Photo © by CTS/Craig Griffin

whole-grain breads and cereals, you can choose bulgur wheat, quinoa, oatmeal, pearl barley, whole-grain corn, or whole oats to fill the bill. In some cases, the caloric value of these alternative carbohydrate sources is equal to that of normal spaghetti, but their different tastes, textures, and common uses in recipes may keep your nutrition program from getting stale. Also, because of their high fiber content, whole grains promote proper bowel function and provide a feeling of fullness with fewer calories.

Breakfast cereal is a staple in many people's nutrition programs and can be a major source of carbohydrate. Determining whether your breakfast cereal is a quality, empty, or pollutant carrier begins with looking at the degree to which the grain portion of the cereal was processed. As an athlete, you want cereals made from whole grains that have been cracked, split, or even puffed. The best of these include muesli, served cold, and oatmeal, served hot. These two cereals are almost entirely comprised of rolled oats and often contain very little added sugar or preservatives. The best varieties add nuts and dried fruits, including almonds, walnuts, raisins, and/or dates; you can add them on your own as well. Pre-packaged oatmeal comes in a variety of flavors, and the addition of a little flavoring and some dehydrated fruit pieces rarely detracts from the benefits of the whole, rolled oats. These packets can be easily prepared in the microwave at work, providing a great breakfast or midday snack. Add some walnuts and raisins to further boost the nutrient density.

Cereals made from whole-grain flour or meal, including corn, wheat, and brown rice, are also very good choices. Even though they may have been ground and cooked into flakes, the nutritional value of the original grains, including the bran and fiber, are still there. Again, the best varieties of these cereals contain nuts, fruits, and a variety of different grains.

Cereal (1-cup serving)	Calories	Carbohydrate (g)	Fiber (g)	Protein (g)	Fat (g)
Post Grape-Nuts	390	90	11	13	.5
Kellogg's Low-Fat Granola	427	89	7	9	7
Quaker 100% Natural Low-Fat Granola with Raisins	389	81	6	9	6
Kellogg's All-Bran Buds	248	72	36	8.5	2
Kellogg's Müeslix with Raisins, Dates & Almonds	300	60	6	7.5	4.5
General Mills Fiber One	123	48	29	5.5	1.5
Kellogg's Raisin Bran	197	47	8	6	2
Kellogg's All-Bran Original	162	45	19.5	7.5	2
Quaker Oatmeal Squares	216	44	5	8	3
Quaker Cap'n Crunch	143	30.5	1	2	2
Kellogg's Product 19	110	25	2	3	.5
General Mills Lucky Charms	116	25	1	2	1
General Mills Multi Grain Cheerios	112	25	2	2.5	1
Kellogg's Rice Krispies	100	23	.5	2	.5
Kellogg's Special K	115	23	1	7	.5

Source: Compiled from information on cereal boxes and corporate websites, 2003.

Empty and Pollutant Carriers

Too Sweet for Your Own Good

While it is theoretically possible to meet your carbohydrate requirement with only Mountain Dew and Pixy Stix, doing so would be a decidedly poor choice. These and other foods like them are referred to as empty carriers because all they deliver is processed sugars. There are no beneficial vitamins or minerals included, no fiber or phytochemicals, just sugar.

Another concern is that the ingestion of sweets (cola, cake, cookies, candy) often displaces more nutritious foods. By replacing milk with a cola at a meal, you are losing out on the beneficial calcium, protein, and other vitamins and minerals available in the milk. This is especially disconcerting with children and adolescents who are still growing and tend to choose sodas over more nutritious choices (see Chapter 12 on sports nutrition for adolescent athletes).

Some empty-carrier carbohydrates masquerade as quality carriers. Choosing fruit juice over cola and granola bars over cookies seem like good ideas, but depending on the ingredients, your fruit juice and granola bars could be nearly as devoid of nutrients as the cola and cookies. Some juices contain very little actual fruit juice, meaning they are nearly equivalent to cola: high-fructose corn syrup, flavoring, and water. Similarly, many granola bars contain a lot of added sugar, as well as fillers that reduce the actual amount of oats in the bar. Take a minute to look at the ingredient panels on your snack foods; there might be a more nutrient-dense choice on the shelf.

Empty-Carrier Carbohydrate	Replace with these better choices . . .
Cola	Quality fruit juice
Kool-Aid	Vegetable juices
Cookies	Milk
Sugar wafers	Low-fat fig bars
Cupcakes	Granola bars
Low-fat candy	Sports drinks
	Nuts
	Energy bars

Sugar Cereals

Breakfast cereals can be a major source of empty carbohydrates. Most of these products are commonly referred to as "sugar cereals," colorful boxes promising magical adventures, free toys, marshmallows, and tastes and shapes similar to cookies, French toast, and chocolate bars. The grains used to make the cereal were processed to remove the bran and germ that contained the fiber and phytochemicals. Most manufacturers fortify their cereals with vitamins and minerals to replace a portion of what processing removed. Then they add a lot of refined sugar, along with the crunch berries and dehydrated marshmallows. It's the addition of sugar and the removal of beneficial components of the grain that lead people to demonize sugar cereals, but again their advice is aimed more toward sedentary individuals and children than toward athletes.

Sugar Cereal (1-cup serving)	Calories	Carbs (g)	Fat (g)	Fiber (g)	Protein (g)
Kellogg's Frosted Flakes	156	37.5	0	0.5	1.5
General Mills Cinnamon Toast Crunch	165.5	32	4	2	2
Smacks	133	32	0.7	1.3	2.7
General Mills Reese's Peanut Butter Puffs	172.5	30.5	4.5	0.5	3.5
Quaker Cap'n Crunch	143	30.5	2	1	2
Quaker Cap'n Crunch's Crunch Berries	138.5	29.5	1.5	1	1.5
General Mills Boo Berry	116.5	27.5	0.5	0.5	1
General Mills Franken Berry	117	27.5	0.5	0	1
Post Fruity Pebbles	129.5	27.5	1.5	0.5	1.5
Kellogg's Apple Jacks	115.5	27	0.5	0.5	1.5
General Mills Cocoa Puffs	119	26.5	1	0	1
General Mills Count Chocula	117.5	26.5	1	0.5	1.5
Kellogg's Froot Loops	117.5	26.5	1	0.5	1.5
General Mills Lucky Charms	116	25	1	1	2
Post Honeycomb	86	19.5	0.5	0.5	1.5

Source: Compiled from information on cereal boxes and corporate websites, 2003.

Sugar cereals can be a fun way to add some variety to your nutrition program, but they should not significantly displace more nutrient-dense cereals. Some athletes like to mix a sugar cereal in with more nutritious cereals, like Smacks mixed with Grape-Nuts. If your favorite cereals don't taste good together, pour smaller portions of each and have them both for breakfast. Some sugar cereals are so sweet that athletes eat them for dessert after lunch or dinner. There's a lot of carbohydrate in sugar cereals, and not much fat. Remember, your body breaks all carbohydrates down to monosaccharides before absorbing them anyway, so if you're looking to replenish depleted energy stores, sugar cereals work pretty well. This doesn't mean you should stock your cupboards with only Cocoa Crispies, Lucky Charms, Smacks, and Fruit Loops; your primary cereal choices should be the whole-grain cereals mentioned above.

Give a Hoot, Don't Pollute

While some sweets are empty carriers in that they are generally devoid of beneficial micronutrients, others fall into the pollutant carrier category because they contain high amounts of saturated fat and trans-fatty acids. These types of fat contribute to the development of cardiovascular disease and should be consumed sparingly. Saturated fat is found in butter, cream, lard, and shortening; and trans-fatty acids are saturated fats made from vegetable oils (both will be discussed in more detail in Chapter 8). Since you get some of each in other parts of your nutrition program, the easiest way to reduce your overall consumption of saturated fat and trans-fatty acids is to sparingly eat sweets and desserts containing them. This includes some candies, cheesecake, and many pre-packaged baked goods like muffins and crackers that are high in trans-fat.

Minor Sources of Carbohydrate

While there are carbohydrates in foods other than fruits, vegetables, and grains, these represent the major sources of carbohydrate in an athlete's nutrition program. Nuts, for instance, contain carbohydrates, but people rarely eat nuts as a means of supplying the majority of their carbo-

Pollutant Carrier Carbs	Serving Size	Calories	Carbs (g)	Total Fat (g)	% Calories from Fat
Cheesecake	100 grams (approx 3.5 oz)	321	26	23	64
Cheese Danish	100 grams	374	37	22	53
McDonald's French Fries (medium)	5.2 oz	450	57	22	44
McDonald's Baked Apple Pie	2.7 oz	260	34	13	46
Dunkin Donuts Powdered Cake Stick	1	450	42	29	58
Dunkin Donuts Plain Cake Stick	1	420	35	29	62
Krispy Kreme Original Glazed Doughnut	1	200	22	12	55
Krispy Kreme Powdered Creme Filled Doughnut	1	340	36	21	56
Little Debbie Honey Bun	1 (3 oz)	360	43	19	48
Hostess Ding Dongs	2 cakes	360	44	19	48
Frito-Lay Cheetos	15 puffs	150	16	9	54
Frito-Lay Ruffles Cheddar and Sour Cream Potato Chips	1.5 oz	240	21	15	56
Keebler E.L. Fudge Sandwich Cookies	2 cookies	120	17	6	45

Source: Compiled from information on packaging and corporate websites, 2003.

hydrate energy. Rather, nuts are a minor carbohydrate source, more suitable for snacks and sought after for their healthy balance of mono-unsaturated fat, protein, and vitamins. Dairy products like milk and yogurt also contain some carbohydrate, but their primary contribution to an athlete's diet is protein, and I'll discuss them more fully in Chapter 7. Meat, poultry, and fish are not really even considered minor sources of carbohydrate because they contain little or none. Their main contributions are protein and fat, and I'll cover them in Chapters 7 and 8.

These carriers...	Contain, in addition to the desired carbohydrate...	Such as...	As found in...
Quality carriers	Beneficial components	Vitamins, minerals, carotenoids, phytochemicals, antioxidants, dietary fiber	Dark-colored fruits and vegetables, brown rice, whole grains
Empty carriers	Things that are neither beneficial nor detrimental	Refined sugar, artificial or non-caloric sweeteners	Cookies, cake, some candies
Pollutant carriers	Components that are harmful or hinder performance	Saturated fat, trans-fatty acids, preservatives	Colas, french fries, highly processed "convenience" foods

Food Properties Influence Effectiveness

A food's quality as a carrier of nutrients should be your first method of determining its suitability to be part of your nutrition program. After you've decided to include a food, it's then time to consider how and when to eat it. The characteristics of the food, and the methods used to prepare it, influence how effectively that food can be used for fuel.

The speed with which you digest a starch doesn't make one vegetable or grain better or worse than another, but it can affect your meal choices before and after exercise. When you are looking for quick carbohydrate energy, as you would from a meal one or two hours before training, you want to eat starches and vegetables that break down quickly into absorbable monosaccharides, such as rice and barley. Some vegetables, such as peas and beans, take longer to break down, so while they are still great sources of carbohydrate and quality carriers, they may not be your best choice when you need energy quickly. Rice or pasta would be a better bet and provide you with energy more quickly. It would be better to eat lentils, peas, and beans as part of a post-exercise meal, or a meal three to four hours before training.

The way you cook or prepare a carbohydrate can improve its effectiveness as a fuel. When starches are heated or boiled, they tend to soften

Good pre-exercise starches (i.e., break down to usable energy quickly)	Good post-exercise starches (i.e., slower to digest, but very good for replenishing fuel stores)
Potatoes Pasta Rice Barley	Peas Beans (black beans, pintos, kidney, etc.) Lentils

or become gelatinous because the cell walls burst and expose their carbohydrate contents. This means your digestive system can get to the starch more easily and break more of it down to usable energy. There is a tradeoff, however, to cooking vegetables. While it is necessary to cook potatoes, rice, and yucca to make their starches accessible, it's better to consume other vegetables raw or steamed. Since boiling a vegetable significantly reduces its vitamin and mineral content, you're better off eating less starchy, more vitamin-rich vegetables raw or lightly steamed. This would apply to vegetables like peppers, broccoli, and spinach.

Grinding or crushing food also makes it more readily available for digestion. The acids and enzymes in your digestive system struggle to break through the skin of corn kernels, peas, and most beans. In order to get as much usable carbohydrate from them as possible, it is sometimes good to break the skins in the process of cooking or preparing meals, as with refried beans, split-pea soup, and creamed corn.

Should be cooked to make carbohydrate available	Should be eaten raw or lightly cooked to preserve vitamin and mineral content
Potatoes Corn Beans Lentils Peas	Broccoli Peppers Spinach Tomatoes

6

SETTING THE RECORD STRAIGHT ON LOW-CARB DIETS FOR ATHLETES

IN AN EFFORT TO REDUCE THE NUMBER OF OVERWEIGHT AND obese people in our society, researchers, doctors, and celebrities have been devising new and innovative diets for decades. Their intentions are honorable, but their methods miss the mark. By focusing on the particular foods they feel should be eliminated, they have put too much emphasis on energy intake and too little on energy expenditure. Diets very low in carbohydrate gained widespread popularity in the late 1990s, promising fast and significant weight loss. Ever since reports of rapid weight loss on the high-protein, low-carb diets have hit the newsstands, active people have been shunning their old reliable sources of muscle fuel (bagels, bananas, and pasta). While these diets have their merits for a *select* population, a nutrition program higher in carbohydrate is much more appropriate for you as an athlete.

How Low-Carb Diets Work

There's no doubt that people who stick to a low-carbohydrate diet can lose weight, but their weight loss has less to do with carbohydrate and more to do with behavior and physiology.

1. Initial Weight Loss Is Due to Lost Glycogen and Water Weight

When you stop eating carbohydrate, you burn through all of your stored glycogen reasonably quickly. It may take a sedentary person two days to deplete his or her energy stores, and an athlete less than one day. Glycogen stores three times its weight of water with it, meaning one gram of glycogen is worth a total of four grams of body weight. The majority of the initial weight loss (4 to 6 pounds) people see with a low-carb diet is due to glycogen depletion and water loss. This doesn't mean a person is necessarily dehydrated, because the water lost was the water stored within the muscle with glycogen. Water content in other tissues and in the blood may remain normal.

Of additional concern to athletes is the fact that in the first few days of carbohydrate deprivation, during the transition from burning stored glycogen to producing ketones (byproducts of fat metabolism) for energy, your body creates as much glucose as it can from skeletal muscle proteins. Your muscles are broken down to supply amino acids, which the liver then uses to produce glucose. Over the course of a few days, muscle-protein loss contributes to initial weight loss, but it also robs you of power and muscle mass that you worked so hard to gain.

2. Cutting Carbohydrates Reduces Snacking, Which Reduces Caloric Intake

When people try to eliminate carbohydrates from their diets, cookies, candy, soda, and crackers are some of the first things to go. These are easily identifiable as high in carbohydrates and are easily removed because doing so doesn't disrupt normal meals or recipes. By simply reducing the number of snacks you eat, you reduce your daily caloric intake, and if you reduce intake below expenditure, you have created the conditions necessary for weight loss.

3. Foods Higher in Protein and Fat Are More Filling, So You Stop Eating Sooner

This is one of the topics that can be spun to the benefit of either the high- or low-carb community. The argument seems reminiscent of an advertising campaign used by Miller Lite in the '80s: Remember those ads where a bar/stadium/living room was split down the middle between groups chanting "Tastes Great" and "Less Filling"? The low-carb community points to the less-filling nature of carbohydrate-rich foods as the reason people eat portions that are too large, and in some cases, they're correct. Some sweets and crackers lack both the fiber that make fruits and vegetables more filling and the caloric density that makes starches more filling. When your carbohydrates come primarily from sources that are quality carriers, however, you shouldn't have trouble feeling full after eating appropriately sized portions.

To argue the tastes-great side of the argument, advocates of nutrition programs based on higher carbohydrate intakes, myself included, say that foods high in protein and fat are more satiating than high-carbohydrate foods. Chefs, including CTS head chef Greg Brown, are fond of saying that the way to make any recipe taste better is to add butter or cream. These and other foods high in fat and/or protein taste richer and lead people to feel full after eating smaller portions. This is partially due to the fact that fatty foods stay in your stomach longer than less-fatty foods. Thus, by eating meals that feel filling but contain fewer calories, people lose weight. If they were to eat the same number of calories as the result of a more balanced diet, even one relatively high in carbohydrate, they would achieve the same caloric deficit.

Insulin and the Athlete

Insulin is one of the most powerful and most misunderstood hormones in the body. For most people, diabetes is the reason they recognize the

Ketones and Exercise

One of the main premises of low-carb diets is that depriving the body of carbohydrates will force it to switch to using fat for fuel. Your body's number-one priority is to provide the brain and central nervous system with a steady supply of energy. Since it can't supply enough energy from carbohydrate (it's not available), or from protein (production of glucose through gluconeogenesis is limited), your body transports fatty acids to the liver so they can be converted to ketone bodies. Ketones can provide energy because, when broken down by muscle and nerve cells, they produce two compounds that are intermediates in normal aerobic metabolism. Your cells don't necessarily care how the intermediates were created, but once they're present, they can be burned aerobically for energy. Athletes should note, however, that ketone bodies break down to intermediates that can only be used by the aerobic system. You can't generate energy anaerobically with ketones, which is one of the reasons athletes on low-carbohydrate diets struggle to sustain even moderate-intensity exercise (50 to 65 percent of maximum effort) when ketone levels are high.

word, and consequently they figure anything having to do with insulin must be connected to disease. As a result, fear has made athletes worry, mostly unnecessarily, about this very important hormone.

Insulin becomes a problem when either you cannot produce enough of it, or your cells become resistant to its effects. In some cases, it is believed that the pancreas just wears out over time, and after years of producing higher-than-normal amounts of insulin, it gradually produces less and less and may eventually stop altogether. This is more often the case in Type II diabetes, and poor nutrition and lack of exercise play integral roles in the development of the disease. Chronic overeating, coupled with inactivity, forces the pancreas to secrete more insulin in order to move a given amount of glucose and fatty acid out of the blood. After a long time, the pancreas wears out.

In a discouraging turn of events, adolescents and children are being diagnosed with Type II diabetes in ever increasing numbers. The number of overweight children and adolescents in the United States had risen to approximately 15.3 percent of children (ages 6 to 11) and 15.5 percent of adolescents (ages 12 to 19) as of the year 2000. An additional 15 percent of children and 14.9 percent of adolescents were at risk for becoming overweight (body-mass index for age between the 85th and 95th percentile). Many young children have such poor nutrition and exercise habits that they're developing largely preventable diseases twenty years earlier than normal.

Some people develop a resistance to the effects of insulin, which leads to chronically high insulin and glucose levels in the blood. The trouble isn't with the insulin itself but with the receptors that are normally sensitive to it. When insulin receptors lose their sensitivity, in part as the result of excessive eating and lack of exercise, it takes more of the hormone to activate the receptors and allow glucose to pass into cells. As a result, insulin levels remain high for longer periods of time, further reducing the receptors' sensitivity and leading to a condition known as insulin resistance. In some cases, the receptors simply stop reacting altogether.

Exercising regularly increases insulin's effectiveness by improving the way cells react when insulin binds to its receptors, thereby promoting more efficient uptake of glucose. This means less of the hormone needs to be secreted to achieve the desired result. Athletes, therefore, are at a lower risk of developing Type II diabetes, since they reduce the strain on the pancreas. This is true even in light of the fact that post-exercise recovery nutrition is often aimed at causing a significant increase in blood glucose, which increases insulin production and secretion. Your body is reacting to low glycogen stores as a result of prolonged exercise, and is only secreting the appropriate amount of insulin to move glucose into muscles and replenish those stores. Insulin levels don't stay elevated for prolonged periods of time, either; they fall as the ingested food energy is absorbed into cells to replenish depleted glycogen stores.

Insulin also has an important anabolic (muscle-building) function. Not only does insulin facilitate the uptake of glucose and triglycerides (fat) from the bloodstream; it also increases the amounts of amino acids absorbed into muscle. Amino acids from protein are the building blocks of muscle and connective tissues. After training applies stress to your muscles, amino acids are necessary to achieve some of the physiological adaptations you're aiming for. They are responsible for building additional muscle tissue, maintaining the muscle you have, and repairing damaged tissue to better prepare you for more exercise.

Sedentary people run into trouble because they usually have full glycogen tanks. When you burn a significant amount of energy as the result of exercise, the energy-storing function of insulin acts to replenish depleted glycogen stores, transporting amino acids into muscle for repair and maintenance. Since sedentary individuals don't expend much energy, they require less food to replenish these stores. Insulin, however, seeks to store energy regardless of how active you have been. If, and only if, energy stores are already full, insulin will facilitate the storage of excess energy in adipose tissue.

The Strengths and Weaknesses of the Glycemic Index

The Glycemic Index has received a lot of attention in recent years, mostly in the context of diabetes and low-carbohydrate diets. The index was originally developed by clinical nutritionists to help diabetics plan their nutrition programs, but athletes have different nutritional goals and needs than do diabetes patients. While low-carb dieters and diabetics see the glycemic index as a means of separating foods into "good" and "bad" categories, athletes see it as a means of determining the best foods for quick energy, long training sessions, and/or replenishing glycogen stores.

A high glycemic-index food quickly raises blood sugar to high levels, while low glycemic-index foods raise blood-sugar levels to a lesser extent. The trouble is, the glycemic index looks at foods in isolation, and it falls short as a practical guide to eating because it doesn't correlate well to the way we *actually* consume food. Most people combine several foods to make a meal or snack, rather than eating a single food. For instance, potatoes have a high glycemic-index value, but when you add some eggs and buttered toast to make breakfast, the fat and protein from these foods blunts the increase in blood sugar (and consequently slows the increase in blood-insulin level) that you would normally see from the potato alone.

Since athletes view food as fuel, they are more likely to eat a single food, like cereal, in order to fuel up before a workout or replenish fuel supplies after one. When you need a quick snack 30 minutes before a one-hour exercise class, try to get 30 to 60 grams of carbohydrate from a food with a medium glycemic-index value (50 to 70 out of 100), including: PowerBar Performance bar, raisin bran cereal, rice, instant oatmeal, Snickers bar, bran muffins, or trail mix with nuts and dried fruit. If you're eating prior to a longer exercise session, your meal should include lower glycemic-index carbohydrates, like pasta and beans.

During your workout, a combination of moderate- and high-glycemic-index foods works well to supply your muscles and brain with the carbohydrates they need. Good choices include PowerBar Endurance sports drink, ripe bananas, granola bars, and energy bars and gels. Studies suggest that after your workout, glycogen replenishment may occur at a higher rate by eating foods with high glycemic-index values, including potatoes, breads, recovery drinks (including PowerBar Recovery) that contain glucose, and breakfast cereals.

The table on page 97 shows foods that have high, moderate, and low glycemic-index values.

Who Benefits from Low-Carb Diets?

There is evidence that low-carb diets can effectively help overweight and obese people lose significant amounts of weight, as long as they can stick to the diet. Some studies have shown that low-carb diets more effectively reduced weight than conventional low-energy, calorie-restricted, low-fat diets. However, these same studies found that people were not able to comply with the necessary dietary restrictions in the long term. Compliance is one of the biggest factors in the success of any nutrition or exercise program. A program can only work as long as you can stick with it

Table of Glycemic Index of Commonly Eaten Foods

High > 80	
Waffles (Aunt Jemima)	Healthy Choice Hearty 100% Whole Grain bread
Doughnut	Couscous
Cheerios (General Mills)	Hamburger bun
Bagel	Bran muffin
Wonder Bread	Corn Chex
Sports drinks	Orange juice (from concentrate)
Oatmeal	Ocean Spray Cranberry Juice Cocktail
Coca-Cola	
Moderate 55-80	
PowerBar Performance bar	Soy milk, low-fat
Banana	Rye-kernel bread, pumpernickel
Brown rice, steamed	Apple
Oranges	Strawberries
Low < 55	
Skim milk	Chickpeas
Ice cream, premium, ultra chocolate, 15% fat	Yogurt, low-fat
Peanuts, cashews	Lentils
Kellogg's All-Bran	

for a long time, and in the best-case scenario, this means permanently changing nutrition and behaviors. For active people and sports enthusiasts, our athletic activities influence the ways we spend our leisure time, the foods we eat for fuel, the equipment we choose to spend our money on, and the kinds of relationships we make. Being physically active profoundly and positively impacts many seemingly unrelated aspects of our lifestyles, making an athletic lifestyle easier to stick with than conventional diet plans.

Low-Carb Diets Are *Not* Suitable for Athletes

Low-carbohydrate diets serve a specific purpose for a distinct portion of the population. They were devised to help overweight and obese people lose body mass in order to improve their health. They were not devised with the intention of improving performance. You, the athletic community, were not the audience those diets were targeting. Sometimes, ideas are good enough to help people beyond those they were intended for, but unfortunately, in the case of low-carbohydrate diets, this isn't so.

One of the goals of low-carbohydrate diets is to chronically deprive the body of carbohydrates. However, we know that when you do not consume enough carbohydrate, you deplete your energy stores and cannot work out effectively. The idea of a low-carb diet is to force the body to rely on fat for energy, thereby burning away stored adipose tissue. As explained in Chapter 2, athletes can't rely on fat for the majority of their energy because their activity level demands energy faster than it can be supplied by fat. Although fat is a contributor to all exercise intensities, it only supplies the majority of your energy for low-intensity (< 50 percent of maximum intensity) exercise. Many recreational and moderately trained athletes work at intensities higher than that during their pre-workout warm-ups. Full stores of glycogen are needed to support the intensity levels that recreational and moderately trained athletes regularly experience during their workouts and athletic activities. When active people attempt to work out in a glycogen-depleted state, as happens when they are eating a low-carb diet, they cannot sustain the exercise intensity or duration as well as they could when they were eating more carbohydrate.

Considering the facts that low-intensity exercise can be beneficial for primarily sedentary people and that low-intensity exercise may be sustainable on a low-carb diet, sedentary people may be the population to benefit from low-carb diets. These people should have enough energy to support the American College of Sports Medicine exercise recommendation of 30 to 60 minutes of walking, three to five days per week. This level of activity may be enough to induce a training effect and reduce cardiovascular disease risk for sedentary people. Active people and athletes, on the other hand, need more food energy to support a higher level of activity, and much of this increased energy needs to come from carbohydrates.

Not only do power, endurance, stamina, and strength decrease as a result of carbohydrate depletion; athletes sometimes feel nauseated, dizzy, and/or lightheaded, too. While most endurance athletes have experienced these symptoms associated with "bonking" or "hitting the wall" at some point, bonking usually occurs hours into a long workout as the result of low blood sugar. The symptoms of bonking catch athletes off-guard when they appear within the first 30 minutes of exercise, but the body is reacting to the same scenario. Glucose is the primary fuel your brain and central nervous system can directly use for energy, so your body acts defensively to preserve whatever glucose it has left. Bonking is your body's way of forcing you to stop exercising while there is still enough glucose in your blood to maintain normal bodily functions. Athletes eating low-carbohydrate diets bonk much earlier than normal because they start workouts glycogen-depleted. As a result, they have far less fuel than they need to supply energy for muscles and the central nervous system.

In addition to glycogen depletion, cutting out essential carbohydrates can lead to a significant deficit in essential vitamins, minerals, fiber, and other nutrients our bodies need to function normally. Consumption of whole grains, fruits, and vegetables has a strong link to cancer prevention. The National Cancer Institute and the American Heart Association (AHA) recommend five servings of fruits and vegetables each day as the minimum amount one should eat in order to help significantly reduce the risk of developing cancer. Studies have shown that approximately 35 percent of all cancer deaths in the U.S. may be related to poor dietary habits. Fruits and vegetables contain literally thousands of compounds that show promise for possibly preventing cancer and many other chronic diseases. Finally, it has been shown that people who eat generous amounts of fruits and vegetables are less likely to suffer from heart disease, high blood pressure, and stroke. Fortunately, many of the books advocating low-carb diets do recommend that the limited amount of carbohydrate participants consume should come from whole grains, fruits, and vegetables.

In a coaches' roundtable discussion about nutritional challenges facing CTS members, the struggle to support training while eating a low-carbohydrate diet received a lot of attention. The CTS director of coaching, James Herrera, MS CSCS, described a typical scenario:

> I watched Paul B, a fellow cyclist who frequently attends my indoor power cycling classes, "hit the wall" like no one I've ever seen before. After the class, we discussed his situation, and he described the low-carb weight-loss methods he had been utilizing for a while. I explained the importance of carbohydrates to athletic performance, and the following week, he was carbed up and riding like a champ. One of the professional mountain bikers I coach, Blair Matheison, "bonked" several times during his early spring training. As we discussed his goal of shedding a few pounds and his recent bonking episodes on just about every training ride, he revealed to me that he'd been experimenting with the low-carb method of losing weight. A week after getting back on a nutrition program rich in high-octane carbohydrate, he placed third in a 55-mile ultra-endurance mountain-bike event. Case closed. Athletes need carbs to fuel working muscles.

Sugar Alcohols and Net Carbs

With the popularity of low-carbohydrate diets and the relative difficulty people experience complying with their restrictions, it was inevitable that food producers would market pre-packaged, low-carb snacks and meals. One of the challenges to removing carbohydrates from foods, though, is compensating for their bulk. If you were to replace the sugar in a cookie with artificial sweetener, it would take up a minuscule fraction of the space the sugar occupied before. You would have to find some way to replace that mass, because otherwise your cookie wouldn't look, feel, or stay together the way you'd expect it to. For better or worse, carbohydrates themselves offer a solution to this problem: sugar alcohols.

Easily produced commercially from regular sugar, sugar alcohols were originally used in sugar-free gum (to prevent tooth decay), and in foods marketed to diabetics (because sugar alcohols are not as readily digested or absorbed as normal sugar). Foods containing sugar alcohols don't supply as much glucose, fructose, or galactose as normal foods do, meaning diabetics can enjoy them without raising blood-glucose levels too high. This same mechanism appeals to the low-carb community because less blood glucose means less secretion of insulin, the hormone they see as responsible for weight gain.

Sugar Alcohols and Athletes

Sugar alcohols can be very beneficial to diabetics' quality of life by increasing the variety of food products they can eat while controlling their blood-glucose levels. It's difficult to advocate their widespread consumption by athletes or non-diabetic, overweight adults because consuming 50 grams or more per day can have a significant laxative effect. Since it is not digested and not much of it is absorbed, most of it reaches the large intestine and colon untouched, where it is then fermented by bacteria. Foods containing significant amounts of sugar alcohols, like low-carb candy and snack bars, are also highly processed, and in some cases they contain lots of preservatives and synthetic ingredients to make them more palatable.

What Net Carbs Mean for Athletes

The phrases "net carbs," "active carbs," and "impact carbs" have become part of the American lexicon as food manufacturers and restaurants try to attract low-carb dieters to their products. An "active" or "impact" carb

Sugar Alcohol*	Digested	Absorbed	Metabolized	Usable Energy*
Mannitol	No	About 25%	Negligible	2.8 kcal/g
Sorbitol	No	About 50%	Up to 85% of absorbed	2.6 kcal/g
Xylitol	No	25%	100% of absorbed	2.4 kcal/g

*Sugars have 4 kcal/g
Adapted from *Present Knowledge in Nutrition*, 7th Ed. Edited by Ekhard E. Ziegler and L. J. Filer, Rr. (Chapter 59 by John W. Finley and Gilbert A. Leveille). 1996 International Life Science Institute Press, Washington, D.C., page 583, table 2.

is one that raises blood sugar, so to arrive at a food's "net carb" count, you subtract the carbohydrates that have minimal impact on blood sugar, like fiber and sugar alcohols. So, while there might be 20 grams of carbohydrate listed on the Nutrition Facts label, if the product contains 15 grams of sugar alcohol, you're only getting five usable grams of carbohydrate: good for the low-carb dieter, bad for the athlete.

The Subway restaurant chain took the "net carb" idea in another direction; their low-carb wrap is mostly indigestible fiber. Honestly, it's great for everybody, not because it's low in "impact carbs," but because fiber may help prevent colon cancer and most of us don't eat enough of it. The tortilla wrap shell alone has 11 grams of fiber in it, compared to 3 grams in their six-inch rolls. When you pile on fresh vegetables, one Subway Wrap can provide more than half of the National Cancer Institute's recommendation of 25 to 30 daily grams of fiber. All the same, if you're looking for carbohydrate fuel, the Subway Wrap won't help you much.

Overall, athletes should be wary of foods produced specifically for low-carb dieters; the fuel you need is exactly what they're trying to avoid. You need digestible, absorbable, and usable carbohydrate to power your muscles with energy far beyond what fat and protein can provide on their own.

AN ATHLETE'S GUIDE
TO PROTEIN

THOUGH CARBOHYDRATE AND FAT ARE BOTH VERY VERSATILE nutrients, neither has as wide-ranging a role as protein does. While the primary roles of carbohydrate and fat are to provide energy, protein provides the building blocks for tissues, enzymes, and hormones that control metabolism and movement. It also provides immune structures that protect your body from infections, in addition to between 10 and 15 percent of your energy during exercise. Protein is an integral part of every athlete's nutrition program, and both power and endurance athletes need to consume more protein than do sedentary people.

Basic Facts About Protein

The structure of protein enables it to fulfill many diverse roles in the human body. A protein is made by linking amino acids together into a

Essential Amino Acids	Nonessential Amino Acids	Conditionally Essential Amino Acids
Must be obtained from food	Can be made in the body	Can be made in the body, but may become essential for growing young people
Histidine	Arganine	Taurine
Isoleucine	Alanine	Cysteine
Leucine	Aspartate	Tyrosine
Lysine	Glutamate	Glycine
Methionine	Glutamine	Proline
Phenylalanine		Serine
Threonine		
Tryptophan		
Valine		

long chain, the sequence and shape of which determines its function. Beyond linking together to form complicated protein structures, amino acids themselves can be used to provide immediate energy or can be converted to either glucose or fatty acids to be stored and then used for energy later.

While all of the proteins your body needs can be constructed from the 20 identified amino acids, your body can't make all of the amino acids it needs. Of the 20, nine are considered *essential* because they have to be supplied from outside the body. It is necessary to obtain these amino acids from your food, but you do not have to include them in every meal. You should try to consume foods that contain the essential amino acids at least once about every 48 hours to prevent deficiencies, and this is rarely a problem for athletes consuming a variety of foods and a relatively high caloric intake.

The Role of Protein in Exercise

More important than its contribution to energy is protein's role in creating enzymes, hormones, lipoproteins (good and bad cholesterol), muscle tissue, connective tissue, red blood cells, and immune-system cells.

Training applies a stress to the body that leads to many positive adaptations that involve protein. Some of these are clearly visible, like the growth of muscle tissue. Others, like the increased production of hormones and neurotransmitters, are not directly visible, but are noticeable as improved performance.

Increasing Fat Oxidation

One of the adaptations to endurance training is an increase in the number of mitochondria in muscle cells and a subsequent increase in the manufacture and storage of carnitine, a protein responsible for transporting fatty acids into mitochondria to be burned for energy. Together, these factors increase the rate at which the cell can produce energy aerobically, which means it can continue burning fat at higher exercise intensities than before. The majority of your carnitine is made in your body from the essential amino acids lysine and methionine.

Increasing Oxygen Delivery

Hemoglobin is a protein found in red blood cells that is responsible for binding oxygen. As blood travels through the lungs, oxygen diffuses into the blood and is picked up by red blood cells. The blood then travels to all tissues, including working muscles, where the oxygen is used by the aerobic system. Adequate protein intake is essential because aerobic training results in increased production of red blood cells, and these cells wear out and need to be replaced constantly.

Strengthening Muscle Contractions

About 20 percent of muscle tissue mass is protein, including the mechanical parts (myosin and actin) responsible for contraction. When these filaments slide over one another, they cause the muscle fiber to shorten, or contract. Both endurance and strength training increase the amount of force you can produce with a muscle by increasing the number of myosin and actin filaments in muscle.

Sparing Glycogen

During exercise, protein can account for 10 to 15 percent of total energy expenditure, and that may help prolong the life span of liver- and muscle-glycogen stores. Some protein can be stripped down and thrown into the aerobic engine right in muscle cells while other amino acids are converted to glucose through gluconeogenesis in the liver. These processes continue when you're at rest, too, providing 5 to 10 percent of your total daily energy expenditure.

Providing Energy

Three of the essential amino acids—leucine, isoleucine, and valine—are also referred to as branched-chain amino acids (BCAAs) due to the way their carbon skeletons are formed. These amino acids are special in that they can be broken down and used for energy within a muscle cell more easily than others, while other amino acids travel to the liver to be converted to glucose, ketones, or fatty acids before being used for energy.

Sustaining Aerobic Metabolism

The entire process of breaking nutrients down to usable energy is lengthy and requires many steps and ingredients (enzymes and intermediates). During sustained exercise, you could actually run out of some of these intermediate ingredients if you couldn't make them from amino acids. To perform optimally, you want your aerobic engine to produce the maximum amount of energy from every bit of carbohydrate and fat, and that can only happen if you have all the intermediates to complete the process. When even one is missing or its supplies are low, you either liberate less energy than you possibly could have from a nutrient, or you limit your ability to burn that nutrient as quickly.

Enhancing the Immediate Energy System

The first 8 to 10 seconds of activity are powered by your immediate energy system, otherwise known as the ATP-CP system. As discussed in

Chapter 2, before either the anaerobic or aerobic system can provide energy, you can use intramuscular stores of ATP and creatine phosphate (CP) to power muscle contractions. This system is limited by the stores of CP in your muscles; stores that can be increased as the result of training. Increasing the capacity of the immediate energy system doesn't significantly extend the length of time it can operate, but it does increase the force you can generate while it is operating. Creatine can be obtained directly from animal foods, but it would take consuming 250 grams of red meat to get one gram of creatine. Considering that the daily requirement for a 150-pound male athlete is thought to be about 2 grams, it's a good thing your body can produce it on its own. The liver, kidneys, and pancreas can make creatine from the amino acids glycine, arganine, and methionine.

Quality-Carrier Protein Sources for Athletes

When choosing protein sources, you have to consider the amino acids the food contains as well as the vitamins, minerals, carbohydrate, and fat it also carries with it. Your body doesn't really require whole proteins per se, but rather specific amounts of essential amino acids.

It's not necessary for every protein source to contain all the essential amino acids. A normal, varied nutrition program supplies all of the essential amino acids from a combination of different foods. You might get some of your essential amino acids from cereals, others from legumes (beans and peas), and still others from animal products. Each food has its own amino-acid profile, and blending these sources in your daily diet provides a suitable balance of amino acids.

Foods that contain all of the essential amino acids, in amounts sufficient to meet your metabolic demands, are referred to as *complete proteins*. Eggs have long been considered the best source of complete protein, and other sources include meat, fish, poultry, and some dairy products. Whey protein, which is found in milk but not in some cheeses, is another great source of compete protein.

An *incomplete protein* is missing at least one essential amino acid.

Protein found in vegetables, with the exception of soybeans, is incomplete, but you can easily obtain all the essential amino acids by including a variety of protein-rich vegetables in your nutrition program.

Soy protein is the only vegetable source of complete protein, making it an important part of a vegetarian nutrition program. Soy products also contain flavonoids, which have been shown to increase levels of good HDL cholesterol and lower levels of bad LDL cholesterol, so they are also a healthy addition to everyone's diet. Because of their health and performance benefits, and their increased presence in grocery stores, foods containing soy protein will be covered in more detail later in this chapter.

While eating foods containing complete proteins is the easiest way to ensure you're meeting your protein requirements, it's also easy to get all your essential amino acids from combinations of incomplete proteins. These combinations are often referred to as *complementary proteins,* and include rice and beans, cereal and milk, whole-grain bread and cheese, bean or split-pea soup and a sandwich, oatmeal made with milk, or a cheese pizza. Again, you don't need to consume all the essential amino acids in one meal. As long as you consume them within the same day, your body will be able to make all the protein it needs.

Animal Protein Sources

Red Meat

Meat is a great source of complete protein and can be a healthy component of an athlete's nutrition program. The important thing in choosing and preparing meat is to watch the amount of fat it contains. In addition to supplying protein, red meat (beef, lamb, venison, and buffalo) is a great source of zinc, especially because zinc is more readily absorbed when it comes from meat than when it comes from vegetable sources. Meat is also high in iron, which plays a critical role in binding oxygen to red blood cells, and in B vitamins, which are important for energy production. The cuts of meat with the least fat are quality carriers, and include those with the words "loin" and "round" in the name (tenderloin, sirloin, top round, eye of round, etc.). Fattier meats include filet mignon and prime rib.

An ounce of red meat contains about seven grams of protein, meaning that the *standard* serving size (3 ounces) contains about 21 grams of protein. Most people, including athletes, consume at least twice the standard portion size in a normal meal. In fact, it's difficult to find a steak in a restaurant that's less than six ounces. A good way to estimate a three-to-four-ounce portion of meat, chicken, or fish is to eat a portion roughly the size of the palm of your hand or a deck of playing cards. The reason portion size is increasingly important in conjunction with meat intake is that consuming large amounts of meat can greatly increase your total caloric intake and saturated-fat intake. Since meat is dense, even a standard portion is a lot higher in calories than it looks.

While steaks and hamburgers are obvious meat choices, you should also look to alternative meals that contain additional nutrients. For in-

Meat (3 ounces, cooked)	Calories	Protein (g)	Fat (g)	Saturated Fat (g)
Quality Carrier (low in fat)				
Chicken breast	142	27	3	1
Pork tenderloin	171	25	7	3
Pork sirloin	177	26	7	2
Beef brisket	183	26	8	3
Beef sirloin	183	25	9	3
Top-round beef	195	26	9	3
Less Desirable (higher in fat)				
Pork center loin	204	24	11	4
Veal sirloin	214	27	11	4
Filet mignon (beef)	200	23	11	4
Lamb sirloin	200	22	12	6
T-bone steak (beef)	210	21	14	5
Beef hamburger	213	21	14	5
Ribs	242	21	17	7

stance, a sandwich made with lean roast beef from the deli counter supplies the protein, zinc, and B vitamins from the meat, additional protein from cheese, and complex carbohydrates and some protein from the bread. Chili is another great way for athletes to include meat in their nutrition programs. Since it often contains a variety of beans, meat, and a tomato base, chili can be absolutely packed with nutrients.

Chicken and Turkey

Chickens and turkeys are the most commonly eaten birds, and they and other fowl are great sources of complete protein. White meat, commonly from chicken and turkey breasts, may be a healthier alternative to red meat because it is lower in saturated fat. However, chicken and turkey contain ⅓ to ½ as much zinc and iron than does red meat. One way you can tell that chicken is lower in saturated fat than red meat is by comparing the consistency of their fats. At room temperature, chicken fat is soft and gelatinous. Beef fat is solid because it is higher in saturated fat. White meat (breasts and most of the meat on the body) is lower in fat than dark meat (legs, thighs, wings), but the protein content is the same.

Chicken and turkey are such good protein sources for athletes, and are so easily combined with other great foods, that they sometimes become staples of athletes' diets. This can be good and bad. The nutritional value of chicken is great, but you also need variety in your diet to ensure optimal nutrition. Overloading on chicken breasts, especially cooked the same way all the time, is not wise.

A few years ago, I was asked to provide a training-and-nutrition consultation for a player in the National Football League. Like many players in team sports such as football and basketball, his training program was less than optimal because the workouts were designed for the entire team, not for him as an individual. Managing the fitness part was relatively easy compared to suggesting changes to his diet. This 275-pound (125 kg) athlete was consuming an average of 12 chicken breasts *every day.* At a conservative average of four ounces per breast, this added up to 48 ounces of chicken and 336 grams of protein. That's nearly 1.25 grams of protein per pound of body weight per day, far more than his body could use. What's more, his primary method of preparing the chicken was a George Foreman Grill, which worked well for removing some of the fat in the chicken, but didn't do anything for adding additional nutrients to his meals. He also wasn't eating much in the way of pasta, rice, potatoes, fruit, or vegetables to increase his carbohydrate intake because he didn't want the additional calories. After I'd looked at his dietary-recall information, the reason for his lack of energy and lower-than-expected performance was clear: his diet was providing insufficient carbohydrate fuel and energy, and far too much protein. Over the next few weeks, he reduced his chicken intake and increased his carbohydrate intake, and the team trainers reported significant improvements in his performance in both practices and competitions.

I have nothing against chicken breasts; it's just important to look beyond them for protein sources in order to add variety and additional nutrients to your nutrition program. Consider buying canned chicken (look for white meat only, packed in water) and adding it to a can of soup or using it to make chicken salad. For the latter, you can even use plain yogurt instead of mayonnaise to further lower the fat content. Purchase sliced turkey breast from your deli counter and use it with lettuce, tomato, and cheese to make sandwiches on whole-grain bread. This quick meal is great after training, because it provides protein and carbohydrate to replenish depleted energy stores.

Eggs

Eggs are a great quality carrier for athletes and have long been considered one of the best and most complete sources of protein. Although they were vilified for their cholesterol content, recent research suggests that eggs are not as bad as they were made out to be. While it's true there is cholesterol in egg yolks, eggs are one of the best and most affordable sources of protein, containing all nine essential amino acids. Eggs are naturally rich in vitamins A and D, as well as in choline—an essential nutrient that plays a role in brain development and memory. In addition, they are a source of carotenoids that reduce the risk of cataracts and other age-related eye problems. And don't worry: Eating just the egg whites and discarding the yolks doesn't greatly diminish the egg's protein contribution to your diet. If you already have high levels of LDL cholesterol in your blood, you may want to consider removing the yolks and making omelets out of egg whites, or buying Egg Beaters, which only contain egg whites.

Cooked vs. Raw

Egg whites and yolks solidify during cooking as the protein gets denatured by the heat, but this doesn't reduce their nutritional quality. In fact,

Free-Range Chickens and Eggs

A few years ago, an athlete I was working with asked me if there was a nutritional benefit to eating "free-range" eggs rather than conventional ones. I'm glad he asked, because many other people have inquired since then. Free-range chickens are raised on farms where they have more freedom to move about, as opposed to hens in factory farms that are confined to cramped cages. While this would definitely seem to improve the hens' quality of life, neither I nor the FDA—the government agency tasked with protecting food safety—have found any evidence that shows there is any difference in the nutritional quality of their eggs.

Some chickens and other livestock animals are given antibiotics and hormones to keep them healthy, increase their milk production, or increase their size. Some people believe that antibiotics, hormones, and pesticides (on crops) end up in the foods we eat and have a host of effects, including earlier onset of puberty, toxicity from pesticides, and the reduced effectiveness of pharmaceutical antibiotics. These claims are still under investigation, and the FDA continues to say that their tests reveal no adverse health effects from consuming animal or vegetable foods treated with antibiotics, hormones, or pesticides. Purchasing organic, free-range, or hormone-free foods, then, remains a personal choice based more on your ethical beliefs about the way food should be produced than on the safety and nutritional quality of the food.

you may be able to absorb more of a cooked egg's amino acids than a raw one's. (Sorry, Rocky, but it's true.) The "unraveling" of complex protein structures makes the individual amino acids more susceptible to digestive enzymes, making it easier for your body to digest and absorb them. Perhaps more important, cooking eggs properly kills any salmonella bacteria that may be present. Whipping egg whites denatures protein by physically breaking it apart, which provides chefs with some interesting possibilities. When air bubbles get trapped in it, you end up with a white, fluffy mixture that can be used to make meringue.

Just to clear up a minor point of confusion for some people: There is no nutritional difference between eggs with white shells and those with brown shells. Different breeds of hens lay eggs with different-colored shells; it has nothing to do with bleaching or processing the eggs. Often, brown eggs cost a little more than white eggs, but as it turns out, this is only because the hens that lay them are bigger; hence, they are more expensive to raise because they eat more chicken feed.

Dairy Products

Low-fat dairy products, including milk, yogurt, and cheese, can be an important part of an athlete's nutrition program because they contain complete proteins and are significant sources of vitamins A and D, riboflavin, and calcium. Yogurt also provides bacteria that are beneficial for your intestinal tract.

Soy Milk vs. Cow's Milk and Yogurt

Soy milk has become increasingly popular and widely used; the perception is that it is healthier than milk and yogurt made from cows because soy milk lacks milk fat and cholesterol. While this is true, soy milk is also naturally lower in protein and riboflavin, and it contains little vitamin A or D. Many brands are fortified with these nutrients to make them comparable with cow's milk, so you should read the Nutrition Facts panel to make sure your favorite brand has these nutrients. Soy milk also naturally contains less calcium than cow's milk, and when it's fortified, it

Cheese (1-ounce serving)	Calories	Protein (g)	Fat (g)	Saturated Fat (g)
Parmesan (grated)	129	12	9	5
Swiss	107	8	8	5
Cheddar	114	7	9	6
Colby	112	7	9	6
Gouda	101	7	8	5
Monterey Jack	106	7	6	5
Mozzarella (skim)	72	7	4	3
Muenster	104	7	9	5
Provolone	100	7	8	5
American	106	6	9	6
Blue	100	6	8	5
Brie	95	6	8	5
Goat (semisoft)	103	6	8	6
Cottage (1% fat)	20	4	0.3	0.2
Feta	75	4	6	4
Ricotta	164	3	2	1
Cream cheese	99	2	10	6

usually contains a different form of calcium than that in cow's milk, one that is not as easily absorbed by the body. While one cup of cow's milk provides 300 milligrams of calcium, you may need to drink enough soy milk to consume 500 milligrams of calcium in order to match the amount of calcium absorbed from cow's milk. Depending on the brand, soy milk can also contain more calories per serving than cow's milk due to added sugar.

While fish is a great source of protein and essential fatty acids, the FDA has issued guidelines for fish consumption based on the presence of heavy metals, primarily mercury, in some species of fish. Women of childbearing age, and those who plan on becoming pregnant, should avoid four fish that contain especially high levels of mercury: shark, swordfish, king mackerel, and tilefish. In addition, tuna has been found

Milk Products (8-ounce serving)	Calories	Protein (g)	Carbohydrate (g)	Fat (g)	Saturated Fat (g)
Yogurt (non-fat)	137	14	19	0	0
Yogurt (low-fat)	154	13	17	4	2
Skim milk	86	8	12	0	0
1% milk	102	8	14	3	2
2% milk	122	8	12	5	3
Whole milk	148	8	11	8	5
Buttermilk (low-fat)	98	8	12	2	1
Goat milk	168	9	11	10	7
Soy milk	81	7	4	5	0.5

to contain relatively high levels of mercury, and the FDA advises limiting your consumption of tuna, as well as other cooked fish, to 12 ounces or less per week. That's about 2½ cans of tuna or 3 to 4 servings of fish.

People who have high levels of LDL cholesterol in their blood may be able to lower them by consuming soy milk and other soy products. These products contain isoflavones, substances that may prevent the body from producing as much bad LDL cholesterol while stimulating it to make more good HDL cholesterol. The American Heart Association recommendation for lowering LDL cholesterol is to eat 25 or more grams of soy protein (which is what soy milk is primarily made of) per day. Soy products are covered in more detail later in this chapter.

Fish and Seafood

Fish surpasses other animal products as a great source of complete protein because it carries additional health benefits. The fat in fish, especially fish that live in cold water, is predominantly unsaturated and is high in omega-3 and omega-6 fatty acids. As I'll explain in more detail in Chapter 8, these fatty acids have been shown to decrease your chances of having a heart attack. The cholesterol levels in fish are also lower than those in red meat and the dark meat portions of chicken and turkey. Shellfish, once considered high in cholesterol, has been shown more recently to be lower in cholesterol than previously believed, and probably contains about the same amount as dark-meat chicken does. Shrimp are higher in cholesterol than other shellfish, but they're still a good choice because they are low in saturated fat. The protein content of fish is roughly the same as that of red meat and poultry at 7 grams per ounce. A three-to-four-ounce serving of fish is also rich in B vitamins, especially B6 and B12, thiamine, and niacin.

Fish can be eaten cooked or raw, although it is very important that raw fish come from reputable stores and restaurants. There isn't any nutritional difference between eating raw fish and cooked fish. However, the manner in which fish is cooked and prepared can make a major difference in its nutritional value. When fish is breaded and fried, drowned in butter, or included in a rich, cream-based soup, you're consuming a lot of additional fat.

Even though there isn't really any evidence that raw fish is any better

Fish and Seafood (3-ounce serving, cooked unless noted, approximately 7 grams of protein per ounce)							
Fish	Calories	Fat (g)	Saturated Fat (g)	Monounsat. Fat (g)	Polyunsat. Fat (g)	Omega-3 (g)	Omega-6 (g)
Lobster	83	0.5	0.09	0.14	0.08	0.07	0.004
Cod	90	0.7	0.1	0.1	0.2	0.14	0.03
Shrimp	84	0.92	0.25	0.17	0.37	0.28	0.08
Tuna	118	1.04	0.26	0.17	0.31	0.25	0.04
Crab	82	1.3	0.11	0.16	0.46	0.36	0.05
Clams	126	1.66	0.16	0.15	0.47	0.25	0.1
Halibut	119	2.5	0.35	0.82	0.8	0.47	0.18
Salmon	93	3.76	0.61	1.02	1.47	1.13	0.14
Tuna (raw)	122	4	1	1	1	0.195	0.031
Swordfish	132	4.4	1.2	1.68	1	0.9	0.11
Caviar (raw)	210	5	1	1	1	1.859	0.116
Trout	144	6	1.79	1.78	1.98	1.05	0.84
Whitefish	146	6.38	0.99	2.18	2.34	1.57	0.54
Salmon (raw)	155	9	2	3	3	1.704	1.447

than cooked fish for athletes, I've known several athletes who swear by the regenerative powers of sushi. After particularly long training rides in the mountains outside of Boulder, Colorado, U.S. Under-23 Cycling Champion Will Frischkorn can often be found downing salmon and tuna sashimi, spicy tuna rolls, and California rolls. Sashimi is just pieces of raw fish, as opposed to rolls, of which there are hundreds of kinds, with different combinations of fish, fish eggs, seaweed, rice, and vegetables. Will has repeatedly told me that when he eats sushi the night after a long training session or race, he feels stronger and less tired the next day. Nutritionally, the meal aids in recovery because of the fish's high protein content, the complex carbohydrates from the rice, and the host of vitamins and minerals from the fish, fresh vegetables, and seaweed. Will understands the nutrition side of things, but he prefers to believe that sushi has magical recovery powers. Honestly, that's fine with me, so long as he doesn't suddenly decide there are "magical" nutritive properties in deep-fried pork rinds.

Plant Protein Sources

Since athletes need a steady supply of dietary protein, we're fortunate that it's available to us from both animal and plant sources. With the exception of soybeans, the protein found in vegetables is incomplete, but it is very easy to obtain all the essential amino acids by consuming a variety of vegetables and grains during the day.

Legumes

Legumes are among the top foods for athletes. Not only are they one of the best plant sources of protein, they are also packed with complex carbohydrates, vitamins, minerals, and fiber. Legumes include beans, peas, lentils, and even peanuts, and there is so much variety in this power-packed family of vegetables that you could probably eat a different dish every day of the year.

Economically, beans are a great way to get the most nutrition for the

Legumes (4-ounce serving)	Calories	Protein (g)	Fat (g)
Soybeans	471	41	23
Peanuts	644	29	56
Lentils	324	27	1
Split peas	336	24	1
White beans	361	23	1
Kidney beans	304	22	0
Black beans	331	21	1
Pinto beans	328	20	1
Chickpeas	364	19	6
Baked beans	191	7	7
Refried beans	118	7	2
Lima beans	88	5	1
Green peas	62	4	0

least cash. Buying dried beans is most cost-effective, and you can cook a giant pot of pinto beans, kidney beans, or black beans and eat them in a variety of ways throughout the week. I used to make huge pots of pinto beans when I was racing. I'd let the beans soak overnight, then cook them for hours the next day. A few years ago, one of my athletes clued me in to a better way, one that I wish I'd known about years ago. It turns out you can drastically reduce the preparation time by boiling a pot of water, turning off the burner, and then adding the dry beans. Instead of soaking them overnight, they'll be ready for cooking in one hour. Using this shortcut, you can make an entire pot of beans, start to finish, in about three or four hours.

Since learning about the bean shortcut, I've come up with a great way to train and prepare beans at the same time: When you get up on a Saturday or Sunday morning to get ready for a workout, boil the water and soak the beans for an hour. By the time you're ready to leave the house for a ride, run, or soccer game, the beans will be ready to go into a crock pot, and by the time you get home, they'll be ready to eat.

If you're not interested in cooking large pots of dried beans, there's nothing wrong with beans from a can. In most cases, there are few or no additives to canned beans, and they've already been cooked for you. Be careful to read the nutrition-information panel on cans of refried beans, however, because different varieties contain varying amounts of fat. Many traditional refried-bean recipes include lard, animal fat that is high in saturated fatty acids. Vegetarian refried beans are a good alternative because they are not prepared with any animal fat or lard.

When I was coaching Jim Rutberg, who now works at CTS, he told me about one of the staples of his nutrition program. He definitely fit the profile of an athlete who was low on cash and attempting to get the best nutrition for the least money. He made black beans and rice by combining a can of Progresso Black Bean Soup with one cup of instant rice and $1/2$ cup of water. He threw the whole thing in the microwave for five to six minutes, added some shredded cheese over the top, and voilà, a power-packed performance meal. In this case, the ratio of percentages of carbohydrate to protein to fat is 62:17:21. The whole recipe has 604 calories, 93 grams of carbohydrates, 26 grams of protein, and only 14 grams of fat. While it would normally serve four people, Jim usually ate the whole thing in one sitting. He estimated that when he could buy the soup on sale, the whole meal cost less than $2.00. When money wasn't so tight, he would add a 4-ounce can of chicken to increase the protein content of the recipe to a total of 57 grams.

Cooking, grinding, or mashing is essential for obtaining the nutrients from beans and peas because your body can't break down their outer coatings by itself. This leads to the overly obvious statement that you should chew your food, but also to the less-obvious benefits of hummus, refried beans, and split-pea soup. Hummus is a spread made by mashing garbanzo beans (chickpeas), and it has long been a popular part of Greek and Mediterranean dishes. Spread on pita bread or a whole-grain bagel, or used as a dip for vegetables, hummus is a delicious, healthy snack.

Breads and Cereal

Though their primary contributions to your diet are in the form of carbohydrate, whole grains also contribute some protein. The degree of processing, however, affects the amount of protein in flour. Dark rye bread has more protein in it than light rye bread because one cup of dark rye flour contains twice as much protein as an equal amount of light rye flour. While the differences aren't as dramatic between whole-wheat and white all-purpose flour, whole-wheat flour still has more protein. A common slice of whole-wheat bread has between 2 and 3 grams of protein and between 10 and 20 grams of carbohydrate. Some breads have a little more protein in them because they have seeds or nuts, like sesame and sunflower seeds, flaxseed, almonds, or walnuts, baked in.

Beyond bread, whole-grain cereal can also contribute some protein to your nutrition program. An ounce of a multigrain cereal contains between 3 and 6 grams of protein, whereas an ounce of a more processed cereal may only contain 1 or 2 grams. Of course, with cereals, you have to look closely at the serving sizes because they're affected by the nature of the cereal. I remember two athletes who were living together as roommates and following very similar training programs. I was only coaching one of them, Andy, but as often happens, the roommate began incorporating large portions of Andy's training program. To save money, the two men pooled their grocery money and cooked almost every meal at home. This meant their nutrition and training programs were virtually identical, except for breakfast. Andy liked Post Grape-Nuts, a bulgur-wheat, whole-grain cereal, while his roommate bought Kellogg's Raisin Bran, also a whole-grain cereal. Over a period of several weeks, Andy's roommate started losing weight and his performance began to decline, and although two different people will always react to training in individual ways, this difference in performance seemed odd. It turns out both men were eating one bowl of their preferred cereal each morning before training, but consuming an entirely different number of calories. Since Grape-Nuts resembles pebbles and Raisin Bran is flakes, you can fit more Grape-Nuts into a bowl than you can Raisin Bran. Therefore, a cup of Raisin Bran contains 197 calories and 6 grams of protein, whereas a cup of Grape Nuts contains 390 calories and 13 grams of protein. Considering that most athletes eat more than one cup of cereal in a sitting, this was leading to significant differences in the amounts of carbohydrate, energy, and protein in their nutrition programs.

Cereal (1-cup serving)	Calories	Protein (g)	Carbohydrate (g)	Fiber (g)	Fat (g)
Post Grape-Nuts	390	13	90	11	.5
Quaker 100% Natural, Low Fat, Crispy Wholegrain w/raisins	389	9	81	6	6
Kellogg's Low-Fat Granola	427	9	89	7	7
Kellogg's Bran Buds	248	8.5	72	36	2
Quaker Oatmeal Squares	216	8	44	5	3
Kellogg's All Bran	162	7.5	45	19.5	2
Kellogg's Müeslix— Apple Almond Crunch	281	7	55	6	7
Kellogg's Special K	115	7	23	1	.5
Kellogg's Raisin Bran	197	6	47	8	2
General Mills Fiber One	123	5.5	48	29	1.5
Kellogg's Nutrigrain Wheat	134	4	32	5	2
Kellogg's Product 19	110	3	25	2	.5
General Mills Multigrain Cheerios	112	2.5	25	2	1
Quaker Cap'n Crunch	143	2	30.5	1	2
General Mills Lucky Charms	116	2	25	1	1
Kellogg's Rice Krispies	100	2	23	.5	.5

Source: Compiled from information on cereal boxes and corporate websites, 2003.

Nuts and Seeds

Nuts and seeds are good sources of protein, but they are more of a complement to a normal, varied nutrition program as opposed to a primary source of protein. They can be considered quality carriers for protein due to the fact that they contain primarily unsaturated fat in addition to protein, as well as folate and magnesium. However, since they are high in fat and calories, they should not be your primary source of protein. Nuts pack a lot of calories and fat into a small package, making it very easy to add hundreds of calories to your daily intake.

Nuts (1 oz serving)	Calories	Protein (g)	Total Fat (g)	Monounsat. Fat (g)	Niacin (mg)	Folate (mcg)	Magn. (mg)
Peanut	161	7	14	7	3	68	48
Pine nut (pignolia)	160	7	14	5	1	16	66
Walnut	172	7	16	4	0.2	19	57
Butternut	174	7	16	3	0.3	19	67
Almond	169	6	15	10	1	9	81
Pistachio	158	6	13	7	0.37	14	34
Sunflower seed	165	5	14	3	2	67	37
Hickory nut	186	4	18	9	0.26	11	49
Cashew	163	4	13	8	0.4	20	74
Brazilnut	186	4	19	7	0.46	1	64
Macadamia	204	2	21	17	0.7	3	37
Beechnut	163	2	14	6	0.25	32	0
Chestnut	103	2	0.5	0.3	0.37	31	39

Peanuts are actually legumes, but I don't think they'd be as appealing if they were called "peagumes," and they're consumed more like nuts than like beans or peas. Peanut butter is the most common way peanuts are consumed in the U.S., comprising about 52 percent of the four million pounds of peanuts we consume every day. According to the makers of Skippy brand peanut butter, Americans eat about 500 million pounds of peanut butter a year, or about three pounds per person per year. Most national brands of peanut butter contain added sugar and some trans-fatty acids (which maintain the consistency), although natural brands containing just peanuts and salt are also available.

For an alternative to peanut butter, consider other nut butters, including almond butter and Nutella. The latter is a spread made primarily from hazelnuts and cocoa, and although it too contains additional sugar, it has as much protein and less fat per serving than peanut butter. For anyone who loves chocolate and has a sweet tooth, a Nutella-and-honey sandwich on whole-grain bread is a real treat and an energy-packed snack. Add banana slices to the sandwich for even more vitamins and potassium.

Minor Sources of Protein

Fruits are considered a very minor source of protein. For instance, bananas, strawberries, blueberries, oranges, and apples contain only trace amounts of protein. Half a cantaloupe contains 2 grams, and one medium-sized avocado contains 4 grams of protein. Likewise, vegetables that have high water contents are often low in protein. A whole bell pepper (green, red, or yellow) contributes only 1 gram of protein. Celery and cucumbers contain almost none, and an entire head of iceberg lettuce contains just 5 grams of protein.

The Vegetarian Athlete

Soy products feature heavily in the nutrition programs of vegetarian athletes because they're such a great way to get both carbohydrate energy and all the essential amino acids necessary for optimal performance. Well-planned vegetarian diets are not only nutritionally sound, they also provide many health benefits. They include lower levels of saturated fat, cholesterol, and animal protein as well as higher levels of whole-grain carbohydrates, fiber, and antioxidants such as vitamins C and E. Several of the coaches at CTS, including Jim Lehman and Kathy Zawadzki, are vegetarians, and they have been instrumental in educating our coaches about the benefits and the nutritional challenges that vegetarian athletes face.

The trend toward a more plant-based diet may be a good one, although there are special concerns for the vegetarian athlete. Vegetarian athletes may be at risk for low intakes of vitamins B12 and D, riboflavin, iron, calcium, and zinc, because many of these nutrients are found in high concentrations in animal products. However, the increased availability of new vegetarian products and fortified foods, such as soy milks, meat substitutes, and breakfast cereals, can add substantially to vegetarians' intakes of these vitamins and minerals. Vegetarian convenience

Soybeans: One Powerful Little Bean

When you're looking for a plant source of complete protein, a lot of carbohydrate, vitamins, minerals, and compounds that can lower your cholesterol and protect your heart, look no further than soy. The diminutive soybean is one of nature's most power-packed sources of nutrients, and its versatility as a food makes it easy and convenient to consume.

Soy products gained popularity in the United States at an astonishing rate during the 1990s, as consumers learned about their health benefits and food companies realized how easy soybeans were to work with. By themselves, soybeans have little taste, meaning they provide a perfect base to build on—you can make sweet milk or spicy burgers out of soy, and both maintain the bean's nutritional quality.

Soy foods are the richest dietary source of isoflavones, a type of phytochemical. Phytochemicals are plant compounds that have biological effects in the animals or humans that consume them. Typical soy foods like tofu might provide 40 to 100 milligrams of isoflavones per ounce. An 8-ounce glass of soy milk provides about 100 to 150 milligrams of isoflavones. Many scientific studies have been conducted to examine the effects of soy protein and cardiovascular disease. To get the heart-healthy benefits of soy protein, the FDA recommends a total of at least 25 grams each day. Fortunately, finding soy products has never been easier. Some commonly available soy foods include:

Green Vegetable Soybeans (Edamame): These large soybeans are harvested when the beans are still green and sweet-tasting, and they can be served as a snack or a main vegetable dish after boiling in slightly salted water for 15 to 20 minutes. They are high in protein and fiber and contain no cholesterol. Edamame can be found in the frozen-food section of your grocery and natural food stores, shelled or still in the pod.

Soy Milk: This is the liquid filtered from soybeans that have been soaked, finely ground, cooked, and strained. Fortified soy milk is high in protein, isoflavones, calcium, and many B vitamins. Soy milk is an excellent substitute for cow's milk. See the section on soy milk vs. cow's milk earlier in this chapter for a more in-depth comparison of the two.

Tofu and Tofu Products: Also known as soybean curd, tofu is a soft, cheese-like food made by curdling fresh, hot soymilk with a coagulant. Tofu is a bland product that easily absorbs the flavor of other ingredients. Tofu made with calcium sulfate (gypsum) has the highest amount of easily assimilated calcium per serving. Extra-firm and firm tofu have more protein than soft or silken varieties because they contain less water.

Soy Nuts: These are soybeans that have been soaked in water and then baked or roasted until lightly browned. They are high in protein, isoflavones, and soluble fiber. Soy nuts make a great portable snack when you're in a hurry, traveling, or relaxing in front of the television.

Miso: Miso is a smooth soy paste made from ground soybeans inoculated with a beneficial bacteria (*Aspergillus orzyae*). Miso is a rich, salty condiment with a strong taste that is popular in Japanese cooking. Grain, like barley or brown rice, is usually added and the paste is aged in cedar vats for one to three years. Miso enhances the flavor of cooking and provides isoflavones as well.

Tempeh: This is a tender, chunky soybean cake. Tempeh is a fermented soy product made from cracked soybeans inoculated with a beneficial bacteria (*Rhizopus oligosporus*) and formed into flat blocks. This process makes it meaty/mushroom tasting and chewy. Sometimes one or more grains, like millet, brown rice, barley, or quinoa, are added to the soybeans. Tempeh is easy to digest and extremely high in protein, isoflavones, and soluble fiber.

Textured Soy Protein: Also known as Textured Vegetable Protein or TVP, this is defatted and dehydrated soy flour that has been compressed into granular or chunk-style shapes. Textured soy protein is high in protein, isoflavones, and soluble fiber. When hydrated, it has a chewy, meat-like texture.

foods, including veggie burgers and veggie dogs, frozen entrées, and soy milk can make it much simpler to be a vegetarian today than it was in the past. According to marketing studies, the U.S. market for vegetarian foods (foods like meat analogs, non-dairy milks, and vegetarian entrées that directly replace meat or other animal products) was estimated to be $1.5 billion in 2002, up from $310 million in 1996. This market is expected to nearly double by 2006 to $2.8 billion.

Are You Sure You Get Enough Protein?

The number-one question that most vegetarian athletes get asked is, "How do you get your protein?" As we have discussed in this chapter, it is possible to obtain *all* of the essential amino acids by consuming a variety of plant foods. If dairy products and/or eggs are included in the diet, then it's even easier. Vegetarian diets that meet energy needs and contain a variety of plant-based protein foods such as soy products, other legumes, grains, nuts, and seeds can provide adequate protein without the use of special foods or supplements. Isolated soy protein can meet protein needs as effectively as animal protein can.

Because we typically think of dairy products as the main source of calcium, ovo-lacto vegetarians (vegetarians who don't eat meat, fish, or poultry, but do eat dairy products and eggs) have no problem getting enough calcium in their diets. For those who consume *no* animal products, it is still possible to get enough dietary calcium from many fortified foods and plant foods. These days it is hard not to purchase a wide range of calcium-fortified products from the supermarket, even if you aren't looking for one. Many juices, cereals, and soy products have been fortified so that they can contribute to your calcium intake. Many greens, including bok choy, broccoli, kale, and okra, provide calcium with a high bioavailability, meaning it is readily absorbed by the body.

Because of the lower bioavailability of iron in plant-based diets, the iron stores in vegetarians are generally lower than those of meat eaters, despite total iron intakes that are similar or even higher. The ADA recommends iron intakes for vegetarians to be 1.8 times those of non-vegetarians because of this lower bioavailability. This means that instead of 8 milligrams for men and 18 milligrams for women, male vegetarians should shoot for 14 milligrams and female vegetarians should shoot for 33 milligrams. Research has also shown that consuming vitamin C along with iron will increase the iron's absorption. So having a piece of fruit along with an iron-rich meal will help to boost the amount of iron that is actually absorbed.

The number-one recommendation for vegetarian athletes is the same that we give to meat-eating athletes: Make sure you are consuming adequate calories to meet your energy needs, and make sure that you are consuming a *variety* of foods. No one food is the "perfect" food, but by consuming a wide range of healthy foods, you will be supplying your body with all of the essential nutrients it needs.

8

AN ATHLETE'S GUIDE TO FATS

THERE WAS A TIME WHEN FAT WAS ABSOLUTELY DEMONIZED by doctors and health professionals. Fortunately, researchers have learned a great deal in the past few decades about the way fat is utilized and stored, and it's emerging as a much more versatile and beneficial nutrient than was previously believed.

Fat Should Not Be Feared

Lipids (fats) are essential parts of cell membranes, are necessary for the production of sex hormones like testosterone and estrogen, and carry and store the fat-soluble vitamins A, D, E, and K. Just as there are different types of carbohydrates, there are also different types of fats, and some can be beneficial while others are harmful.

Foods that are significant sources of fat can also be quality carriers, or pollutant carriers depending on the types of fat and other compounds they contain. For instance, a cold-water fish like salmon contains fat, but it is a great source of omega-3 and omega-6 fatty acids, which may reduce your risk of suffering a heart attack. Dairy products naturally contain fat, but they are also carriers of valuable vitamins and minerals. However, most commercial baked goods, like muffins and cookies, contain trans-fatty acids. These fatty acids may actually be worse for your health than saturated fat, and processed foods that contain a lot of trans-fats often fall into the pollutant-carrier category.

People fear fats because they don't understand that the processes of liberating energy from carbohydrate and fat are so intimately interrelated. When you're optimally utilizing your carbohydrate stores to fuel your workouts and energize your brain, you are simultaneously burning fat. In order to burn fat, you have to have carbohydrate in your body as well; fat burning would completely halt if carbohydrate were not being burned at the same time.

Basic Facts About Fats

Saturated and Unsaturated Fatty Acids

Fatty acids are packed with energy, and completely burning one fatty acid yields three to four times the energy liberated from burning one molecule of glucose. Fatty acids are almost always delivered to the body as triglycerides: three fatty acids held together by a glycerol molecule. It is the degree of each fatty acid's saturation that determines whether it is beneficial or dangerous. A fatty acid is saturated when it is carrying as many hydrogen atoms as it can, and foods that are high in saturated fatty acids tend to be solid at room temperature. As mentioned earlier, the fat on the edges of a beefsteak is solid at room temperature, but the fat on chicken breasts is more gelatinous because it is lower in saturated fatty acids. High concentrations of saturated fatty acids are found in animal fat (beef, poultry, pork, dairy products) and some vegetables (palm-kernel oil and coconut oil). Your intake of saturated fatty acids should comprise no more than 10 percent of your total daily caloric intake. It is well documented that consuming large amounts of saturated fat is a contributing factor in the development of coronary artery disease, hypertension, and some forms of cancer.

When a fatty acid is carrying fewer hydrogen atoms than it could, it is said to be unsaturated. These fats are liquid at room temperature, and consuming them in place of saturated fats has been shown to decrease your risk of developing several diseases. Unsaturated fatty acids fall into two categories, monounsaturated and polyunsaturated, based on their degrees of saturation. A high percentage of the fat in olive oil, peanut oil, peanuts, almonds, and avocados is monounsaturated. Nuts and most vegetable oils, including corn, sunflower, and soybean oil, are high in polyunsaturated fatty acids. Two unsaturated fatty acids, omega-3 and omega-6, are considered *essential fatty acids* because they can't be made in the body and have to be obtained from food. More on these later.

Trans-Fatty Acids

All of the fatty acids mentioned up to this point are naturally occurring, but trans-fatty acids are manmade. Through a process known as hydrogenation, food processors can add hydrogen to unsaturated fatty acids. If you're reading a Nutrition Facts panel on a package and see the words "partially hydrogenated" or "hydrogenated" in reference to an oil, that food contains trans-fatty acids. In 2003, the U.S. Food and Drug Administration decided that food producers will need to list the amount of trans-fat in foods by the beginning of 2006. This information will be found in the Nutrition Facts panel of packaged foods on a separate line, under saturated fat. Trans-fats are found in vegetable shortening and many crackers, cookies, snack foods, pre-packaged baked goods, salad dressings, and other processed foods. Foods that are designed to have a long shelf life, such as Twinkies and similar cake-like products stacked on convenience-store shelves, almost always contain trans-fatty acids. Be sure to read the nutrition labels on your favorite crackers and cereals; even some whole-wheat crackers and whole-grain cereals contain trans-fatty acids.

It turns out that trans-fatty acids may be more detrimental to your health than saturated fatty acids from animal products. Fatty acids are used in the structure of cell membranes in your body, including the membranes of blood vessels. Trans-fatty acids stiffen cell membranes in blood vessels, may affect the way cholesterol gets removed from the bloodstream, and decrease the level of good HDL cholesterol in your blood.

An Athlete's Sources of Fat

Fat is by far the easiest of the three macronutrients to find, as it is present in various forms in almost every meal, recipe, and snack. Fat helps food taste better and richer, and makes food feel better in the mouth by making it moister and creamier. CTS Coach Greg Brown, who is also the professional chef who contributed the recipes to this book, is fond of saying that you can make anything taste better by adding butter or cream. Fats are an important part of an athlete's diet because they transport the vitamins A, D, E, and K; supply fatty acids that are used for building and maintaining cell membranes; and produce energy for working muscles.

Even though all athletes, even the leanest ones, have tens of thousands of calories' worth of fat stored in their bodies, it is critical that they include healthy fats in their nutrition programs. Some of the fat stored in your body is not readily available for use, including the fat that surrounds and cushions the internal organs. There is also fat stored within muscle cells, and strenuous exercise may actually deplete these stores of intramuscular triglycerides (IMTG). What's more, it's unclear whether IMTG stores can be completely replenished by existing stores of fat from adipose tissue, especially before your next strenuous workout. Regardless, ingested fat can be and is definitely used to replenish IMTG stores.

Fat Is Either Good or Bad

There really aren't too many empty carriers when it comes to fat-rich foods. Since fats can either be beneficial or detrimental to your health on their own, the type of fat in a food determines that food's overall quality. Foods high in saturated fat are pollutant-carrier foods, even if they contain valuable vitamins and minerals. The beneficial nutrients can be obtained from other foods, and oftentimes the saturated fat can be more harmful than the vitamins are beneficial.

It is possible, however, for a fat-containing food to be a quality carrier. Foods like nuts, avocados, olive oil, and fish contain monounsaturated and polyunsaturated fats, which have been shown to reduce your risk of heart disease, especially when they displace saturated-fat intake. Foods that are quality carriers for fat also bring vitamins, minerals, phytochemicals, and fiber with them. Red meat, for instance, can be a quality carrier or a pollutant carrier, depending on the cut and method of preparation. Lean cuts of meat are great sources of zinc, iron, and protein, and they are relatively low in saturated fat. Cooking in ways that allow melting fat to drip away or be drained from the meat further reduces its fat content. Fattier cuts of meat, like filet mignon, prime rib, and regular ground hamburger, are still great sources of zinc, iron, and protein, but the higher concentrations of saturated fat make them less desirable.

Meat, Fowl, and Fish

As well as being very good sources of protein for athletes, animal foods can also be good sources of fat. Sometimes the fat can be beneficial, as in the case of omega-3 and omega-6 fatty acids from fish; and sometimes the fat can be harmful, as in the case of saturated fat in bacon. There are even differences in the amount and type of fat found in different parts of the same animal.

One of the biggest differences between animal and non-animal foods, in terms of fat, is the presence of cholesterol in animal foods. Animals, including humans, produce cholesterol, and when you eat meat, poultry, fish, egg yolks, or dairy products, you consume the cholesterol made by that animal. As you can see in the sidebar about cholesterol, research is still uncertain as to the effect of dietary cholesterol on cholesterol levels in your blood. It appears that in some people, eating more cholesterol leads to higher LDL (bad) cholesterol levels in the blood, but this is not true for all people. Likewise, some people who eat a low-cholesterol diet still have an abnormally high level of LDL cholesterol in their blood.

Meat

Red meat, whether it's beef, lamb, venison, or buffalo, has its place in an athlete's nutrition program. It's a great source of zinc, especially because zinc is more readily absorbed when it comes from meat than from vegetable sources. Meat is also high in iron, which plays a critical role in binding oxygen to red blood cells, and B vitamins, which are important for energy production.

Start out by choosing cuts of meat that are naturally low in fat, like those with the word "round" or "loin" in the name. Some of these include eye of round, top round, tenderloin, and sirloin steak, and you should either ask the butcher to trim the fat from around the edges or do it yourself. Cuts of meat that are higher in fat include filet mignon and prime rib.

Though it's not among the most popular cuts, liver is an organ meat that is very rich in iron. Many of the other organ meats, including heart, kidney, tongue, and tripe (cattle intestine) are higher in cholesterol than lean meats (which are muscle tissue) and often higher in fat as well.

Choosing Your Ground Beef

The beef your butcher or grocery store grinds to make your hamburger makes a big difference in the burger's fat content. Search the meat case for ground round, and if you don't find any, ask the person at the counter to grind some for you, because it's the leanest type of ground beef. If you can't find ground round, go with ground sirloin before ground chuck. To make things even easier, just look at the packaging. Most grocery stores label the ground beef with "Percent Lean" or "Percent Fat" stickers. Select ground beef that's at least 90 percent lean, or has 10 percent fat or less. If the meat ends up too dry after cooking it, consider using sauces during preparation or starting with meat that has a slightly higher fat percentage.

Chicken and Turkey

Chickens and turkeys may be the most commonly eaten fowl, but you can also eat duck, goose, dove, grouse, and a variety of other birds. Duck and goose are higher in fat, while chicken, turkey, and quail are leaner. In any bird, white meat contains less fat than dark meat, and both are lower in saturated fat than red meat. White breast meat is one of the leanest meats there is and also gets high marks for B vitamins, iron, zinc, and magnesium. Don't be afraid to eat chicken out of a can either; after all, you eat tuna from a can. Look for labels saying the chicken is all white meat packed in water. Most of the time, it's extremely low in fat and very easy to add to recipes. Sliced turkey breast is one of the best choices at your local deli counter. Many times, chicken and turkey is cooked in its skin, such as when you roast a turkey for Thanksgiving dinner. The skin is almost entirely fat, so although it is crunchy and tasty, you're better off leaving it on the plate.

As with red meat, the way you prepare chicken and turkey affects its fat content. Baking, roasting, and grilling are generally good ways to reduce the fat content. Rotisserie chicken is a good choice, too, since a lot of the fat drips off during cooking. Rotisserie chicken works well in most chicken-salad recipes, but be aware that it often contains more calories per serving than plain roasted chicken. Because rotisserie chickens are marinated and sometimes injected with seasoned marinades before cooking, the chicken meat is generally higher in calories than standard roasted chicken, containing 250 to 325 calories for a 4-ounce serving, versus 200 calories for the same size serving of plain roasted chicken.

Breading and frying chicken in oil, and the relatively recent phenomenon of deep-frying an entire turkey, are less desirable because they increase the meal's fat content. Also be wary of self-basting turkeys; they're injected with fat, which melts and keeps the meat moist during cooking, but which also adds unnecessary fat to your meal.

Eggs

As I mentioned in Chapter 7, chicken eggs were vilified in the '80s and early '90s due to the amount of cholesterol contained in egg yolks. While it's true that there is a lot of cholesterol in an egg yolk (about 213 milligrams), eggs are one of the best and most affordable sources of protein. They are also naturally rich in vitamins A and D and choline—an essential nutrient that plays a role in brain development and memory. Recent research suggests that the addition of one egg per day to a low-fat diet does not increase your risk of cholesterol-related artery disease.

Fish

As I mentioned earlier, when discussing the different types of dietary fat, fish should be an important part of an athlete's nutrition program.

Fish and Seafood (3-ounce serving, cooked unless noted, approximately 7 grams of protein per ounce)							
Fish	Calories	Fat (g)	Saturated Fat (g)	Monounsat. Fat (g)	Polyunsat. Fat (g)	Omega-3 fatty acids (g)	Omega-6 fatty acids (g)
Salmon (raw)	155	9	2	3	3	1.704	1.447
Whitefish	146	6.38	0.99	2.18	2.34	1.57	0.54
Trout	144	6	1.79	1.78	1.98	1.05	0.84
Caviar (raw)	210	5	1	1	1	1.859	0.116
Swordfish	132	4.4	1.2	1.68	1	0.9	0.11
Tuna (raw)	122	4	1	1	1	0.195	0.031
Salmon	93	3.76	0.61	1.02	1.47	1.13	0.14
Halibut	119	2.5	0.35	0.82	0.8	0.47	0.18
Clams	126	1.66	0.16	0.15	0.47	0.25	0.1
Crab	82	1.3	0.11	0.16	0.46	0.36	0.05
Tuna	118	1.04	0.26	0.17	0.31	0.25	0.04
Shrimp	84	0.92	0.25	0.17	0.37	0.28	0.08
Cod	90	0.7	0.1	0.1	0.2	0.14	0.03
Lobster	83	0.5	0.09	0.14	0.08	0.07	0.004

Essential Fatty Acids: Getting Your Omega-3s and Omega-6s

You need different fatty acids for various purposes, and your body can often make what it needs out of the ones you've consumed. There are two important exceptions that must be obtained from food: omega-3 and omega-6 fatty acids. The omega-6 fatty acid, linoleic acid, plays a large role in maintaining the immune system and vision. Fortunately, it's not very difficult to find, and it doesn't take much to meet your requirement. You need about 1 to 2 percent of your total caloric intake to come from linoleic acid, which is easy to obtain from most vegetable oils, including corn, sunflower, safflower, and peanut oils. For a person on a 2,500-calorie per day diet, it would take about one tablespoon of one of these oils to get the daily requirement.

Omega-3 fatty acids are found in fish, and fish that live in cold water have more of it than other fish. Research has shown that people who eat at least 8 ounces of fish a week are at a lower risk for heart attack than people who rarely eat fish. Part of the reason for this may be that the omega-3 fatty acid, alpha-linolenic acid, tends to keep blood from clotting. Since heart attacks and strokes often occur as the result of a blood clot that starves heart or brain tissue of oxygenated blood, reducing blood clotting reduces the risk of heart attack and stroke. It is possible to consume so much alpha-linolenic acid that normal blood clotting is impaired, but this is rare. The best sources of this important fatty acid include salmon, albacore tuna, mackerel, and sardines. If you don't eat fish, you can get omega-3 fatty acids from flaxseed, soybean, and canola oils.

Finned fish that live in cold water, like salmon, albacore tuna, mackerel, and sardines, are high in omega-3 and omega-6 fatty acids (see sidebar above). As part of a heart-healthy and protein-rich diet, athletes should aim to eat at least eight ounces of fish per week (the normal serving size is 3 to 4 ounces, or a portion the size of a checkbook). Most other finned fish are high in good omega-3 fatty acids, although they contain slightly less than the aforementioned types. The fat in fish is also primarily polyunsaturated. Shellfish, such as crab, shrimp, clams, oysters, scallops, squid, and octopus, contain small amounts of omega-3 and omega-6 fatty acids. They are higher in cholesterol than finned fish, and they contain about the same amount of cholesterol as found in dark-meat chicken.

The table on page 135 lists commonly eaten fish in order of their fat content.

Fat from Vegetables, Fruits, and Nuts

Most vegetables that are significant sources of fat contain monounsaturated and polyunsaturated fats, and no cholesterol. Since only animals can make cholesterol, consuming vegetables and nuts will not increase your blood-cholesterol levels. Since they are also good sources of vitamins, minerals, and phytochemicals, vegetable sources of fat tend to be quality carriers.

Oils

Oils made from fat-containing vegetables, along with nuts, are good dietary choices because they are high in unsaturated fats. Olive, peanut, soybean, canola, corn, and sunflower oils are very low in saturated fats and mostly comprised of a combination of monounsaturated and polyunsaturated fats. Use them for cooking, salad dressings, and sautéing.

Flaxseed oil is also very beneficial for your health. Like most vegetable oils, it contains linoleic acid, an essential fatty acid needed for survival. But unlike most oils, it also contains significant amounts of another essential fatty acid, alpha-linolenic acid (ALA). ALA converts in the body to the same heart-protective omega-3 fatty acids found in salmon, sardines, and mackerel. Although it is not suitable for cooking, flaxseed oil can be used in salads. You can also add it to stir-fries or pasta sauces, but you should stir it in right before serving. One tablespoon (15 milligrams) of flaxseed oil per day is recommended as a supplement (it can be used in salad dressings or on vegetables) to ensure a supply of essential fatty acids.

In comparison to flaxseed oil, it is less expensive to get your omega-3 fatty acids from the actual flaxseed. Flaxseeds are sold whole or ground, but they should be ground before use so they can be digested more readily. You don't need any special equipment for this process either; just throw whole flaxseeds in your coffee grinder. The ancient mortar-and-pestle method works well, too. In addition to sprinkling them on cereals, salads, casseroles, and desserts, ground flaxseed can be used in baking to boost the nutritional content of cookies and brownies. Cooking does not significantly reduce the nutritional value of ground flaxseed, whereas flaxseed oil loses it beneficial properties if it's exposed to too much heat.

Oil (1 tablespoon)	Total Fat (g)	Saturated Fat (g)	Mono-unsaturated Fat (g)	Poly-unsaturated Fat (g)	Omega-3 Fatty Acids (g)	Omega-6 Fatty Acids (g)
Avocado	14	2	10	2	0	0
Olive	14	2	10	1	0.08	1.1
Hazelnut	14	1	11	1	0	1.3
Grapeseed	14	1	2	10	0.01	9.5
Safflower-linoleic	14	1	2	10	0	10
Flaxseed	14	1	3	10	8	2
Canola	14	1	8	4	1	3
Peanut	14	2	6	4	0	4.3
Soybean	14	2	3	8	0.9	7
Corn	14	2	3	8	0.09	8
Wheat germ	14	3	2	8	1	7
Cod liver	14	3	6	3	3	0.3
Salmon	14	3	4	5	4	0.3
Cottonseed	13	4	2	7	0.03	7
Palm	14	7	5	1	0.03	1.24
Palm kernel	13	11	2	0.2	0	0.22
Coconut	14	12	0.8	0.2	0	0.24

Fruits, Vegetables, Seeds, and Nuts

Most fruits and vegetables tend to have very little fat—so little that they can almost be considered fat-free. One fruit that contains high amounts of polyunsaturated fat is the avocado, making it a wonderful quality carrier for fat. A medium-sized avocado contains 340 calories and 30 grams of fat, the vast majority of which is monounsaturated and polyunsaturated fat (19 grams monounsaturated, 4 grams polyunsaturated, and only 5 grams of saturated fat). Made into guacamole by mashing it with a little cilantro, salt, pepper, and hot sauce yields a tasty snack that provides a great source of unsaturated fat as well as about 4 grams of protein, 15 grams of carbohydrates, 10 grams of fiber, and nearly 20 milligrams of vitamin C from the avocado.

Seeds and nuts are also good sources of unsaturated fats, although they are also high in calories and easy to overconsume. Rather than sitting down and polishing off an entire canister of peanuts, you'd be better off sprinkling raw cashews, almonds, walnuts, pine nuts (actually a seed), sunflower seeds, or flaxseeds (see pages 137–138) over a salad, or including them in a bag of trail mix. In addition to monounsaturated fats, you'll also benefit from protein, magnesium, folate, and niacin. See page 122 for a table of nuts.

Peanut butter, in its most natural form, is just peanuts and maybe a little salt. Natural peanut butter usually needs to be stirred before use because the peanut oil rises to the top, and you may find it bland if you're used to supermarket brands. Peanut butter that has been processed, like most of the brands in the grocery store, contains added sugar and some partially hydrogenated vegetable oil. The sugar appeals to our taste buds, and the partially hydrogenated vegetable oil acts as an emulsifier, maintaining the peanut butter's smooth consistency and making stirring unnecessary. Go with the peanut butter you're going to enjoy eating the most, but avoid eating too much of it, since it is high in calories. Two tablespoons have about 200 calories and contain 16 grams of fat, even though only 3 grams are saturated fats. The remaining fats are the heart-healthy monounsaturated and polyunsaturated varieties. A great snack for sustained energy and a lot of vitamins and minerals is a peanut butter,

Brand of Peanut or Other Nut Butter	Type	Calories (2-tablespoons serving)	Fat (g)	Protein (g)	Carbo-hydrate (g)	Added Sugar (Y/N)
Jif	Peanut Butter	190	16	8	7	Yes
Jif	Peanut Butter Reduced Fat	190	12	8	15	Yes
Kettle	Almond	184	16	5	6	No
Kettle	Hazelnut	188	19	4	5	No
Kettle	Sunflower	160	14	6	5	No
Kettle	Peanut Butter	166	14	8	5	No
Maranatha	Almond	220	18	8	6	No
Maranatha	Cashew	190	15	5	11	No
Maranatha	Macadamia	230	24	3	5	No
Peanut Butter & Co	Peanut Butter	200	16	7	7	No
Smuckers	Peanut Butter Natural	200	16	7	7	No
Smuckers	Peanut Butter Reduced Fat Natural	200	12	9	12	No
Wild Oats	Peanut Butter	200	16	9	6	No
Wonder	Peanut Butter Reduced Fat	100	2.5	4	13	Yes
Wonder	Soy	170	11	8	10	Yes

Source: Compiled from information on packaging and corporate websites, 2003.

banana, and molasses sandwich on whole-grain bread. If you're not a fan of molasses, substitute honey. Blackstrap molasses has more nutrients than honey, but honey is still a good choice.

Dairy Products

Dairy products should be one of your sources of quality-carrier fats, since they are also high in protein, calcium, vitamins A and D, riboflavin, phosphorus, and active cultures of beneficial bacteria. The amount of fat in a dairy product has a large influence on its quality as a carrier. Low-fat varieties of milk and yogurt are quality carriers because they contain the most calcium, carbohydrate, and protein, with the least amount of fat. Some brands of fruit-flavored yogurts also have a lot of added sugar, but considering the positive benefits of the bacteria cultures in yogurt, yogurt of any flavor is worth eating.

It's difficult to classify any dairy product as a pollutant carrier since almost all of them contain calcium and vitamins, but it's important to keep in mind that the fat in milk is primarily saturated fat. Whole milk is over 3.25 percent milk fat by weight, whereas lower fat varieties are .5 percent (skim milk), 1 percent, or 2 percent milk fat. Cream, sour cream, and butter should be used sparingly because they are high in saturated fat and not good sources of calcium. And since dairy products are produced by animals, they also contain cholesterol. As the fat content in a dairy product increases, so does the cholesterol content.

Milk, Yogurt, Cottage Cheese Products	Serving Size	Calorie	Fat (g)	Calcium (mg)	Vitamin A (IU)
Non-fat cottage cheese	8 oz	160	0	160	400
Skim milk	8 oz	80	0.4	300	16
Yogurt (skim)	8 oz	127	0.4	200	16
Low-fat buttermilk	8 oz	98	2	285	81
1% fat cottage cheese	8 oz	162	2	140	85
1% chocolate milk	8 oz	143	2	285	453
1% milk	8 oz	102	2	300	500
Low-fat yogurt (fruit)	8 oz	232	2	300	104
Soy milk (Soy Dream)	8 oz	130	4	40	78
Non-fat frozen yogurt	8 oz	200	5	600	400
Frozen yogurt	8 oz	400	9	500	400
Cottage cheese	8 oz	240	10	160	400
Goat's milk	8 oz	168	10	325	451
Sheep's milk	8 oz	245	16	472	333
Chocolate ice cream (Häagen-Dazs)	8 oz	540	18	300	1000

Choosing the Best Cheese

There's a gourmet grocery store in Colorado Springs that boasts more than 200 different kinds of cheese, and while I haven't sampled all of them, I can tell you that, nutritionally speaking, some are better than others. Depending on how cheeses are made, the amount of fat and calcium they contain can differ drastically.

Cottage cheese, for instance, is a great source of protein and can be low in fat, but it is lower in calcium than most cheeses. One cup of cottage cheese contains 150 milligrams of calcium, while just one ounce of cheddar cheese contains 205 milligrams. As a means of comparison, consider that one cup of non-fat yogurt contains 450 milligrams of calcium.

Ice Cream vs. Frozen Yogurt

Although ice cream and frozen yogurt are tasty treats, neither should be your primary dairy source. Neither one is very high in calcium or vitamins, and regular ice cream contains a significant amount of saturated fat. Some people, in an effort to avoid the fat in ice cream, switch to non-fat frozen yogurt. While they have sidestepped the fat, frozen yogurt is not nearly as nutrient-dense as many people believe it to be. It is high in sugar and calories, and low in calcium and vitamins. It qualifies more as an empty carrier because it is mainly sugar with a little yogurt. Ice cream and frozen yogurt should be consumed sparingly and considered only minor sources of quality nutrients. In truth, when athletes are craving a frozen dessert, I'd rather see them enjoy a small bowl of ice cream, with its rich, full, fat-influenced taste and consistency, than bother with frozen yogurt. It tends to be a more satisfying treat, a more fulfilling reward for hard work.

Butter vs. Margarine

A stick of butter or margarine is entirely fat. Either should be used sparingly rather than slathered on everything you eat. However, since butter is made from milk fat and margarine is made from vegetable oil, butter

Type of Cheese (1-ounce serving)	Calories	Fat (g)	Calcium (mg)
Non-fat cream cheese	27	0.3	52
Cottage cheese (1% fat)	20	0.3	17
Low-fat colby/cheddar	49	2	118
Cottage cheese	29	2	17
Ricotta	49	4	59
Mozzarella (part skim)	72	5	183
American spread	82	6	159
Mozzarella	80	6	147
Feta	75	6	140
Goat (soft)	76	6	40
Parmesan	111	7	336
Camembert	85	7	110
Romano	110	8	302
Swiss	107	8	272
Provolone	100	8	214
Gouda	101	8	198
Caraway	107	8	191
Blue	100	8	150
Brie	95	8	52
Gruyere	117	9	286
Monterey Jack	106	9	211
Cheddar	114	9	204
Muenster	104	9	203
Colby	112	9	194
American	106	9	175
Pimento	106	9	174
Fontina	110	9	156
Goat (hard)	128	10	254
Cream cheese	99	10	23

has cholesterol and margarine doesn't. Unfortunately, being cholesterol-free doesn't make margarine any healthier than butter. Many stick margarines sold in stores are high in trans-fatty acids. To limit the intake of trans-fats, the American Heart Association recommends choosing liquid or soft tub margarines, and using them in moderation as well. In general, the softer the margarine, the less trans-fat it contains. Margarines made without trans-fat are now available, so be sure to look for butter-type products that say "no trans-fatty acids" on their labels.

If you already have high levels of LDL cholesterol in your blood, you may want to consider replacing both butter and margarine with spreads that contain plant stanol and sterol esters. These substances have been shown to reduce LDL cholesterol levels, although they do not increase HDL cholesterol levels. A product called Benecol is a spread that contains these ingredients and is meant to replace butter and margarine, and it can be used in cooking as well.

Cooking sprays are another way to reduce the amount of butter and/or margarine in your diet. Most cooking sprays are simply some form of vegetable oil in an aerosol can, and you can also purchase refillable, non-aerosol oil atomizers in many kitchenware stores. You simply add oil, operate a built-in pump to pressurize the canister, and then spray the oil into pans or over salads. The advantage of these aerosol and non-aerosol cooking sprays is that they usually cause you to use less oil in cooking. Instead of melting a few teaspoons of butter in a pan before cooking vegetables, meat, or a grilled cheese sandwich, using cooking spray reduces the amount of fat in your meal while still keeping your food from sticking to the pan.

Utilizing Fat: Your Endless Supply of Aerobic Energy

Controlling Fat in the Body

Some of the same hormones that influence carbohydrate usage also control the breakdown and storage of fat in the body. Insulin, for instance, is the primary storage hormone and facilitates the uptake of glucose into muscle cells. When you eat a high-carbohydrate meal, insulin is secreted to move glucose out of the blood and into muscle tissue. Glucagon, on the other hand, is one of several mobilizing hormones. Its goal is to make energy available for the brain and for muscle tissue. When glycogen stores are nearly depleted, glucagon and epinephrine are released to stimulate lipolysis (fat breakdown) and preserve the remaining glucose. To do this, it acts one way in regard to carbohydrate and another way in regard to fat. Glucagon inhibits the uptake of glucose into muscle cells in an effort to preserve blood glucose for the brain. At the same time, it stimulates lipolysis so your muscles can continue to get adequate fuel.

Excess Carbohydrate Is Rarely Stored as Fat

Science is beginning to show that the common belief that excess dietary carbohydrate is stored as fat may not be entirely true, or at least show that less carbohydrate is stored as fat than previously thought. Studies show that when glycogen tanks are only partially full, carbohydrate will be stored as glycogen until your muscle stores are completely replenished. When glycogen tanks are full and there is still more carbohydrate available, or if excess carbohydrate is consumed, you burn less fat until the excess carbohydrate is burned off. Even at rest, your body can downregulate the oxidation of fat in the presence of excess carbohydrate. This means you use the extra carbohydrate to fuel normal bodily functions rather than storing it as fat.

While the mechanism is different from what was previously believed, the end result is the same. Since overeating carbohydrate reduces fat oxidation, you end up burning less fat than normal for a given period of time. This means that less of your already-existing fat stores will be broken down, and possibly that more of the fat you consumed in the previous meal will be stored as well. As a result, you may end up gaining weight. The important distinction is that the weight gain is the result of reduced fat oxidation as opposed to the conversion of carbohydrate to fat.

This has important implications for the way we percieve the relationship between carbohydrates and fat. When we believed the usage of fat and carbohydrate at rest were mainly independent of one another, it was easy to blame carbohydrate for significantly contributing to fat storage. Now that overeating carbohydrate has been shown to reduce fat oxidation, it's clear that the carbohydrate itself is not the problem, but rather the problem is not burning off *enough* carbohydrate during the day. When a high-carbohydrate meal is consumed, fat oxidation only decreases when you already have full glycogen stores. After acitivity, you continue burning fat to supply energy for normal activities as you store the glucose in your post-exercise meal. Athletes, therefore, should not fear carbohydrates because an athlete's activity level leads to glycogen depletion. The carbohydrates you eat will then be stored as glycogen, and if you eat more than is needed to fill the glycogen tanks, most of the excess will be used to fuel normal daily activities and will not be stored as fat.

Cholesterol and Heart Disease

There is significant evidence that carrying excess fat mass also correlates with increased risk of developing coronary heart disease, due in part to high levels of low-density-lipoprotein (LDL) cholesterol and high levels of total cholesterol. However, it is important to note that being slim doesn't guarantee a good blood cholesterol profile.

Slim people, and even athletes, can have high LDL cholesterol levels because of the types of fat they consume. Diets that are high in saturated fats and cholesterol raise the levels of LDL cholesterol in the blood. Athletes, however, are more fortunate than sedentary people when it comes to dietary fat and cholesterol. Exercise can increase the level of beneficial high-density-lipoprotein (HDL) cholesterol in the blood. In addition, estrogen increases a person's HDL cholesterol, which explains why women generally have higher HDL levels than men do.

HDL cholesterol is known as the "good" cholesterol because it seems to protect against heart attack. Medical experts think that HDL tends to carry cholesterol away from the arteries and back to the liver, where it's passed from the body. Some experts believe that HDL removes excess cholesterol from plaque in arteries, thus slowing the buildup. Your liver produces about 1,000 milligrams of cholesterol a day, and another 200 to 500 milligrams can come from the food you eat. There are many factors that come into play when looking at how cholesterol can lead to heart disease. If you take in more cholesterol than your body can use or excrete, then you are at higher risk. However, even if you eat right and exercise, you could have abnormal cholesterol levels. Some people have an inherited tendency for high cholesterol levels—their bodies either make too much cholesterol or are not able to remove the excess. So, regardless of your good eating and training habits, it is a good idea to have your cholesterol tested.

The American Heart Association recommends that adults over the age of 20 have their cholesterol measured every 5 years. When measured, your total blood cholesterol will fall into one of these categories:

Desirable—Less than 200 mg/dL
Borderline high risk—200–239 mg/dL
High risk—240 mg/dL and over

Not only do you want to get your total cholesterol measured, but also a breakdown on your LDL and HDL levels. An LDL level less than 100 mg/dL is optimal, while HDL levels should be at a minimum of 50 to 60 mg/dL. In addition, some physicians will use your cholesterol ratio as a determination of your cardiovascular risk. The ratio is obtained by dividing the HDL cholesterol level into the total cholesterol. For example, if a person has total cholesterol of 200 mg/dL and an HDL cholesterol level of 50 mg/dL, the ratio would be stated as 4:1. The goal is to keep the ratio below 5:1; the optimum ratio is 3.5:1.

Liberating Energy from Fat

Beta-Oxidation

Technically, lipolysis is the breakdown of triglycerides (fat) in the adipose or muscle tissue to free fatty acids and glycerol, and results in an increase of free fatty acids in the bloodstream.

When a fatty acid enters a muscle cell, it is carried into one of the cell's many power plants, the mitochondria. Once inside the mitochondria, enzymes begin the process of beta-oxidation. This is the same place that carbohydrate is broken down for energy, but a single glucose molecule only yields 36 to 38 adenosine triphosphates (units of energy) via aerobic metabolism, whereas a fatty acid with 16 carbons (glucose has six) yields a whopping 129 ATP.

Beta-oxidation of fatty acids obviously has an advantage over glucose metabolism when it comes to energy production, but unfortunately it has some serious limitations that prevent it from being a high-performance fuel. For one thing, liberating energy from fat as opposed to carbohydrate takes longer due to the increased number of steps involved. This means that your demand for energy, especially during moderate and intense exercise, can easily exceed the rate at which you can produce it from fat.

Fat as a Fuel During Exercise

One of the many benefits of training is an increased ability to mobilize and use stored fat during exercise. Your fitness level, the intensity and duration of exercise, carbohydrate availability, as well as your pre-exercise meal will all have effects on how much fat is utilized, and also on where the fat comes from.

Low- and Moderate-Intensity Exercise

During low-intensity exercise, fat oxidation supplies a majority of your energy. At this intensity level, the demand for energy is slow enough that beta-oxidation can keep up reasonably well. As exercise intensity increases, however, the demand for energy overwhelms your ability to produce it from fat. You reach the point where you are breaking down fat as rapidly as possible, and covering the additional energy requirement by burning carbohydrate. Even though the vast majority of your energy for high-intensity efforts comes from carbohydrate, fat still supplies a significant amount.

Long Endurance Exercise

When your athletic activities last more than about 90 to 120 minutes, your body begins to run low on stored glycogen. As previously mentioned, in order to preserve glucose for use by the brain and central nervous system, the hormone glucagon is released into the bloodstream. This hormone stimulates adipose tissue to release more fatty acids so they can be used as fuel, and it inhibits the absorption of glucose by muscle cells in an effort to keep blood glucose levels stable.

While consuming food during exercise will help maintain blood-glucose levels and provide carbohydrate fuel for muscles and your brain, you can't consume enough to completely compensate for depleted glycogen stores. Eating during exercise can extend your glycogen stores' life span to about 3 or 4 hours, maybe more in highly trained endurance athletes; but once these stores are gone, the exercise intensity you can maintain decreases.

9

VITAMINS AND MINERALS: SPARK PLUGS THAT IGNITE YOUR PERFORMANCE

VITAMINS AND MINERALS ARE THE SPARK PLUGS IN YOUR EN-gine. The key difference between these substances and carbohydrate, protein, and fat is that vitamins and minerals do not provide energy. Rather, they allow you to burn your fuels most effectively and cleanly. If your spark plugs are not firing properly—or vitamins and minerals are not present in adequate amounts for your needs—you won't be running your best.

It is important to realize that vitamins and minerals impact both performance and overall health. You may not see any appreciable change in your performance tomorrow by consuming vitamins today, but their influence on your ability to remain healthy, active, and injury-free will be become evident as months turn into years. There is no reason why you can't be as active at 65 as you are or were at 35, and good nutrition is the key to a long and healthy life. I see evidence of this every day with CTS members. Our coaches work with athletes ranging from teenagers to senior citizens, and some of our older athletes are performing better now than they did twenty and even thirty years ago.

Needs of Active Individuals

Research suggests that the established Recommended Dietary Allowances (RDAs), standards set by the Food and Drug Administration, for certain vitamins and minerals are on the low side for active adults. This is likely to be even more prominent in endurance athletes.

Frederick T. Sutter, MD, a sports-and-rehabilitation physician in Maryland and an avid amateur athlete, addresses the nutrition and supplement needs of the patients he treats. He helps them understand that the RDAs define the *minimal* level of consumption of a nutrient, below which deficiency diseases occur; that they were established to create public-health guidelines; and that they were *not* established to suggest the optimal intake for individual needs or for those who are stressed or ill, nor have they been evaluated for athletic performance. As an athlete, your goals are more ambitious than preventing deficiency; you want to perform at your best.

While at Johns Hopkins University, Dr. Sutter studied health promotion extensively. His research led him to overwhelmingly conclude that diet is a lifestyle choice that plays a major role in an individual's health and longevity. As he is fond of saying, food is not just something to fill you up, but is a type of information that you are giving your body. While genetics play a large role in determining your long-term health, some estimates that lifestyle accounts for about 75 percent of the influence on our destiny. With this in mind, strengthening the nutrition component of your training program can pay more than just performance dividends.

Increased intake of vitamins and minerals may not improve your performance as much as a deficiency of these substances may harm performance. Therefore, if vitamin supplements are provided to eliminate a known deficiency, they will lead to better health and provide a foundation for better training and improved performance. Athletes who are most likely to experience vitamin deficiencies include those who restrict caloric intake in order to maintain a low body weight, such as wrestlers, runners, dancers, and gymnasts.

Inadequate consumption of fresh vegetables and fruits may be the most common vitamin-related dietary problem, and it results in potential deficiencies of B-complex vitamins and of the antioxidant vitamins E, C, and beta-carotene. We often see this illustrated when our athletes complete their nutritional analyses. The most frequent recommendation CTS nutrition coaches make to their athletes is to consume more vegetables and fruits. For most active people, eating more whole, unprocessed foods will cover the additional requirement for some vitamins and minerals. While supplementation can be safe and effective, I recommend that athletes interested in increasing their dietary intake of micronutrients learn to find most of what they are looking for in foods rather than pills.

Categorizing Vitamins and Minerals

The best way to understand the sophisticated interactions of micronutrients is through a functional classification. Traditionally, vitamins are classified as fat- or water-soluble. Fat-soluble vitamins are stored by your body in fat cells and include vitamins A, D, E, and K. These vitamins are stored in the liver, and if taken in excess (usually through supplementation), they can produce toxic effects. Therefore, be very careful with taking higher than recommended amounts of fat-soluble vitamins. Water-soluble vitamins include thiamine (vitamin B1), riboflavin (vitamin B2), niacin (vitamin B3), pantothenic acid (vitamin B5), pyridoxine (vitamin B6), cobalamin (vitamin B12), biotin, folic acid, and ascorbic acid (vitamin C). These vitamins are not stored in large amounts; therefore, regular consumption is necessary. These are safer than the fat-soluble vitamins, as excesses are easily eliminated.

Functionally, we group micronutrients according to what they do for us as athletes. The table below presents the roles of some common vitamins and minerals. While there's no doubt that micronutrients are critical to energy production, bone health, and blood formation, I've found that athletes consuming a varied diet and adequate energy intake almost always get enough micronutrients to cover their energy production, bone health, and blood-formation needs, especially those who take a daily multivitamin. Out of all the vitamins and minerals out there, antioxidants, calcium, and iron are the micronutrients I believe you need to focus most intently on.

What Are Antioxidants? Why Are They Important?

Understanding Free Radicals

Just as an apple slice turns brown in the presence of oxygen, certain body tissues become oxidized as well. Several conditions may contribute to increased oxidative stress, including consuming diets low in antioxidant nutrients, smoking cigarettes, living in areas with significant air pollution, or having certain diseases associated with elevated oxidative stress status, such as diabetes. Antioxidants are critically important to athletes, not necessarily because they improve performance, but because they counteract a potentially harmful side effect of high activity levels. Although regular exercise produces many positive benefits, your high activity level as an ath-

Antioxidants	Energy Production	Bone Health	Blood Formation
Zinc	Biotin	Calcium	Iron
Selenium	Thiamine (B1)	Phosphorus	Copper
Coenzyme Q	Riboflavin (B2)	Magnesium	Folate
Beta-carotene/ Vitamin A	Niacin (B3)	Vitamin D	Pantothenic acid (B5)
Ascorbic acid (C)	Pantothenic acid (B5)		Pyridoxine (B6)
Vitamin E	Pyridoxine (B6)		Cobalamin (B12)

lete may also put you at greater risk than your sedentary counterparts for producing higher levels of cell-damaging free radicals.

Free radicals are not a new terrorist group, but they are just as dangerous as one. Under normal conditions, most of the oxygen used by the aerobic system is reduced to form water along with energy. However, about 2 to 5 percent of available oxygen becomes converted to free radicals, which can move freely about the cellular structures and cause damage to cell membranes, enzymes, and protein structures. They are dangerous in that their presence can create a chain reaction to produce even more of themselves. Free radicals have been implicated in most diseases associated with aging. This consideration is of particular importance to the more "mature" or aging athlete (see Chapter 14).

Interestingly, the mitochondria, the part of your cells responsible for producing energy, are among the most susceptible structures to damage from free radicals, and the damage can actually impair the cell's ability to produce new, more effective mitochondria for itself. This has been suggested as one of the primary causes of the diminished ability to produce energy associated with aging.

Antioxidants

Given that free radicals are produced during normal metabolism, it is not surprising that our bodies are equipped to manage them. Antioxidants are nutrients that deactivate these dangerous byproducts and help repair the cellular damage they cause. They keep the damage from getting out of control in your body by (1) neutralizing free radicals, (2) minimizing the formation of new free radicals, and (3) repairing the damage from oxidation.

Think of antioxidants as "traffic lights" for your cells. Traffic lights work to keep order and prevent destruction and mayhem in a maze of cars and traffic. The more "traffic" (free radicals) there is, the more traffic lights (antioxidants) you need. Several studies have shown that training enhances an athlete's antioxidant-enzyme defense system. However, you can't take advantage of this increased capacity unless you consume more foods that contain antioxidants. The most important vitamins and minerals that function as antioxidants in the body are vitamin E, vitamin C, beta-carotene, vitamin A, selenium, and zinc. By relying on a well-balanced diet with a variety of fresh fruits and vegetables, you can ensure that you will be getting a good balance of these antioxidants. Take care when consuming multiple supplements that contain vitamins A and E, as these are fat-soluble and can accumulate to toxic levels in the body.

Vitamin E

Vitamin E is an essential vitamin that is actually a family of related compounds and is considered one of the safest fat-soluble vitamins. One of its primary roles is to protect the polyunsaturated fatty acids in cell membranes against oxidative damage. Vitamin E will interrupt the chain reaction of free radicals to help maintain membrane stability and fluidity; this in turn protects other cellular structures against damage.

Vitamin E is mainly found in high-fat foods, which means that individuals who drastically restrict fat intake may also take in less vitamin E. Primary food sources include vegetable oils, although there is very little vitamin E in either corn oil or soybean oil. Avocados, nuts, seeds, wheat germ, and whole grains are also good sources. The natural form is clearly superior in terms of absorption and retention in the body, although less effective synthetic forms of vitamin E are found in many supplements. If you're taking a supplement that contains vitamin E, look for the "d-" form instead of the "dl-" form of "d-alpha tocopherol," the name of the natural form of the vitamin.

The recommended daily intake of vitamin E from food now stands at 15 milligrams from food, 22 international units (IU) from the natural-source vitamin E, or 33 IU from the synthetic form. However, several experts, including Bruce Ames (professor emeritus of biochemistry and microbiology at the University of California at Berkeley) and member of the editorial board of the U.C. Berkeley *Wellness Letter,* increased their recommendations for vitamin E intake up to 200 to 400 IU a day for both athletes and sedentary people. Daily intake of 400 IU or more is recommended during prolonged periods of intense exercise (i.e., Specialization Period), and for athletes who are routinely exposed to air pol-

Sources of Vitamin E

Food	International Units
Wheat germ oil, 1 tablespoon	26.2
Almonds, dry roasted, 1 oz	7.5
Safflower oil, 1 tablespoon	4.7
Corn oil, 1 tablespoon	2.9
Soybean oil, 1 tablespoon	2.5
Peanuts, dry roasted, 1 oz	2.1
Mixed nuts w/ peanuts, oil roasted, 1 oz	1.7
Broccoli, frozen, chopped, boiled, 1/2 cup	1.5
Dandelion greens, boiled, 1/2 cup	1.3
Pistachio nuts, dry roasted, 1 oz	1.2
Spinach, frozen, boiled, 1/2 cup	0.85
Kiwi fruit, 1 medium	0.85

Source: National Institutes of Health. *Facts About Vitamin E.* Updated 12/9/02. Accessed 1/5/04. http://www.cc.nih.gov/ccc/supplements/vita.html

lutants during exercise. It is safe to take up to 1,000 IU of natural E, or d-alpha tocopherol. However, you would need to consume approximately 400 almonds, 1 to 2 pounds of sunflower seeds, or 2 quarts of corn oil to get over 200 IU of vitamin E! Realistically, it is difficult to get more than the RDA from your diet, so supplementation is quite common. Since standard multivitamins usually contain about 30 IU, a separate vitamin E supplement is needed to achieve this level.

Vitamin C

Vitamin C, also referred to as ascorbic acid, is an essential water-soluble vitamin. As an important antioxidant, it specializes in scavenging oxidants and free radicals, aids in regenerating vitamin E, and has many other important functions, including enhancing iron absorption, improving gum health, assisting wound healing, and stimulating the immune system.

Vegetables and fruits are the best sources of vitamin C. Broccoli, oranges, strawberries, grapefruit juice, and red bell peppers are excellent

Sources of Vitamin C

Food	Milligrams
Yellow/red pepper (1/2 large pepper)	160
Broccoli (1 stalk)	115
Broccoli (1 cup chopped)	82
Chili pepper (1 pepper)	109
Strawberry (1 cup sliced)	105
Orange (1 large)	97
Orange juice (1 cup 100% juice)	96
Spinach (1 bunch)	95
Papaya (1 small fruit, 4.5" long)	93
Kiwifruit (1)	89
Cantaloupe (1/4 large melon)	86
Honeydew (1/4 large melon)	62
Green pepper (1/2 large pepper)	73

Source: Nutribase Nutrition Database

sources. Raw foods have the highest amounts of usable vitamin C, as it can be destroyed by exposure to heat. By limiting cooking time, you can preserve a lot of the vitamin C in your vegetables.

Vitamin C gained popularity when Nobel laureate Linus Pauling promoted daily megadoses of vitamin C as a way to prevent colds and protect the body from other chronic diseases. While the scientific community is still split over the effectiveness of megadoses of vitamin C for the prevention or treatment of the common cold, Dr. Sutter prescribes vitamin C in doses of 500 to 1,000 milligrams, depending on age, activity, and tolerance. Though the vitamin is not a magical cold-prevention pill by any means, his patients have consistently reported the absence of the usual two or three winter colds per season. More than cold prevention, Dr. Sutter sees the best results from vitamin C therapy in accelerating wound healing.

While most plants and mammals can make their own vitamin C, we must consume it. The current recommended dietary intake for vitamin C is 90 milligrams for men and 75 milligrams for women. However, for vitamin C to effectively serve as an antioxidant, prevent cell damage, prevent heart disease, and help prevent cancer, many researchers believe significantly larger daily intakes are needed. Considering the safety and potential benefits of relatively large doses of vitamin C for athletes, I agree with Dr. Sutter and recommend 500 to 1,000 milligrams per day.

Beta-Carotene and Vitamin A

Beta-carotene is part of a large family of colored compounds known as carotenoids (which includes more than 600 members, such as lycopene in tomatoes and lutein in spinach). Carotenoids are widely found in fruits and vegetables and are responsible, along with flavonoids, for contributing the color to many plants. While not a vitamin itself, beta-carotene is a plant pigment that is converted to vitamin A once inside your body. When you eat a carrot or an orange, part of the beta-carotene is converted to vitamin A. The remaining beta-carotene acts as an antioxidant, dousing free radicals and preventing oxidative damage.

Beta-carotene

Most scientific evidence for the health benefits of beta-carotene came from studies that looked at food sources of beta-carotene, not supplements. Since food sources contain beta-carotene and other carotenoids, fruits and vegetables are often referred to as sources of "mixed carotenoids." Many carotenoids have antioxidant properties, and some are known for targeting different areas of the body (e.g., lycopene for the prostate; lutein for the eye). Managing oxidant stress with one high-dose antioxidant is like thinking that a Mozart concerto played with a single instrument will sound the same as when it's played by an orchestra. From population studies, we know that a high consumption of vegetables and fruits is associated with a significant reduction of many diseases—especially several forms of cancer (lung, stomach, colon, breast, prostate, and bladder). So, if you opt to take beta-carotene as a supplement, look for a product that includes all of the carotenoids, or says "mixed carotenoids" on the label, and use it with a full complement of other antioxidants.

The best way to get your beta-carotene and other carotenoids is by eating a wide variety of fruits and vegetables. There is no RDA for beta-carotene, and the best sources of beta-carotene are plants with dark, rich colors such as carrots, pumpkin, sweet potatoes, winter squashes, cantaloupe, pink grapefruit, apricots, broccoli, spinach, and most dark-green, leafy vegetables. By including several servings of vegetables and fruit in your sports-nutrition program, you can easily get at least 10 milligrams per day. For instance, one sweet potato contains almost 15 milligrams, and one cup of winter squash contains 3 milligrams.

Vitamin A

All of your body's tissues need vitamin A for general growth and repair, and it is especially important for bone formation, night vision, and healthy skin and hair. Most important to athletes is that it helps your body resist infection, something we all need during a hard training phase. The newly revised daily RDA for vitamin A is 2,333 IU daily for women and 3,000 IU for men. Many labels on foods and supplements, however, still refer to Daily Value (%DV) requirements, which includes

Sources of Beta-Carotene/Vitamin A

Food	International Units
Liver, beef, cooked, 3 oz	30,325
Carrot, 1 raw, 7.5 inches long	20,250
Carrot juice, canned, 1/2 cup	12,915
Sweet potatoes, canned, drained, 1/2 cup	7,015
Spinach, frozen, boiled, 1/2 cup	7,395
Mango, raw, sliced, 1 cup	6,425
Cantaloupe, raw, 1 cup	5,160
Spinach, raw, 1 cup	2,015
Oatmeal, instant, fortified, plain, prepared with water, 1 packet	1,510
Tomato juice, canned, 6 ounces	1,010
Fat-free milk, fortified with vitamin A, 1 cup	500
Cheese pizza, 1/8 of a 12"-diameter pie	380
Milk, whole, 3.25% fat, 1 cup	305
Cheddar cheese, 1 ounce	300
Whole egg, 1 medium	280

Source: National Institutes of Health. *Facts About Vitamin A and Carotenoids.* Updated 10/6/03. Accessed 1/5/04. http://www.cc.nih.gov/ccc/supplements/vita.html

Teamwork: Antioxidants Support One Another

There's a delicate balance between free radicals and antioxidants in the body, and antioxidants work together to maintain that balance. It's well known that vitamins C and E work together and protect each other from oxidation. Recent research strongly suggests that these vitamins can also help limit the oxidation of beta-carotene, or recycle it after it is oxidized, so that it won't damage cells.

5,000 IU for vitamin A. If you take a multivitamin, check the label; it should contain no more than 5,000 IU of vitamin A. Since vitamin A is a fat-soluble vitamin and can be stored in the body, excessive supplementation can be toxic (signs of toxicity include an orange-yellow tint to the palms and feet). The safe upper limit for vitamin A is 10,000 IU.

Selenium

Selenium works synergistically with other antioxidant nutrients such as vitamin E, zinc, and vitamin C to combat cellular damage caused by free

Sources of Selenium

Food	Micrograms
Brazil nuts, 1 oz	840
Tuna, canned in oil, drained, 3.5 oz	78
Cod, cooked, dry heat, 3 oz	40
Noodles, enriched, boiled, 1 cup	35
Turkey breast, oven-roasted, 3.5 oz	31
Spaghetti with meat sauce, 1 cup	25
Chicken, meat only, 1/2 breast	24
Beef chuck roast, oven-roasted, 3 oz	23
Bread, enriched, whole-wheat, 2 slices	20
Oatmeal, 1 cup, cooked	16

Source: National Institutes of Health. *Facts About Selenium.* Updated 12/9/02. Accessed 1/5/04.
http://www.cc.nih.gov/ccc/supplements/selen.html

radicals. As a trace mineral, selenium travels through the food chain in soil and water. The mineral content of foods is dependent on the soil that it is grown or raised in. The same vegetable grown in different geographic regions can have quite different mineral contents. Areas known to have soil depleted of selenium include New Zealand and parts of China and Finland. Selenium deficiency is rare in the U.S., since we eat foods from so many geographical regions. The most important food sources of selenium include nuts, unrefined grains, brown rice, wheat germ, and seafood.

The RDA for selenium is 70 micrograms per day for men and 55 micrograms per day for women. Daily selenium intake should be limited to 200 micrograms, and multivitamins typically contain 50 to 200 micrograms per dose.

Zinc

Zinc is an essential trace mineral that is part of about 300 different enzymes. As such, zinc plays a role in almost every process in your body. It plays a large role in supporting the immune system, and it is also important for prostate health, particularly with benign prostate enlargement.

Sources of Zinc

Food	Milligrams
Beef shank, cooked, 3 oz	8.9
Beef tenderloin, lean only, cooked, 3 oz	4.8
Pork shoulder, lean only, cooked, 3 oz	4.2
Breakfast cereal, fortified with 25% of the DV for zinc per serving	4
Chicken leg, dark meat only, roasted, 1 leg	2.7
Yogurt, plain, low-fat, 1 cup	2.2
Baked beans, canned, plain or vegetarian, 1/2 cup	1.7
Cashews, dry roasted without salt, 1 oz	1.6
Yogurt, fruit, low-fat, 1 cup	1.6
Swiss cheese, 1 oz	1.1
Chicken breast, meat only, roasted, 1/2 breast	0.9

Source: National Institutes of Health. *Facts About Zinc.* Updated 12/9/02. Accessed 1/5/04.
http://www.cc.nih.gov/ccc/supplements/zinc.html

Soil is frequently deficient in zinc, thereby limiting this mineral's availability from some foods. Zinc deficiency is not uncommon, and Dr. Sutter sees it as the most common of all mineral imbalances. Mild-to-moderate zinc deficiency can lead to significant reductions in the ability to take up and use oxygen, remove carbon dioxide, and generate energy during high-intensity exercise, all crucial elements in your lifestyle as an athlete. The RDA for zinc is 15 milligrams, and Dr. Sutter recommends that athletes take 30 milligrams per day of elemental zinc, as well as 1 milligram of copper for every 30 mgs of zinc consumed. Usually, this amount of copper can be found in a good multivitamin. Higher doses of zinc (more than 50 milligrams per day) for prolonged periods should be

Impending Cold? Try Zinc Lozenges

In other news . . . There is certainly sufficient evidence supporting the use of zinc lozenges in reducing the duration and severity of colds. Although zinc gluconate lozenges can help kill cold viruses in the mouth and throat, you must begin using them as soon as possible following the onset of cold symptoms. Sometimes, just a single tablet taken very early can ward off problems—like after a hard training session and your throat is starting to have that warning feeling. Test-tube studies have shown that zinc can block the cold virus from replicating—an effect that could help the body's natural immune defenses "get a jump on" killing the viruses. The distinct flavor of zinc, which is notoriously difficult to cover, can leave a bad taste in your mouth. For many people, however, the slightly metallic taste is a small price to pay for the quicker relief from cold symptoms. Studies in which sugar was used with zinc to cover the taste showed that the zinc was much less effective, so look for lozenges that have no sugar. As therapy for colds, levels in the range of 13 to 23 milligrams (in lozenge form) taken every two hours for no more than two weeks have been shown to be effective for reducing the duration and severity of cold symptoms.

avoided; they can disrupt the natural balance with copper, since zinc and copper compete for absorption in the gut. The most typical side effect of too much zinc is abdominal distress and pain.

Bone Health

We typically think of our skeletons as being fully developed after puberty. However, there is an ongoing process, known as *remodeling*, that maintains our structural skeleton. Bone remodeling is regulated by many factors, including hormonal status, weight-bearing exercise, and calcium bioavailability. It has been well established that weight-bearing exercise (weight training, walking, or running) results in an increase in bone density. Population studies have shown that active adults who participate in these types of activities have a higher bone density than their sedentary counterparts. In addition to exercise, one has to have an adequate macronutrient energy intake to maintain bone. This relationship between energy intake and physical activity is evident when looking at the high incidence of osteoporosis in young female athletes (more on this in Chapter 13). The important nutrients for not only forming bone, but for maintaining bone in adults are calcium, phosphorus, magnesium, and vitamin D. Most athletes get enough phosphorus, magnesium, and vitamin D from food and multivitamins, but many athletes I've worked with have had trouble getting enough calcium.

Calcium

Calcium is the most abundant mineral in the human body, and an average adult has about 2 to 3 pounds of it in his or her body. Since the main function of calcium is structural, about 99 percent of calcium is found in the bones and teeth. The remaining 1 percent of body calcium is found in the blood and within cells, where it helps with dozens of metabolic processes. Calcium is required for blood clotting, muscle contraction, nerve transmission, and maintenance of normal blood pressure. There is

Daily Reference Intakes (DRI) for Calcium According to Age and Gender*

1,300 mg for ages 9–18
1,000 mg for adults age 19–50
1,200 mg for older adults
1,500 mg for postmenopausal women not taking hormone-replacement therapy

*The Upper Intake Level (UL) for calcium is 2,500 mg per day. Intakes above 1,500 mg per day have not been associated with any greater benefits than more moderate intakes in the 1,200-to-1,500-mg-per-day range.

continuous movement of calcium between the skeleton and blood and other parts of the body. This 1 percent of calcium is so important to maintain that the body will draw on calcium stores in the bones—even at the expense of causing osteoporosis—to keep blood and cellular calcium levels within the proper range.

Dairy products are the most common sources of calcium consumption in the U.S. Skim milk and other low-fat dairy sources, including cheese and yogurt, are some of the best sources of dietary calcium. The calcium in milk has the highest absorption rate for food groups, at 27 percent. This means that nearly a third of the calcium available is absorbed by the body. This is high when you compare it to spinach, from which only 5 percent of the calcium is absorbed. In addition to dairy, other good sources of calcium include fortified juices, tofu (fortified with calcium sulfate), kelp, kale, and kidney beans. If you don't regularly

Sources of Calcium

Dairy sources	Milligrams	Non-dairy sources	Milligrams
Yogurt, non-fat (1 cup)	490 mg	Collard greens (1 cup, chopped)	350 mg
Cow's milk (1 cup)	321 mg	Orange juice (calcium-fortified, 1 cup)	350 mg
Swiss cheese (1 ounce)	270 mg	Dried figs (4)	168 mg
Ice cream, light (1/2 cup)	200 mg	Instant oatmeal (1 packet)	163 mg
Cottage cheese (1 cup)	150 mg	Refried beans (1/2 cup)	94 mg
American cheese (1 ounce)	140 mg	Brown bread (2 slices)	70 mg
Cream cheese (1 ounce)	100 mg		

consume dairy products or green vegetables, it can be difficult to get the required amounts. Many active individuals rely on calcium supplements to make up the difference.

When selecting a calcium supplement, you want to pick the one that will provide the most absorbable form of calcium. Studies on chelated calcium have demonstrated higher absorption rates than milk, and animal studies showed that over 50 percent more calcium from the chelates found their way to bone tissue compared with calcium carbonate. Similarly, there is competition for available absorption sites in the greater intestinal tract when higher doses of multiple minerals are consumed in their inorganic form. You can limit the challenges of competitive absorption of minerals by taking chelated mineral products. In addition, taking calcium with other trace minerals (zinc, copper, manganese) was shown to arrest bone loss in elderly women, whereas calcium alone just slowed the process. Also, be aware that taking calcium and iron together can inhibit absorption of the iron and of several other minerals.

Timing Is Everything

What you eat or drink along with supplements and foods high in calcium can affect its absorption into the body. The calcium in dairy products is readily available because proteins, lactose, and vitamin D all increase

Foods and Situations That Decrease Calcium Absorption

These things decrease calcium absorption...	Because...
Rhubarb, Swiss chard, spinach, beet greens, cocoa, soybeans, cashews, and kale	They are high in a compound called oxalate, which binds to calcium and makes it unavailable to the body
Alkaline foods, antacids	An acidic environment is needed for calcium absorption, and these products raise the pH in your gut
Carbonated beverages	They contain phosphates, high intakes of which are linked to reduced calcium absorption
Megadosing calcium supplements	You can only process about 400–500 mg of calcium at a time, so instead of taking 1,000 mg all at once, break it into two or three doses

its absorption. Acidic foods, or foods that lead to a more acidic environment in the stomach, also increase absorption. Thirty minutes before or after taking a calcium supplement is the time frame to avoid the bad and seek the good. The table on page 165 describes some foods and situations that hinder calcium absorption.

Blood-Cell Formation

Blood cells are formed in the bone marrow, a spongy tissue inside your bones. This is a constant process, and folic acid, vitamins B5, B6, B12, and the minerals iron and copper are critical to keeping it going. Among many other critical functions, red blood cells carry the oxygen necessary to fuel the process of energy production in muscles. Developing anemia, or low red-blood-cell count, is one of the faster routes to poor performance. Menstruating women are at increased risk of anemia and may benefit from iron supplementation. For more information on iron intake for women, see Chapter 13.

Should I Supplement?

Given the scientific knowledge today, it makes sense to give your body the best support and protection from the self-induced stress of training so that you can actively participate 20 years from now. Individuals who use the correct training methods actually support the body's ability to manage free-radical stress much more effectively than those who don't exercise. Couple this with the right diet and performance-supplementation program, and you're headed for your personal best. If you are pregnant or nursing, do not take any supplements unless they're prescribed by your physician, as performance levels of the nutrients we have discussed may not be appropriate.

There have been concerns in the media about supplementation with vitamins and minerals and a variety of other substances to aid in performance enhancement. It is generally recommended by knowledgeable sources that the average person will benefit from supplementation with a multivitamin. Eating right, training right, and supplementing right will all benefit the athlete. CTS took this recommendation one step further by developing CTS Powermix™, a daily multivitamin supplement designed to meet the increased needs of endurance athletes.

Considerable press has been given to the discovery of Union Cycliste Internationale (UCI)–banned substances in the urine of professional athletes who had unwittingly consumed them in a contaminated or inappropriately labeled product. This raises serious questions about supplement content, quality, and purity. Dietary supplements are not regulated by any oversight agency, so I've provided some guidelines to consider when shopping for a quality supplement.

- "GMP" or "cGMP" on the label means current Good Manufacturing Practices, which relates what guidelines the manufacturer uses to produce supplements. These were developed using an integration of references from the FDA and International Conference on Harmonization (ICH) guidance documents, United States Pharmacopoeia (USP), and the Code of Federal Regulations (CFR). These are consistent with the quality controls of the pharmaceutical industry, and manufacturers who use them produce the highest quality of supplements you can get. Fewer products will meet the quality standards beyond USP, since they are more expensive to produce, and their cost will reflect this.
- Watch for unreasonable claims on the label or in testimonials. Federal law does not allow medical claims on the labels of nutritional supplements.
- When looking for chelated minerals, which are more absorbable than non-chelated minerals, the industry leader is Albion. They have gone to great lengths to study mineral metabolism and bioavailability. They only provide "fully reacted" chelates, or minerals that are completely chelated (i.e., no inorganic salts present) in the preparation. If a product uses a mineral provided by Albion, the name will usually be somewhere on the label.
- Make sure that it at least has "USP" on the label, which indicates that

the product has passed minimum standards on how fast it dissolves (yes, some vitamin products will come out the other end, intact!). USP "grade XXIII" is the highest grade available for the USP method of rating and represents a "pharmaceutical" grade.

- Some products have been formulated specifically for the endurance athlete. These will usually include amounts of nutrients beyond the DRIs and RDAs. Using these preparations will provide levels that you as an athlete need in order to combat oxidative stress. All of these issues have been addressed in our reformulated CTS Powermix formula.

10

FOR BEST RESULTS, WATER FREQUENTLY

WATER IS ABSOLUTELY ESSENTIAL FOR LIFE AND FOR OPTIMAL performance. Every cell in your body contains water, and it is the medium through which you transport oxygen and nutrients, to your cells and waste products away from them. It also plays a central role in maintaining your body temperature, which is critical for athletes. Over the years, I've seen athletes lose when they should have won, and win when they should have lost, as a result of the amount of water in their bodies.

Avoiding Your Achilles' Heel

Hydration, or more precisely, dehydration, is every athlete's Achilles' Heel. Lance Armstrong provided a clear illustration of this during Stage 13 of the 2003 Tour de France. From the time he woke up to the end of his 47-kilometer individual time trial, a mere eight hours, his body weight had dropped 13 pounds and he nearly lost the entire Tour de France. To understand fully how something so dramatic could happen to a man whose meticulous nature led his teammates to nickname him "Mr. Millimeter," you have to back up several days.

During the week leading up to Stage 13, several factors set the stage for this crisis. During the summer of 2003, France and much of Europe experienced one of the worst heat waves in the past 50 years. In France alone, more than 10,000 people died from heat-related causes. Temperatures were nearly 100 degrees Fahrenheit day after day, and every rider in the Tour de France was suffering. Whereas the riders normally consume about two 16-ounce bottles of fluid per hour of racing, the team cars following the racers reported that they were handing out nearly twice that to their riders. In the spirit of goodwill, and for the safety of all the riders, team cars even distributed bottles to riders on rival teams. The team directors knew there would be a time later in the race when a rival team would return the favor.

As careful as Lance, his teammates, and his support staff were, he started slowly losing body weight during the second week of the Tour. Lance typically weighs himself after he goes to the bathroom in the morning, and again following his training rides or races. During this short span of time, any weight he gains or loses would be due to water weight. It is normal for riders, including Lance, to lose one to three pounds during a day of racing, slightly more when it is especially hot. By eating meals and drinking water and/or sports drinks throughout the evening, riders replenish the lost fluids and wake up the next day the same weight they were the morning before.

When athletes push their limits in extreme conditions like those endured during the 2003 Tour, strange things begin to happen. There's a limit to how much fluid your body can process in the roughly 18 hours between the end of one stage and the beginning of the next, and Lance's body wasn't able to keep up anymore. It didn't matter how much fluid he consumed, nor the amount of carbohydrate, sodium, or other nutrients the drinks contained; his body wasn't absorbing as much as he needed to fully replace the water he was losing through sweat. He was heading

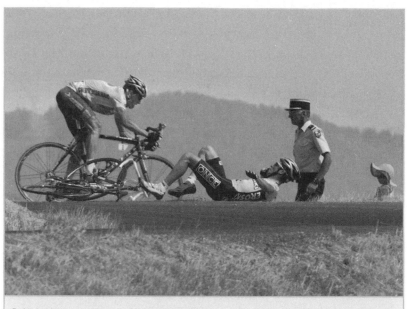

Dehydration was only one of several challenges Lance overcame on his way to his fifth consecutive Tour de France victory. Photo © by AFP

into a scenario of chronic dehydration, and his team director, Johan Bruyneel, his teammates, support staff, and I were doing everything we could to find a solution.

For his part, Lance made the best of a situation he knew to be dangerous. As an elite athlete, he knew how important hydration is to optimal performance. He understood that losing as little as 2 percent of his body weight due to dehydration could hinder overall performance by 10 to 15 percent; and I didn't need to remind him that losing over 5 percent of his body weight could drop his performance by 30 percent. The difference between winning and losing the Tour de France is less than a 1 percent difference in performance. In other words, Lance knew any edge he had over the competition at the beginning of the Tour was gone. Superman was wearing a cape of kryptonite.

In cycling, a team director is analogous to the head coach of a football team, only the sidelines are moving at 30 miles per hour. Johan

Bruyneel drives one of the team's two cars in the race caravan, devises the team's strategy, and communicates with his riders via radio throughout each stage. Johan changed the team strategy to take as much pressure as possible off of Lance. He called upon other team members to do more work so Lance could do less, and thereby let him save the power he had left for when he needed it most: the big mountain passes and the individual time trial. With the race heading toward the individual time trial on Stage 13, Johan's strategy had worked beautifully; Lance had survived the Alps and was still wearing the race leader's yellow jersey. Unfortunately, that's just when the bottom dropped out.

July 19 was unbearably hot, and Lance started the day under his optimal weight. Though he drank a lot of water and sports drink throughout the morning, the situation hadn't improved by the time he needed to start warming up for the time trial. An individual time trial is called the "race of truth" because each rider must cover the distance alone. There are no teammates to draft behind, and your team car can't help you unless you have a mechanical problem. It is each man for himself, against the clock, and the rider who covers the distance the fastest wins. Lance excels in this discipline, having won eight individual time trials in his four previous Tour de France victories and a bronze medal in the time trial at the 2000 Olympics. His primary Tour de France rival, the German Jan Ullrich, was also an ace in time trials, with six Tour time-trial victories and a World Championship to his credit.

Warming up is essential to performing optimally in short, intense efforts like time trials, and even though the air temperature was nearly 100 degrees, Lance performed his normal 45-minute warm-up on a stationary trainer. There were massive fans blowing on him and his teammates as they warmed up, but the environment was still too hot. By the time he rolled into the start house to begin the time trial, we knew he was in trouble. His core temperature was high, his heart rate was high, he was feeling lethargic, and his weight was too low.

He was carrying as much water as he could on his bike, easily enough to get through a 47-kilometer time trial under normal conditions, but by the halfway point of the race, he was out of water. While riders are allowed to get bottles from the team car during regular road stages, it is against the rules to do so during a time trial. No one in the team car following just feet behind him could do anything to help him—Lance just had to keep the pedals turning over until he reached the finish line. A few minutes ahead of him on the road (the top riders leave the start house at two-minute intervals), Jan Ullrich was tearing up the pavement. Low and smooth over his bike, the German powered over the second half of the course, reducing the time gap between himself and the yellow jersey with every pedal stroke. By the time Lance crossed the finish line, cotton-mouthed and overheated, lips encrusted with dried mucus, he had lost one minute and 36 seconds to his German rival. Jan Ullrich's margin of victory was more time than anyone had taken from Lance in a time trial since his comeback from cancer.

Lance Armstrong should have lost the Stage 13 time trial by more than three minutes, and with it, the entire 2003 Tour de France. The fact he only lost 1:36 is a testament to his will power and courage. When he stepped on a scale following the time trial, we realized that he had lost 13 pounds of water that day, an astonishing 8 percent of his body weight. His power output should have been so drastically reduced that he shouldn't have been able to ride nearly as fast as he did. Similar levels of dehydration have sent athletes to the hospital, and Lance had just 18 hours to get ready for the next four-hour stage of the race.

In the days following the Stage 13 time trial, the Tour riders crossed the Pyrenees in southern France. The heat was on, from both the weather and the competition. Once seemingly invincible, Lance Armstrong had been shown to be vulnerable. His teammate, George Hincapie, saw that his good friend's confidence had been shaken, and told him, "I think yesterday [the time trial] was the best ride I've ever seen you do." It was the right thing to say at the right time. Lance was focused on the time he'd lost, the situation it put him and his team in, and the prospect of losing the Tour. George reminded him of the bigger picture: he'd done something that should have been physically impossible, and he still had the yellow jersey and a team willing to ride themselves into the ground for him.

The attacks came from everywhere, and from riders on several different teams. It takes several days to recover from the effects of severe dehydration, even when you're not trying to continue racing. Against substantial odds, both physiological and competitive, Lance weathered the onslaught. Finally, the day before the Tour de France ended, the weather broke. There was another time-trial stage that day, and this one was going to be longer and in the rain.

The rain was good news for Lance; he excels as the conditions worsen. On the other hand, Jan Ullrich had a history of struggling in wet weather. The stakes were extremely high. Lance's lead over Ullrich was only 1:07, and just days earlier Ullrich had beaten Lance by 1:36 in a time trial 20 kilometers shorter than this one. Ullrich left the start house knowing that if he put everything on the line, and if luck and power were on his side, he still had a chance to win the Tour de France.

The bikes used in time trials are very specialized machines. They are designed to put the rider in a position from which he can generate the most power with the least amount of aerodynamic drag. As a result, the rider's hips are high, his body is rolled forward, and his arms are low and extended onto aerobars. While riders like Lance and Jan Ullrich are highly skilled on time-trial bikes, the rider's body position makes the bike inherently less stable than a normal road bike. Riding in a downpour with the Tour de France yellow jersey in the balance, Ullrich had to test the limits of his bike and his handling skills. He had everything to gain and nothing to lose, so he had to take risks on the rain-slicked corners. Going through a roundabout, Ullrich's wheels slipped out from under him and he and his bike slid across the pavement for what seemed like days. If there's one benefit to crashing in the rain, it's that the same slickness that caused your wheels to lose traction also reduces the friction between your butt and the pavement. You slide a bit longer, but you usually remove less skin.

Skin was less important to Jan Ullrich than time, and he popped back up and onto his bike very quickly. As happens to all riders, though, the crash rattled him a bit, and he struggled to regain the smooth, powerful tempo he had been riding at. Lance, riding a few minutes back on the road, heard about Ullrich's crash through his radio earpiece. Since he already had the yellow jersey, the crash gave him the opportunity to back off the throttle a little bit, enough to reduce his own risks of crashing. He gingerly negotiated the remaining kilometers of the course and flashed a smile of pure joy as he crossed the finish line. He was going to win his fifth consecutive Tour de France, albeit by the smallest margin of the five, and in spite of suffering from the effects of severe dehydration.

You don't have to come anywhere close to the level of dehydration Lance Armstrong experienced to suffer its debilitating effects. Many Americans, perhaps the majority of us, live in a constant and chronic state of dehydration. On a daily basis, we don't consume enough fluids, and those we do consume often contribute to dehydration. Caffeinated drinks are diuretics, meaning they increase urine output. In addition, consumption of carbonated beverages and overly sweetened juices causes athletes to stop drinking well before they have replaced the water they lost through sweating.

Part of the problem comes from the way we approach hydration. Instead of looking at water and other fluids as essential nutrients, we tend to look at them as something we use to satisfy our thirst, wash down food, or complement the taste of a meal. Very few athletes, or sedentary people for that matter, realize how much water they need to consume just to replace the obligatory losses from normal activities of daily life. The human body is about 60 percent water, and about 62 percent of that water is contained in blood and muscle tissue. Dehydration affects these areas the most, whereas water contained in the skin, organs, bones, and adipose tissue is less susceptible. This means that when you lose more water than you are putting in, your blood volume and the water content of your muscles are the first things to decrease. While this prevents minor dehydration from seriously affecting the function of your internal organs, it also means that even minor dehydration can have serious detrimental effects to athletic performance. If the only thing you change about your nutrition and training programs is consuming more fluids, your performance will most likely improve.

The Basics About Hydration

How Much Fluid Do I Normally Need to Be Hydrated?

The exact amount of fluids you need depends on several factors, but a good rule of thumb is to consume 70 to 100 ounces (about ½ to ¾ of a gallon) of fluid each day just to replace normal losses. Exercise increases this amount, so I recommend that athletes consume a full gallon (128 ounces) of fluids each day.

Activity level, environmental factors, and diet also affect water balance. Exercising in dry conditions, cold, and/or high altitude increases the amount of water you lose because it takes more fluid to moisten the air coming into the lungs. Living and/or exercising in warm climates also increases water loss because of the increased need to cool the body. Finally, diets high in protein and sodium lead to increased urine output as the body tries to get rid of nitrogenous waste and keep the sodium content of the blood at proper levels. Putting all of this together, you could say that a lean, muscular athlete training at altitude in the winter, consuming a diet high in protein and sodium, would require the highest amount of fluid, possibly more than 1½ gallons per day, to maintain proper hydration.

How Much Fluid Do I Need to Consume During Exercise?

As with overall daily fluid intake, the amount of water and/or sports drink you need during exercise varies by person, environmental conditions, and activity. Since you most likely exercise in similar conditions from day to day, varying of course with the seasons, you can fairly accurately determine how much water you need to consume by weighing yourself before and following exercise. As I mentioned, this is the primary method I use with Lance to determine if he's getting enough fluids.

While exercising, you should aim to consume 80 to 100 percent of the water you lose. This means that if you lose two pounds (32 ounces) during a workout, the next time you complete a similar workout, you should drink 25 to 32 ounces of water or sports drink. It is also useful to determine how much fluid you lose per hour so you can determine how much you're going to need for a variety of activities. For instance, if you know you lose 16 ounces of fluid per hour of cycling, you know you're going to need nearly 50 ounces of fluid if you plan on being out for a three-hour ride. Backpack hydration systems have made it much easier for outdoor athletes to stay properly hydrated. I've found that athletes tend to consume more fluids when the drinks are more readily available, and hydration packs make drinking very easy because the hose comes right over an athlete's shoulder. You don't have to reach for anything, just bite the valve and suck. These systems have reservoirs that hold anywhere from 50 to 100 ounces of fluid, as well as additional storage space for equipment, clothing, and safety gear.

Your goal is to lose no more than 2 percent of your body weight during a workout or competition, no matter how long it is. For instance, a 165-pound (75 kilogram) athlete who wants to perform at his or her best should weigh no less than 162 pounds after a workout. Losing any more than this from dehydration decreases overall performance and time due to exhaustion.

Jim Lehman, one of the coaches in the CTS office, noticed that another employee rarely drank any water during the day. With the number of athletes and coaches in the office, not consuming water is more conspicuous than carrying a water bottle. He suggested that the employee start drinking more, even setting a watch alarm to reinforce the habit of drinking regularly. In the first few days, the employee joked that he was spending more time walking to the bathroom than working; but once he had maintained this higher fluid intake for about a week, the frequency of his bathroom trips decreased back to normal. He had been chronically dehydrated for so long, his body had adapted as well as it could. When he initially increased his fluid intake, it stimulated increased urine output because his body wasn't able to put the additional water to good use; it was just flowing through him. Interestingly, we all saw other associated benefits once he was properly hydrated. We thought lethargy and grumpiness were just the employee's unfortunate personality traits, but both disappeared as soon as he started drinking more water. We put a sign up in his office: FOR BEST RESULTS, WATER FREQUENTLY.

When Should I Drink During Exercise?

You should actually start drinking before you even begin exercising. Ideally, this means consuming fluids throughout the day, but if you can consume even a little extra fluid in the hour before you start exercising, your performance will most likely improve. Studies have shown that being better hydrated prior to exercise improves performance more than consuming fluids only during exercise. Regardless of your pre-exercise hydration state, it is important to start drinking as soon as you begin exercising and to continue drinking at frequent intervals throughout the workout. Rather than slugging down an entire bottle at once, take a few gulps of water every 10 to 15 minutes during exercise.

Do My Hydration Needs Change When I Train Indoors?

Most indoor training sessions or classes are short, about 60 minutes, and take place in a relatively warm room with poor air circulation, so fluid is more important than energy in your choice of drinks. Water or an electrolyte-replacement drink will work well, and you should aim to consume at least 50 percent of the fluids you lose through sweat. This percentage increases to between 80 and 100 percent for longer training sessions, but consuming that much fluid in a hard, 60-minute workout often leaves people feeling too full to work out.

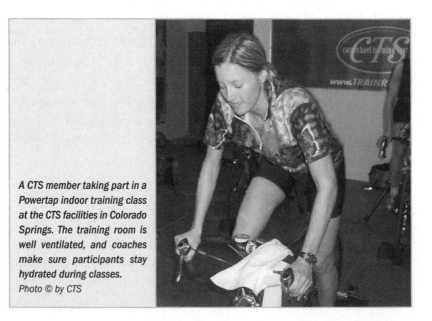

A CTS member taking part in a Powertap indoor training class at the CTS facilities in Colorado Springs. The training room is well ventilated, and coaches make sure participants stay hydrated during classes.
Photo © by CTS

Cranking Up the Heat

Recent trends in exercise classes have leaned toward making the workouts either extremely difficult or conducting them in hot environments to make people sweat more than usual. There are several rationales behind this trend, and I believe people are drawn to these workouts because they have a belief that sweating more means they're doing more work. People like looking down into a puddle of their own sweat or walking out of a workout completely drenched, because it tells them the workout was very effective. This is untrue. Sweating more because you're exercising in a hot environment just means you're struggling to cool your body, not that you're training more effectively. What's more, sweat only helps you if it evaporates off your body; it doesn't do you any good in a puddle on the floor. If you're consuming enough fluids to replace what you're losing through sweat, there's no real problem with these classes. However, considering that amateur athletes usually consume too little fluid, it is far more likely that these classes lead to significant levels of dehydration.

The Bikram style of yoga represents the extreme of this trend. These classes are held in rooms deliberately heated to between 100 and 116 degrees Fahrenheit, and they last up to 90 minutes. While there is evidence that flexibility may increase when muscles are warm, exposure to such extreme temperatures can be dangerous. And while I respect devotees' assertion that there is a spiritual and meditative component to doing yoga in such conditions, it is difficult to place those benefits above the very serious health consequences of exercising in extreme heat.

Signs and Effects of Dehydration

Dehydration can have a wide range of effects, from minor deficits in performance to life-threatening heat illnesses. Performance is dramatically affected by relatively minor dehydration, regardless of whether this dehydration results from exercise or exists prior to exercising. Learning to recognize the effects of dehydration is an important step to avoiding more serious problems.

Increased Exercise Heart Rate

This is one of the most recognizable signs of dehydration and occurs because a good portion of the water you lose through sweat comes from blood plasma. As blood volume goes down, your heart has to beat more quickly to supply oxygen to your entire body.

Sensation of Thirst

For a sedentary individual, this is a reasonably good mechanism for maintaining hydration. Unfortunately, it works too slowly for athletes, and you are already dehydrated by the time you feel thirsty. Interestingly, the sensation of thirst doesn't work as precisely in humans as it does in other species. When we drink water, our sensation of being thirsty disappears before we have consumed enough fluid to be fully hydrated.

Onset of Heat Illness

The onset of heat illness can result from inadequate fluid intake, excessive exercise intensity, exposure to extreme heat and/or humidity, or a combination of these factors. Some of the signs of heat illness include hot, dry skin; a fast, weak pulse; disorientation; dizziness; and nausea. In extreme cases, you can lose consciousness, suffer from heart trouble, or even die. Heat illness is so dangerous because you've dehydrated to the point that your body can no longer cool itself. As a result, your core temperature can rise to dangerous levels. If your body temperature reaches 106 degrees Fahrenheit, you start to damage cells, and at over 107 degrees, the cells begin to die.

During the last few kilometers of Stage 13 in the 2003 Tour de France, Lance noticed he was barely sweating anymore. He knew he was suffering the early stages of heat illness, but also that he was only a few minutes from reaching the finish line and the help of his teammates and support staff. He said afterward that had he reached that condition before the halfway point of the time trial, less than 15 kilometers earlier, he probably wouldn't have finished the stage. As it was, he arrived back at the team bus significantly overheated, and the team soigneurs worked quickly to bring his body temperature back down to normal.

The Great Debate: Water vs. Sports Drinks

Over the past twenty years, sports drinks have moved from a niche market to the mainstream, and they now outperform several other segments of the beverage market. As manufacturers continue to develop new formulas, flavors, and marketing campaigns, the sales of sports drinks continue to rise. The rapid proliferation of drinks with a wide variety of formulas and ingredients invariably raises questions of effectiveness. Is a sports drink any better than water for performance, hydration, or recovery? Are all sports drinks the same, and if not, how are they different?

Sports drinks have been shown to be more effective than plain water in improving performance, hydration, and recovery for athletes participating in activities that last 60 minutes or longer. This means that sports drinks should be part of an athlete's training and nutrition programs, but that they should not displace plain water completely. Both are necessary for optimal performance. All sports are not created equal, and there are four main categories of sports drinks, each with different goals and formulations: electrolyte-replacement drinks, carbohydrate-replacement drinks, protein drinks, and energy drinks.

In 2003, the PowerBar company approached me about formulating two sports drinks with them. They were looking to enter the market with drinks that were scientifically proven to help athletes perform at their best, just as their PowerBar Performance Bar had done for nearly 20 years. This led me to delve deeply into sports-drink research, and I called upon two of the best coaches I know, Dean Golich and Craig Griffin, for invaluable assistance. Prior to CTS, the three of us worked together at USA Cycling on Project '96, a multi-year project with the mission of delivering the most technically, psychologically, and physically prepared athletes to the Atlanta Olympic Games. With the collaborative efforts of coaches, sports scientists, and engineers, Project '96 broke new ground in the science of endurance training, sports drinks, thermal regulation, altitude training, and the monitoring of athletic progress. I knew they were the right people to ferret out the truly essential components of a highly effective sports drink. Likewise, they share my belief that there's no reason to fill a drink with unnecessary ingredients.

I'm extremely pleased with the final products that PowerBar launched in February 2004. PowerBar Endurance and PowerBar Recovery take the science of sports drinks to a new level. Our coaches and the scientists at PowerBar took a wider view than just dumping dissolvable carbohydrate powder into water. They considered the reasons people drink and what they prefer to drink in specific situations, and then they designed products that achieve all the goals of sports drinks.

If you look at sports drinks on the market, almost all are attempting to accomplish the same objectives:

1. Stimulate the drive to drink
2. Accelerate fluid absorption
3. Improve performance by providing carbohydrate
4. Maintain blood volume
5. Quickly restore normal hydration levels

Goal #1: Making People Drink More

While the cynics among you will say this goal is more marketing than science, I strongly disagree. One of the problems with plain water is that it satisfies your thirst before you've consumed enough to meet your hydration needs. One of the goals of a sports drink, then, is to increase the amount of fluid you as an athlete will voluntarily consume, thereby increasing the likelihood you will achieve or maintain an optimal hydration level. This was one of the most interesting parts of the research for me, because it really made me look at all kinds of beverages in a different light. While we concentrated on the factors that made people consume more fluids during exercise, it's easy to see how the same type of thought process can and has been applied to fruit drinks, sodas, beer, and liquor.

What tastes good to a person during exercise is very different than what tastes good at rest. Many sports drinks have been formulated to taste good to a person at rest, but during exercise, the same drink is too sweet or has too strong a taste. Drinks that are overly sweetened often leave a syrupy feel in the mouth, and people describe them as feeling thick, sticky, or viscous. Studies have shown that during activity, people prefer a non-carbonated, citrus-flavored, moderately tart and lightly sweetened drink. If a drink has these characteristics, people tend to drink more and are therefore more likely to stay hydrated.

The right amount of sodium in a sports drink will stimulate people's desire to drink, but it also more or less leads athletes to consume too little fluid to maintain adequate hydration. While there are other electrolytes—potassium and magnesium—that are important for maintaining electrolyte balance in the body, sodium is the only one that has a major effect on the desire to drink.

Goal #2: Get Fluid Into the Body Fast

The biggest determinant of how quickly you can absorb the fluids and nutrients in a sports drink is how quickly you can get the drink out of the stomach and into the small intestine. This is governed, in part, by the drink's osmolality, a complicated word for the number of particles in a given volume. Basically, the thicker the drink, the longer it takes to empty from the stomach and get absorbed in the small intestine. The most effective sports drinks contain a 6-to-8-percent carbohydrate solution because this solution is rapidly absorbed when large volumes are consumed. It also helps for a drink to contain multiple kinds of carbohydrate, like a mixture of glucose, sucrose, maltodextrin, and fructose, because they can activate a variety of transport mechanisms at once instead of depending on one.

Goal #3: Get Carbohydrate to Working Muscles

Even though carbohydrate-replacement drinks are only one of the four types of sports drinks, every one of them accomplishes its goal, to a significant extent, as a result of the carbohydrate it contains. A properly formulated carbohydrate-and-water solution empties out of the stomach faster than water alone. Even more importantly, ingesting carbohydrate during exercise has been shown to delay the onset of fatigue by sparing liver glycogen and maintaining blood glucose for use by the brain and central nervous system. Other additives to drinks, including vitamins, amino acids, and stimulants, may improve performance, but the research is largely inconclusive and the benefits are not as substantial as those derived from the carbohydrate component of the drinks.

Goal #4: Pump Up the Volume

Maintaining blood volume is one of the central goals of consuming fluids at any time, and it is especially important during exercise. Sweating decreases blood volume, and this increases its sodium concentration and leads to a host of reactions. For instance, your blood vessels constrict to maintain adequate blood pressure, and anti-diuretic hormone (ADH) and the steroid aldosterone are released and work together to trigger the kidneys to reabsorb and retain as much water as they can.

Training increases your blood volume so you can supply more oxygen to working muscles and so you have a larger fluid reservoir for sweat production. When this reservoir starts drying up, your ability to cool yourself diminishes, and a rising core temperature is detrimental to performance. Nielson et al. (1993) reported that athletes voluntarily stopped exercising when their core temperatures reached nearly 40 degrees Celsius (104 degrees Fahrenheit). They stopped not because they were physically unable to continue but because their motivation disappeared.

An increased blood volume is also seen in athletes who train and compete in hot climates, and it is an important step in acclimating to heat. Exercising in heat was one of the subjects we researched extensively prior to the 1996 Olympics. Anyone who had been in Atlanta, Georgia, in August knew that heat and humidity were going to be factors in winning medals. Athletes unaccustomed to competing in the heat and humidity overheat quickly because their thermoregulatory systems don't react optimally to the conditions. In 1994, Craig Griffin was the U.S. National Endurance Track Cycling coach, and he decided to test some of the available research in the process of preparing the U.S. team-pursuit squad for the Track Cycling World Championships in Palermo, Italy. The team was training at altitude in Colorado Springs, Colorado, where the air is thin and dry. The competition, however, would be held at sea level in the heat and humidity of Palermo. Craig didn't want to give up the benefits of living at altitude, so he asked U.S. Swimming to let his riders train on the deck inside their Flume, a sealed chamber with an "endless pool" that they use to test Olympic swimmers. The environment in the Flume is computer-controlled, so Craig could program it to replicate the heat, humidity, and even altitude of Palermo. Weeks later, the team traveled to Italy and stunned a lot of people by winning a silver medal in the team pursuit at the World Championships, the first medal any U.S. team-pursuit squad had ever earned at the Worlds.

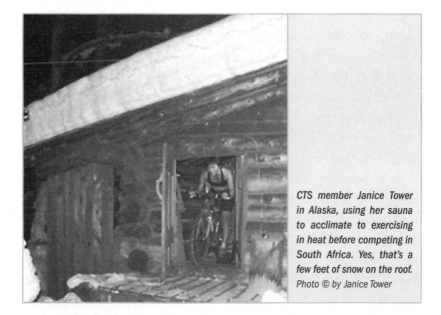

CTS member Janice Tower in Alaska, using her sauna to acclimate to exercising in heat before competing in South Africa. Yes, that's a few feet of snow on the roof.
Photo © by Janice Tower

More recently, CTS Coach Jane Beezer had to find a way to prepare CTS member and experienced ultra-distance athlete Janice Tower for an eight-day mountain-bike stage race in South Africa. In this case, the distance of the event wasn't the biggest challenge; it was finding a way to simulate the heat and humidity of a South African summer while training in an Alaskan winter. Janice was more accustomed to racing cold events like Iditasport Extreme, a 350-mile winter mountain-bike race based on the Iditarod sled-dog race. To prepare for the South African event, she set up a stationary trainer in her sauna and controlled the temperature by opening the door to the negative-15-degrees-Fahrenheit wind.

Goal #5: Quickly Restore Hydration

The final goal of sports drinks encompasses some of those mentioned above. For instance, in order to restore hydration, there has to be a stimulus to drink, and the fluid has to be absorbed. Sodium and carbohydrate in sports drinks accelerate the transport of fluids into the body, and the right amount of sodium also makes people want to continue drinking.

Jim Rutberg, coauthor of *The Ultimate Ride* and this book, tells a story about his father and grandfather that illustrates the effect of restoring hydration. Jim's father, Michael, and grandfather, Franklin, were both doctors, the elder long retired and in his eighties. Franklin was rushed to the hospital one morning after collapsing in his bedroom. Jim recalls that his grandfather didn't look well at all when the family first arrived at the hospital. He was incoherent and pale, and he seemed much more frail than he ever had. Jim's father inquired into his hydration state and was informed that Franklin had just been put on intravenous fluids. Turning to Jim, he said, "Watch this. It's amazing what a bag of saline can do. You get a much better picture of your patient's true condition once you get them hydrated again." Sure enough, less than thirty minutes later and without any other medications, Franklin was lucid again, his color had returned, and he was asking to go home. Michael remarked, as they left the hospital a little while later, "Medicine's come a long way in the thirty years I've been a surgeon, but you can never forget or underestimate the power of water. The human body can endure a lot, but it can't do it for very long without water."

Choosing the Right Sports Drink

Each of the sports-drink types has its place in sports, and choosing the right drink depends on the duration of a particular activity. For instance, the role you're expecting a sports drink to fulfill is different in sports lasting 60 minutes or less compared to sports lasting 3 to 5 hours. Please note that the fluid-intake recommendations below are good starting points, but you should adjust them according to your individual needs.

Drink Recommendation for Events Lasting Less than 60 Minutes

Many amateur team sports like basketball, soccer, and hockey, as well as exercise classes in health clubs, fall into this category. Because the activity is relatively short, athletes can maintain higher intensity levels than during longer activities. This increases the rate of fluid loss, and it also means athletes are less willing to consume a lot of fluid. At high intensities, gastric emptying slows and people sometimes feel like they're too full to perform optimally.

Since the activity is over pretty quickly, it is okay for athletes to consume about half the volume of fluid they lose, as opposed to consuming more during longer activities. There should be a higher priority on fluid and electrolyte replacement due to increased sweat rates; but since energy stores generally aren't completely depleted during shorter events, there is less need for high amounts of carbohydrate in the sports drink. Therefore, 16 to 32 ounces of plain water or an electrolyte-replacement drink is recommended for these activities. An additional 16 to 32 ounces of fluid should be consumed in the hour prior to exercise to offset the fact that fluid intake decreases during high-intensity, short-duration activities.

Drink Recommendation for Events Lasting One to Three Hours

The intensity of these endurance events tends to be lower than during events lasting just 60 minutes. While the total fluid loss will be greater, decreased sweat rate means you are more able to keep up by ingesting fluids during exercise. Glycogen depletion is a big concern in endurance events, and studies have shown that ingesting carbohydrate can delay the onset of fatigue and improve power output, speed, and stamina. Therefore, the best sports drinks for these activities should include both electrolytes and carbohydrate.

Look for sports drinks that contain a mixture of carbohydrates, including sucrose, glucose, maltodextrin, and fructose. Drinks that contain only fructose may lead to gastrointestinal problems, but these problems virtually disappear when fructose is combined with other sugars. For most athletes in most conditions, consuming 24 to 48 ounces of fluid per hour should be adequate to replace at least 80 percent of the fluid lost through sweat. Performance hasn't been shown to improve any more by consuming more than 80 percent of fluids lost. It is also unnecessary to consume only sports drinks during these activities, but 50 to 60 percent of the fluid you drink should contain electrolytes and carbohydrate.

Drink Recommendations for Events Longer Than Three Hours

Many events, including marathons, Ironman and Half-Ironman triathlons, cycling road races, and adventure races can last significantly longer than three hours. In addition, many noncompetitive activities, like hiking and touring, can last several hours. During these events, glycogen depletion is virtually ensured, and the ability to sustain adequate energy output is dependent upon carbohydrate ingestion. A combination of sports drinks, plain water, and solid food is essential for keeping you going.

Since the average intensity for events lasting more than three hours tends to be less than for shorter events, your sweat rates will usually be lower and you will lose less fluid per hour. As mentioned above, 16 to 40 ounces of fluid should be adequate to replace at least 80 percent of the fluid lost through sweat. Also remember that 50 to 60 percent of the fluid you drink should contain electrolytes and carbohydrate.

While less of a concern during shorter events, hyponatremia is a real possibility during long endurance events. Otherwise known as "water intoxication," hyponatremia is a condition characterized by overly diluted bodily fluids as a result of excessive electrolyte losses from sweat and/or overconsumption of plain water. Electrolytes like sodium, potassium, magnesium, and calcium are crucial for transmitting electrical signals in your nerves and muscles. Cases of moderate hyponatremia are associated with loss of muscle control and disorientation, whereas severe cases of this condition can lead to a coma or even death. While it is important for people to learn about it, it should be noted that this condition is relatively rare and very easy to prevent. This is part of the reason that athletes should consume sports drinks and eat solid or gel foods, like PowerBars and PowerGels, during endurance events.

What About Additional Ingredients?

In an effort to improve performance and distinguish themselves in the marketplace, sports-drink manufacturers have added everything from oxygen to ATP to their products. Some of these additional ingredients, including vitamins, may not improve performance while you are exercising, but may be beneficial overall by ensuring that you're getting enough vitamins in your nutrition program. Many others, though, serve little or no use in sports drinks. In some cases, your body makes what it needs, and additional supplementation from foods and drinks has little effect on the amount available for use.

It is also important to note that the FDA does not evaluate sports drinks to determine if their ingredients are effective or live up to the claims made by the manufacturer. Companies are also not required to list the amounts of non-nutrient ingredients they contain, so you don't necessarily know if a drink contains trace amounts of herbs or heaps of them. To ensure that people experience a stimulant effect from herbal ingredients, some companies also include caffeine in their products. The table on pages 190 and 191 includes the claims and truth about some of these ingredients.

Ingredient	Claims	Facts
Guarana extract; kola nut extract; yerba mate extract	Similar to caffeine	Similar to caffeine; often unknown quantities of active ingredients; could lead to anti-doping violation if too much caffeine
Ciwujia, hydroxycitrate, ephedra	Stimulates metabolism and brain function; increases lipid oxidation	Very little evidence of athletic performance effect; ephedra can cause cardiovascular dysfunction and death in sensitive individuals
Ginkgo biloba, ginseng	Boosts memory; enhances endurance; increases peak oxygen uptake	Peak oxygen consumption and endurance at submaximal workloads not increased
Echinacea	Enhances immune-system function	No effect on athletic performance or fighting the common cold
Kava-kava and St. John's wort	Calms the nervous system	No athletic performance effect; kava-kava associated with liver failure
Amino acids from hornet's saliva	Increases endurance; decreases lactic-acid levels in mice	No evidence of effect on athletic performance in humans
Creatine	Delays fatigue in high-intensity exercise; enhances power and sprint capacity	Insufficient amount in energy drinks to be effective. Could cause possible cramping, kidney stress, along with an increased urinary rate
L-Carnitine	Delays fatigue by sparing muscle glycogen; burns body fat; further reduces recovery time by eliminating free radicals; increases the efficiency of the heart; increases respiratory efficiency	No ergogenic effects on athletic performance, enhanced fat oxidation, or sparing of muscle glycogen
Chromium	Maintains stable energy by maintaining stable blood glucose levels; rebuilds muscle tissues and replenishes spent muscle glucose stores	No effect in a sports drink; unlikely to affect C_HO metabolism in lean, fit athletes
Coenzyme Q10	Muscular exhaustion reached at higher workloads; improves heart-rate recovery after intervals; reduces post-exercise soreness; improves overall endurance; powerful antioxidant	No measurable effect on cycling performance, VO_2 max, submaximal parameters, or lipid oxidation

Ingredient	Claims	Facts
Oxygen	Increases aerobic metabolism; decreases lactic acid; improves endurance through elevated oxygen-carrying capacity of the blood	No effect on metabolism or athletic performance in typical athletes who have no deficiency of vitamins; no data available to support claims
Royal jelly/ bee pollen	Improves exercise performance	No effect on performance; dangerous for those allergic to bee stings
ATP	Gives a short-term energy boost without stimulants through increased muscular contractions; maintains and increases replenishment of ATP stores	ATP cleaved in the digestive process, therefore is not effective as a performance-enhancement drink additive
Pyruvate	Enhances aerobic metabolism; delays fatigue; decreases body fat through enhanced lipid oxidation	Performance improved, although amount needed is far in excess of what current products provide; larger quantities cause GI distress

Adapted from Bonci, L. (2002) "'Energy' Drinks: Help, Harm or Hype?" *Gatorade Sports Science Exchange #84*

The "Stimulating" Scoop on Energy Drinks

In the late 1990s, energy drinks emerged as an entirely new breed of beverages in the marketplace. These beverages are mainly consumed as a source of stimulants. If you were to trace the evolution of these drinks, it would probably lead you back to Jolt Cola, a soda that was similar to Coca-Cola but contained a lot more caffeine. The new and "improved" versions of energy drinks still contain a lot of caffeine, but they're also full of herbal ingredients that have similar effects.

When we looked more closely at the ingredients in energy drinks and the claims made by their producers, it became evident that the "energy" these drinks provide comes primarily from carbohydrate and caffeine. Most of the additional ingredients are the same ones that were ineffective in improving performance in other sports drinks. Energy drinks also tend to be more potent, providing more carbohydrate and caffeine in less water. While they can supply athletes with plenty of carbohydrate, the high concentrations of caffeine and lack of water promote dehydration. I'd rather see an athlete consume a carbohydrate-electrolyte sports drink like PowerBar Endurance than an energy drink, because overall performance and training will improve more from carbohydrates and plenty of water than from a stimulant boost. Frequent consumption of high amounts of caffeine also leads to diminishing performance benefits or an increased tolerance to the substance. This means you would have to consume even more caffeine to see an effect.

Overall, energy drinks are not very beneficial for athletes and are more novelty beverages than anything else. There's nothing wrong with drinking them now and then if you like the taste or want the caffeine, but like colas, they shouldn't displace water, fruit drinks, and sports drinks that are more beneficial and have fewer diuretic effects.

Protein Drinks: The New Movement in Recovery

While bodybuilders, weight lifters, and dieters have been consuming protein shakes for many years, protein-containing sports drinks designed for endurance athletes and casual exercisers have only more recently become available. Some of the early research that showed adding protein to sports drinks could be beneficial to all athletes was done by one of my mentors, Dr. Edmund Burke, Ph.D., and by one of the coauthors of this book, Kathy Zawadzki. Their research suggested that a drink containing mostly carbohydrate and some protein increased the rate of glycogen synthesis immediately after exercise.

I still remember Ed sitting down in my office, having dropped by in the middle of his afternoon bike ride, to tell me about this new idea he had. As he explained how adding protein to a carbohydrate drink was going to improve muscle recovery, he became increasingly animated, and that was my first indication that he was really onto something. Having known him as long as I had, I knew he only got this excited after he had examined something from every angle and was absolutely sure he

Energy Drinks	Energy (kcal/12 oz)	Carbohydrate (g/12 oz)	Additional Ingredients
Arizona Extreme Energy Shot	165	42	Caffeine, taurine, ribose, ginseng, carnitine, guarana, inositol, vitamins
Arizona Rx Energy	160	41	Caffeine, ginseng, schizandrae, vitamins
Battery Energy Drink	152	36	Caffeine, guarana
Bawls Guarana	128	36	Caffeine, guarana
Dynamite Energy Drink	126	33	Caffeine, taurine, inositol, vitamins
Hansen's Energy	142	41	Taurine, ginseng, caffeine, ginkgo biloba, guarana, vitamins
Jones Whoop Ass Energy	142	36	Caffeine, royal jelly, guarana, taurine, inositol, vitamins
Mad River Energy Hammer	146	36	Guarana, ginseng, bee pollen
Nexcite	133	28	Guarana, damiana, schizandrae, mate, ginseng, caffeine
Oxytime+ Sports Drink	106	24	"Stabilized oxygen," carnitine, aloe vera, protein
Red Bull	145	36	Taurine, caffeine, inositol, vitamins
Red Devil Energy Drink	106	28	Caffeine, taurine, guarana, ginseng, ginkgo biloba, vitamins
Sobe Adrenaline Rush	179	46	Caffeine, taurine, ribose, carnitine, inositol, ginseng, vitamins
Sobe Energy	150	40	Caffeine, guarana, arginine, L-cysteine, yohimbe, vitamin C
Venom Energy Drink	170	37	Caffeine, taurine, mate, bee pollen, guarana, ginseng, protein, vitamins

Adapted from Bonci, L. (2002) "'Energy' Drinks: Help, Harm or Hype?" *Gatorade Sports Science Exchange #84* was right. In the years since that afternoon, many studies have confirmed Ed's early theories, and the new segment of the sports drink market he envisioned has become a reality.

More recent research continues to show that the addition of protein to a primarily carbohydrate drink can improve recovery by increasing the rate of glycogen synthesis following exercise. The same research, however, suggests that the addition of protein does not increase the total amount of glycogen synthesized. In other words, you can achieve the same results by consuming a lot of carbohydrate or a drink that contains a mixture of carbohydrate and protein. As a result, when CTS coaches and I were working with PowerBar to create PowerBar Recovery, we recommended a ratio of seven parts carbohydrate to one part protein. Based on our research, we believe this to be the optimal ratio for maximizing both the rate and the amount of glycogen synthesis during the recovery period following exercise.

Glycogen synthesis is only one of the goals of recovery drinks; the others include rehydration and the repair and building of muscle tissue. To regain proper hydration levels, athletes should consume 100 to 150 percent of the water they lost through sweat during exercise. The addition of protein to a post-workout drink may provide amino acids that can reduce the breakdown of existing muscle protein. This is part of the reason we included protein in PowerBar Recovery even though some research has shown that consuming carbohydrate alone can lead to maximum glycogen synthesis. The most important factor for optimal recovery is consuming enough calories, because muscle-protein breakdown has been shown to occur when energy intake is too low, regardless of the amount of dietary protein ingested.

The table on page 195 shows a list of recovery drinks that contain enough energy and protein to effectively aid recovery from exercise.

Recovery Drinks	Ingredients (per 12 ounces)			
	Calories	Protein (g)	Carbohydrate (g)	Approximate Carbohydrate/Protein Ratio
Boost	360	22	49	2:1
Endurox R4	280	14	53	4:1
Gatorlode	280	0	71	n/a
PowerBar Recovery	135	4.5	30	7:1
Sustained Energy	171	5	37	7:1
Smartfuel	290	11	59	5:1
Ultra Fuel	300	0	75	n/a

Source: Compiled from information on packaging and corporate websites, 2003.

11

FUELING UP FOR PERFORMANCE: BEFORE, DURING, AND AFTER

Why Fueling Is Essential

There are steps to getting ready for any type of exercise. Runners pay special attention to their shoes, cyclists check the air pressure in their tires, and swimmers make sure they remember their goggles on the way to the pool. When you want to improve your performance and enjoy your workouts in the process, proper fueling prior to, during, and after your workouts should be second nature, like strapping on shin guards before your soccer game.

As we've said already, starting exercise with full glycogen stores will improve performance and increase the amount of time you can exercise before fatigue sets in. To further help you prolong your ability to perform at your best, eating carbohydrate during exercise helps spare glycogen stores by providing blood sugar for your muscles and brain to use. And once you've finished your powerful and successful workout, eating soon afterward accelerates the recovery process, enabling you to more quickly replenish depleted energy stores before tomorrow's training session.

There are no perfect combinations of foods that guarantee optimal performance, but there are undoubtedly some foods that will work better for you than others. Let's also keep in mind that there are many individual factors that affect how each of us digest, absorb, and metabolize what we ingest during training. I know some athletes who can consume peanut-butter-and-jelly sandwiches during a grueling training ride and others who struggle to get down easily digestible sports bars and drinks. While you're going to have to experiment with various foods to find the best combinations for you, the information in the following sections should help you make smart choices.

Nutrition *Before* Training/Competition

What Nutrients You Need, How Much, and When

The meals and snacks you eat prior to exercise play a huge role in the effectiveness of your workouts. Sometimes your pre-exercise meal is eaten minutes prior to the start of a workout; other times hours may transpire between your last meal and your next workout. A late-night dinner could be the pre-training meal for an early-morning workout session; a hearty breakfast will still be working to fuel your body during a lunch-hour run. It could be one hour or ten hours before training, but what you eat and how much you eat will definitely affect your performance during that training session.

The goal is to time your pre-exercise meal so that most of the food is out of the stomach, broken down, and absorbed out of the small intestine by the time exercise starts. Simple sugars are absorbed fastest, followed by low-fiber complex carbohydrates, then high-fiber complex carbohydrates. Foods higher in protein and fat stay in the stomach longest. Based on this, you want to avoid the higher-fat and -protein foods as you get closer to your training or racing time. Ideally, you should try to eat your last full meal at least two and a half to three hours before exercise to allow time for the stomach to empty into the intestines, and for the digestive process to be well under way.

The best foods for pre-exercise meals are easily digestible and not heavy on fat or calories. Your meal should be high in carbohydrate (70 to 80 percent of calories), provide moderate amounts of protein (10 to 12 percent of calories) and fiber, and be low in fat (less than 15 percent of calories). While the exact foods that comprise an optimal pre-exercise meal vary between individuals, the following table shows some examples of common pre-exercise foods, as well as some foods you might want to steer clear of before working out.

Good Foods for Pre-Exercise Meals:	Less Desirable Foods for Pre-Exercise Meals:
High carbohydrate, moderate protein, low fat	1. High fat and/or protein, low carbohydrate 2. Low carbohydrate, low calorie
Pasta, rice, potatoes, sandwiches (roast beef, turkey, peanut butter and jelly), oatmeal, breakfast burrito with eggs and potatoes, pizza (reduced cheese), fruit	1. Steak, bacon, sausage, ice cream, chili dogs, cream sauces 2. Salads (garden, tuna, or chicken), diet soft drinks

Eating regular food is preferable for your pre-exercise meal, but carbohydrate-rich sports-drink beverages like PowerBar Endurance are good to drink within 60 minutes of exercise because they provide calories from carbohydrates, and the added bonus of fluid. If you're on the road, have an early morning race, or need to sneak out of work at lunch to train, carbohydrate drinks can work quite nicely.

Performance often depends on the timing of your carbohydrate intake before and after exercise. Numerous studies published over the last fifteen years have proven that eating between .5 and 2 grams of carbohydrate per pound of body weight between one and four hours before training or competition will maximize the available fuel during exercise. However, the carbohydrate and calorie content of the pre-exercise meal needs to be reduced the closer you get to your exercise session. For example, an hour before training, a meal of .5 grams per pound of body weight would be appropriate, while a meal of 2 grams per pound of body weight would be better if you had four hours to digest the food before training.

Recommended Grams of Carbohydrate in Pre-Exercise Meals

Body Weight (lbs)	3-4 hours prior (1.5-2 g/lb)	2-3 hours prior (1-1.5 g/lb)	1-2 hours prior (0.5-1 g/lb)	0-60 minutes prior (.25-.5 g/lb)
110	165–220	110–165	55–110	30–55
120	180–240	120–180	60–120	30–60
135	200–270	135–200	65–135	30–65
150	225–300	150–225	75–150	35–75
165	250–330	165–250	80–165	40–80
180	270–360	180–270	90–180	45–90
195	290–390	195–290	95–195	50–95

Below are some examples of meals that a 170-pound (77-kilogram) athlete might use prior to exercise. Please note that you would eat *one* of the meals listed, at the appropriate time, as opposed to eating the pancake breakfast three to four hours prior, then eating the bagel sandwich one or two hours later. If you have the three or four hours before training begins, my advice is to eat the larger meal; then, an hour before, top off the tank with the sports drink and bar.

Three or Four Hours Before Exercising, a Large Meal Is Fine:

"Lunch" meal prior to late-afternoon/evening training

Tuna salad pita sandwich
Fruit salad with peach/pear/apricot/pineapple/cherry (2 cups)
Mini pretzels (30 small)
Orange-juice muffins with honey
Skim milk (1 cup)

Calories (kcal)	Carbohydrates (g)	Protein (g)	Fat (g)	Fiber (g)
1168	205	57	15	13.5

Morning meal prior to training or competition

Banana breakfast shake (¹/₂ pint nonfat skim milk, 1 banana, 1 teaspoon vanilla extract, ¹/₄ tsp ground cinnamon)
Whole-wheat pancakes (5 six-inch pancakes)
Maple syrup (3 tablespoons)
100% orange juice (12-ounces)

Calories	Carbohydrates (g)	Protein (g)	Fat (g)
1,285	264 (1.55 g/lb)	30	11

Two or Three Hours Beforehand, a Smaller Meal Is Suitable:

Morning meal prior to training or competition

Whole-grain bagel (1 four-ounce)
Peanut butter (1 tablespoon)
Jelly (2 tablespoons, any flavor)
Banana
Apple-cranberry juice (12 fluid ounces; 100% juice, not from concentrate)
Powerbar Endurance sports drink (12 ounces)

Calories (kcal)	Carbohydrates (g)	Protein (g)	Fat (g)
820	170	18	7

"Lunch" meal prior to late-afternoon/evening training

Chicken salad sandwich with spinach
Cornbread (2 pieces, 2" × 2" each)
Canteloupe, ¹/₂ small melon
Bananerberry Smoothie (1 serving; see page 313 for recipe)

Calories (kcal)	Carbohydrates (g)	Protein (g)	Fat (g)
950	170	40	12

One hour before:

PowerBar Performance or Harvest Bar (65g) PowerBar Endurance sports drink (10 fluid ounces)

Calories (kcal)	Carbohydrates (g)	Protein (g)	Fat (g)
305	66	9	2

There are many other snack combinations that provide 50 to 75 grams of carbohydrate and would work in the hour leading up to training, including:

- 1 cup vanilla yogurt + ½ cup Grape-Nuts + 2 tablespoons raisins
- 1 cup vanilla yogurt + 1 cup fresh fruit
- 1 cup juice + 1 banana
- 1 slice banana-nut bread + 1 cup skim milk
- 1 energy bar + 8 ounces sports drink
- Smoothie: 2 cups skim or soy milk + 1½ cup mango or berries + 2 tablespoons soy protein
- 1½ cup multigrain cereal + 1½ cup skim milk
- 1 bagel + 1 banana + 1 tablespoon nut butter
- 1 cup cottage cheese + 8 whole-wheat crackers + 1 apple

Fueling Your Early-Morning Workouts

I remember when, a few years ago, athletes began to pick up the bad habit of training early in the morning without eating; they were convinced it would help them "train" their bodies to better burn fat for fuel. Fortunately, word got out that this was not a good way to start the day. Training or competing on an empty stomach does *not* improve performance; rather, it may cause additional protein to be sacrificed for fuel. After an 8-to-10-hour overnight fast, you would start exercising with depleted carbohydrate stores. In these conditions, your body converts protein to carbohydrate in order to maintain adequate blood sugar levels. As we learned in Chapter 6, relying on fat and protein for energy is a very inefficient way to burn fuel, and the quality of your training will suffer.

So, what should you do before an early-morning ride or race? Your early-morning meal should be primarily carbohydrate with a touch of protein to help you feel a little more full and satisfied. The meals recommended above for the 60 minutes prior to exercise will also work to get you through most morning workouts that last for less than 90 minutes, especially if you take some carbohydrate to eat during the training session. If your morning workout is going to be over two hours, I recommend waking up early enough to eat a more substantial breakfast between 90 and 120 minutes before training.

Carbohydrate Loading

During the normal progression of your training program, deliberate carbohydrate loading is generally unnecessary. If 65 to 70 percent of your total calories are already coming from carbohydrate as part of your normal sports nutrition program, you don't have to carbo-load for daily workouts. Carbohydrate loading can be useful, however, for athletes participating in longer endurance events, like those lasting from 90 minutes to several hours.

Though the concept of muscle-glycogen super-compensation or "carb loading" has been around for more than 35 years, the classic method designed in the '60s was very hard on the athlete, and interrupted training to the point that the disruption sometimes outweighed the potential benefit of starting an event with greater glycogen stores. Fortunately, the process has become less complicated and stringent over the last decade. This "modified" regimen eliminated some of the classic protocol's problems with interfering with training. Using the modified plan, you consume a 50-percent-carbohydrate diet for three days while training normally, then increase to a 70 to 75-percent carbohydrate diet (about five to six grams per pound of body weight), with reduced training load, for the last three days before competition. During the first three days, you'll deplete your glycogen stores more than normal. In the latter three days, when you consume more carbohydrate, your body super-compensates for the perceived carbohydrate deficiency, and you'll end up with glycogen stores similar to those seen with the classic method. This method has the additional benefit of being less intrusive to an athlete's training during the week leading up to an event.

More recent research (Fairchild et al., 2002) shows that you can ditch the classic and "modified" routines and build maximal glycogen stores in just a day. A speedier carbohydrate-loading regimen has been shown to help cyclists, runners, and other athletes preparing for events lasting longer than 90 minutes, and it causes less disruption to their training.

The high-speed method of carbohydrate loading requires a workout that includes a short (2-to-3-minute), ultra-hard bout of exercise the day prior to your event, followed by rest and a very high carbohydrate intake (approximately 90 percent of calories) for about 24 hours. The next day, you can have glycogen stores as high or higher than levels attained by athletes who ate a high-carbohydrate diet for up to six days. If you choose to try this method, you will need to consume five-plus grams of carbohydrate per pound of body weight (more than 850 grams of carbohydrate for our 170-pound athlete). You're going to need to carefully choose concentrated sources of carbohydrate. Liquid carbohydrate drinks are useful because they lack solid food's bulk: a slice of bread averages 15 grams of carbohydrate, meaning that a 150-pound athlete would have to eat about 50 slices of bread to meet this target!

Nutrition *During* Training/Competition

It is widely accepted that carbohydrate ingestion during exercise leads to improved exercise performance and increased time before the onset of fatigue. For training sessions or competitions that are going to last at least an hour, you should plan to consume carbohydrates while you're exercising so you can train or play longer before running out of gas. Your body uses stored glycogen to fuel working muscles, and most athletes have enough stored glycogen in their bodies to go for 90 to 120 minutes at approximately a 70 percent effort. After that time, when you run out of glycogen, your intensity must drop as you are forced to rely more heavily on fat for fuel. Your brain, however, needs carbohydrate energy, and eating carbohydrate during exercise supplies energy to your central nervous system and working muscles, thereby preserving glycogen stores and reducing the need for the liver to make as much glucose from protein. It is only fair to mention that there are several factors besides glycogen depletion that contribute to fatigue, including psychological factors and changes within the central nervous system. Running low on fuel, however, is one factor to fatigue that you *can* control.

Ingesting carbohydrate also helps keep you more mentally alert. Adequate carbohydrate consumption (in the form of food and sports drinks) helps delay the deterioration of complex sport-specific skills, which is important in endurance sports as well as high-intensity, intermittent-effort sports. Hockey players, for instance, skate and control the puck better in the third periods of games when they consume carbohydrates along with water during the first two periods. There's also an increase in your ability to concentrate and focus on the task at hand. I have found this to be particularly important in high-speed sports that require split-second decisions, such as downhill mountain biking and motocross. Athletes who are running low on blood sugar make poor decisions, while those who have consumed carbohydrate have a better chance of making the decisions that lead to victory.

How Much Is Enough?

To prevent a drop in blood glucose and delay the onset of fatigue during prolonged exercise, you should take in 30 to 60 grams of carbohydrate per hour. Now, I realize that this is a big window—30 to 60 grams. If you're going out for a low-to-moderate-intensity training session during the Foundation Period, you would probably be fine sticking closer to the lower end of the range, about 30 grams. However, since carbohydrate gets burned at a much higher rate when the exercise intensity begins to increase, you may want to ingest closer to the 60 grams during harder, longer training sessions found in the Preparation Period or during the high-intensity training or racing sessions of the Specialization Period.

The recommendation of 30 to 60 grams an hour includes both what you eat *and* what you drink. Nutrition during exercise can include sports drinks, bars, gels, and solid food. Regardless of your pre-exercise hydration state, it is important to start drinking as soon as you begin exercising, and to continue drinking at frequent intervals throughout the workout. (Look for more information on sports drinks in Chapter 10.)

How to Get 30 to 60 Grams of Carbohydrate per Hour

Below are combinations of sports drinks, gels, and solid foods to meet your carbohydrate requirements *during* exercise.

One PowerBar Performance Bar (any flavor)	45 grams
One PowerGel	25 grams
	70 grams
One medium-size banana	30 grams
One PowerGel	25 grams
	55 grams
Two Fig Newton cookies	24 grams
20 ounces PowerBar Endurance sports drink	36 grams
	60 grams

It is important to find a balance between eating enough to prevent hunger and the pitfall of the "if a little is good, a lot is better" philosophy. If you err on the side of eating too much, you run the risk of abdominal cramping and nausea. It is best to eat at the start of the event and continue with small amounts at frequent intervals. That may mean grabbing a few bites of an energy bar at a time, instead of wolfing down the whole thing at once. Since everyone responds a bit differently under the stress of exercise, I cannot emphasize enough how important it is to experiment with different combinations of food, drinks, and other products to find the ones that work best for you.

Energy Gels

One of the easiest ways to get a good dose of carbohydrates while exercising is to suck down a PowerBar PowerGel or other similar product. Gels, which are specially formulated with a combination of simple and complex carbohydrates, are designed to provide quick energy. While some athletes love gels, others don't care for them because they tend to be thick, kind of like cake frosting. Most gels will provide between 90 and 100 calories (approximately 25 grams of carbohydrate) per packet.

For a gel to work properly, it's essential that you drink at least 8 ounces of water or sports drink with it. Combining a gel and sports drink is a very easy way to get your 30 to 60 grams of carbohydrate per hour. The gel has to be diluted in order for you to absorb the carbohydrates quickly, and without water, you may actually slow down this important process. Some gels also contain caffeine, which gives athletes a physical and, just as importantly, a psychological boost toward the end of a training session or competition.

Energy Bars and "Real" Food

While sports drinks and gels are good sources of energy, you can also get the fuel you need from regular food and energy bars. Fig, cereal, and granola bars work very well, as does fruit or even a sandwich. During the Tour de France, Lance and his teammates eat energy bars and gels as they race, but they also augment them with cheese sandwiches, cold baked potatoes, fruit, and pastries.

With all of the bars on the market today, it pays to spend some time reading the labels for information on additives, calorie content, protein, and fats. While there are a lot of protein-heavy bars on the market, you should eat high-carbohydrate energy bars during exercise. Carbohydrate is the fuel your muscles are burning, and eating a lot of protein or fat during exercise doesn't help you spare your muscle- and liver-glycogen stores. The goal of energy bars is to get the glucose into the blood so that your brain and muscles can use it for fuel. Walking down the sports-nutrition aisle of your local supermarket will reveal an entire line of low-carb bars. These bars are being heavily marketed to the millions of Americans on low-carbohydrate/high-protein diets, and they contain high levels of

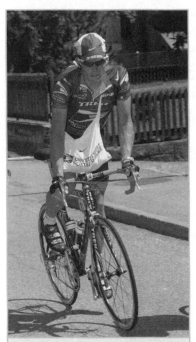

Lance carrying a "musette" bag containing a combination of PowerBars, PowerGels, fruit, pastries, sports drink, and water. Photo © by Graham Watson

sugar alcohols. As you might remember from Chapter 6, athletes should be wary of foods containing sugar alcohols.

Bonking

Upon returning from a particularly long and harrowing mountain bike ride, one of my employees commented, "That was the most fun I *never* want to have again." One trip over that route was enough for him, which is the exact opinion almost everyone shares about bonking.

Every athlete and active person has or will bonk at one point; it's like a right of passage. More accurately, it's part of the natural learning curve. Bonking is the result of making at least one, and possibly several mistakes; and mistakes are the sometimes unpleasant ways we learn a lot of important things.

The experience of bonking varies, and we all have stories of spectacular episodes: blasting through the first half of a marathon, yet barely recognizing your name by mile 17; pushing the pace on a long climb, then a mile later, cracking so hard you can barely keep your bike upright; laughing and kidding with your spouse in the middle of a workout, then less than 30 minutes later being extremely irritable, snapping at her, and having to walk home.

No matter when or how often it happens to you, bonking never gets any more pleasant, so it's best to learn how to avoid it altogether. The important thing is to understand what is happening when you bonk so you're better prepared to prevent it.

In the past, it was thought that running out of muscle glycogen was the primary cause of the weakness aspect of bonking. It turns out there's sometimes plenty of glycogen left in the muscles, but very little left in the liver. Liver glycogen, rather than muscle glycogen, is your brain's primary source of glucose, and when your liver glycogen stores run low, your brain struggles to get enough fuel. Your muscles can't directly release glucose into the blood to alleviate this situation, and the assistance they can offer takes so long that your brain's appetite can far exceed your ability to convert glycogen to blood glucose. Both active and inactive muscles can partially break glycogen down to lactate (the same byproduct you get from anaerobic metabolism) and release it into the blood. Your liver can then convert the lactate to glucose and release it back into the bloodstream for your brain and active muscles to use. This "lactate shuttle" is also one of the theoretical methods by which glycogen from your biceps can provide energy for your quadriceps during prolonged exercise. Gluconeogenesis, using a mixture of protein, lactate, pyruvate, and glycerol to produce glucose in the liver, also aids in providing blood glucose but often falls well short of meeting the demands of your brain's rapacious appetite.

When you deprive your brain of fuel, it leads to a cascade of unpleasantries. The portions of your brain that control decision making, coordination, motivation, and even interpretation of visual images are affected. The resulting combination of confusion, disorientation, nausea, and possibly hallucinations usually accomplishes your brain's goal of slowing you down. Your brain selfishly seeks to stop you from exercising so it can keep you conscious and alive.

The most common cause of bonking is simply failing to consume enough carbohydrate, especially during higher-intensity workouts. You can increase the rate at which you burn through the carbohydrates in your body up to five times as the intensity of your efforts increases. In

Recommended Energy Bars for Carbohydrates During Exercise

Energy Bars	Serving Size (1 bar)	During or After Exercise	Calories (g)	Carbohydrate (g)	Protein (g)	Fat (g)
PowerBar Performance	65g	During	230	45	10	2
PowerBar Harvest	1 bar	During	240	42	7	4
PowerBar Pria	28g	During	110	16	5	3
Clif Bar	68g	During	250	45–52	4–10	2–4
Clif Luna	48g	During	180	24	10	5
Balance Bar	50g	During	200	22	14	6
Kellogg's Nutrigrain bar	37g	During	140	27	2	3
Nature Valley Granola Bar	48g	During	180	29	5	6

Source: Compiled from information on packaging and corporate websites, 2003.

other words, you might be fine eating 35 grams of carbohydrate per hour during an interval workout at moderate intensity, but the same amount of carbohydrate may not be enough to support the same workout at a higher intensity. The best strategy to prevent bonking is to start your workouts with full glycogen tanks and start eating and drinking early.

Consuming carbohydrates in the form of energy bars, gels, and sports drinks are effective ways to prevent bonking, and they are equally effective at helping you recover from it. When you do bonk, as you inevitably will at some point, getting some carbohydrate into your body is the only thing that will make you feel better and enable you to get home safely. This isn't a time to be picky, either; it's an emergency, so grab whatever you can (see Chapter 15 for more on emergency foods).

Even the best athletes in the world aren't immune to the devastating effects of bonking. U.S. Postal Service strongman George Hincapie missed an opportunity to win one of the most prestigious one-day classic races, Paris-Roubaix, as the result of bonking. In 2002, the 260-kilometer (160-mile) race began under a clear sky, but a cold rain began falling a few hours later. Perceiving that going back to the team car for warmer clothing was too risky, George pressed on and made the critical selections that put him in good position at the front of the race. Unfortunately, fighting to stay warm led him to burn through his energy faster than normal, and he bonked just 25 kilometers (less than 20 miles) from the finish. He lost control of his bike on a muddy, slick section of cobblestones and flipped head over heels into a ditch.

Nutrition *After* Training/Competition

Paying attention to what you eat after a training session or a race is critical in maximizing recovery. This is especially important in the first 15 to 60 minutes after exercise, because your body is most efficient at replenishing energy stores during this "glycogen window." I always tell my athletes that they will *eventually* recover even if they do nothing to enhance the process, but they may have to wait 48 to 72 hours for their bodies to replenish depleted muscle-glycogen stores. Optimizing the rapid resynthesis of muscle glycogen is critical for peak performance the next day and those following.

The rate of muscle-glycogen synthesis is highest immediately after exercise; your muscles are empty and blood flow is still high. This is the optimal time to consume carbohydrate-rich foods. By eating or drinking about .75 grams of high-glycemic-index foods (recovery drink, rice, cereal, honey, potatoes) per pound of body weight within 15 to 30 minutes after exercise and every two hours for the next four to six hours, you can maximize the replenishment of glycogen stores. Think of it as having more "windows" open into the muscle. The longer you wait after a training session, the fewer of these windows will be open to transport fuel back into your muscles. When you want to have energy for exercise on back-to-back days, take advantage of these windows to accelerate the recovery process.

The rate of muscle-glycogen resynthesis depends on a number of factors, including the extent of the depletion, the amount of carbohydrate available, and the timing of the carbohydrate intake. The number-one factor in determining how fast your glycogen will be replaced is the availability of carbohydrate. The recent research that has focused on the addition of protein to carbohydrate recovery drinks has concluded that, regardless of the protein content of the drink, there must be sufficient carbohydrate available to maximize glycogen resynthesis. The protein may affect the rate at which this replenishment occurs, but adequate carbohydrate is necessary to completely refill glycogen stores.

There has been a lot of research on the combination of protein and carbohydrate in recovery drinks, and Kathy Zawadzki did some of the early work on the subject. Recent research suggests that protein ingested in the immediate post-exercise window (15 to 60 minutes) may help the absorption of carbohydrates and may also aid in stimulating amino-acid transport, protein synthesis, and muscle-tissue repair. However, the same research also shows that protein is not the most important part in this process, but rather that the most important goal is to maximize carbohydrate intake during this time. If adequate carbohydrate is not ingested, the additional protein will do nothing to enhance muscle glycogen resynthesis. In other words, you can achieve the same results whether you consume a lot of carbohydrate or a mixture of carbohydrate and protein. However, if no food or too little carbohydrate is consumed, ingestion of protein or specific amino acids during recovery from prolonged exercise may not accelerate glycogen resynthesis.

Typically, eating a high-carbohydrate meal right after training or competition is not feasible. Many times, runs and training sessions are far from home or the convenience of a good restaurant. As a result, high-carbohydrate recovery drinks have become very popular. (See Chapter 10 for more details on recovery drinks.) While recovery drinks are convenient and have the added benefit of providing fluids as well as nutrients, research has shown that there is *no* difference in recovery between liquid supplements and a "real food" meal, so long as the carbohydrate content is the same. Solid and liquid forms of carbohydrate replace muscle glycogen equally well.

Beyond solid and liquid, simple and complex carbohydrates, including glucose, sucrose, and maltodextrins, all appear to replace muscle glycogen equally well. They all increase insulin levels, which in turn stimulates glucose transport into the muscle cells, glycogen synthesis, and even the transport of amino acids into muscle cells.

If you only eat enough to partially refill your energy stores, you are more likely to run out of fuel during the following day's workout. If you experience several days or even weeks where you feel sluggish or lethargic, or if your perceived effort during workouts is higher than normal, you may be chronically glycogen-depleted. Taking a week of active recovery may help alleviate this problem by allowing you to fully replenish your energy stores.

Post-Workout Recovery Meal for a 170-Pound Athlete

Cashew Crusted Chicken (1 serving)
Tomato Florentine Recovery Soup (1 serving)
Long-grain and wild rice (2 cups)
Italian garlic bread (1 serving)
Steamed broccoli (4 spears)
Skim milk (1 cup)

Calories (kcal)	Carbohydrate (g)	Protein (g)	Fat (g)
1,425	221	63	38

Putting It All Together

So, what happens when you eat properly before, during, and after exercise? Let's say Joe, a 150-pound male runner, is in the Preparation Period and is planning on running for two hours on a Sunday afternoon. As you may recall, the periodization plan for nutrition calls for increased amounts of carbohydrate when training volume and intensity are high. The increased intensity from the Foundation Period to the Preparation Period causes an increase in carbohydrate usage.

Carbohydrates in Grams per pound of body weight for the Entire Day During the Preparation Period

Weekly Training Hours	< 8	8-12	>12
Carbohydrate (g/lb body weight)	3	3.25	3.5

For Joe, an entire day's consumption would average around 500 grams of carbohydrate. Three to four hours prior to exercise, he might eat a meal that contains 225 to 300 grams of carbohydrate (1.5 to 2 grams per pound). Then, during his two-hour training session, he might consume 40 grams of carbohydrates an hour, or 80 grams total (30 to 60 grams per hour). Following training, Joe should take in another 110 grams of carbohydrate (.75 grams per pound of body weight) as soon as possible after his run—ideally in the first 30 minutes. After the first carbohydrate is consumed, it is important that he continues to consume high-carbohydrate foods for the remainder of the day.

Pre-Exercise Meal	225–300 g
Carbohydrate Intake During Exercise	80 g
Post-Exercise Meal	110 g
Sub-Total	415–490 g
Remainder of the Day	35 g

PART

Sports Nutrition
from All Angles

3

THE YOUNG AND RESTLESS:
THE ADOLESCENT ATHLETE

IN MY WORK AS A COACH, I'VE NOTICED THAT IF SEASONED athletes in their twenties and thirties could use a little education to help them fuel their workouts and reach their goals, adolescents could use that information even more. They've been left virtually in the dark as to how to best maintain their energy levels and what foods to eat at their age—to say nothing of the fact that the adolescent years offer unique challenges, and often obstacles, both to their physical development and their personal development of life-long, healthy habits.

Participating in after-school sports or on school-sponsored sports teams is very beneficial to adolescent development. Physically, these activities enhance the development of motor skills and reflexes and help with balance and muscle control. Sports also strengthen an adolescent's aerobic engine and provide a healthy means for burning off excess en-

215

ergy. Young people who become interested in sports and exercise tend to establish healthier habits than their more sedentary peers; they are less likely to smoke, they spend less time lazily watching television or playing video games, and they establish friendships with other athletic, goal-oriented kids.

Healthy Adults Start as Healthy Kids

The subjects of sports and nutrition for adolescents are very important right now because the beginning of the twenty-first century has seen a dramatic increase in childhood obesity and the premature development of Type II diabetes. Improving long-term health by encouraging adolescents to be physically fit is a much better, and more cost-effective, option than depending on the medical community to fix their health problems years from now. Before I address the nutritional challenges facing adolescent athletes, I want to briefly discuss the role of sports in an adolescent's life and suggest some ways parents can guide their children toward a healthier, more active lifestyle.

Team sports offer benefits far beyond physical fitness and conditioning. These activities are important for teaching teenagers communication skills, the value and necessity of teamwork, and the concept that hard work and practice lead to the accomplishment of goals. Since adolescents are still growing, it's best for them to be involved in several different types of sporting activities to encourage balanced muscular and skill development. Even when I work with adolescent cyclists, I make sure they spend a portion of the year participating in other sports. As endurance athletes, they excel in cross-country running or soccer during the fall, and some play basketball or are on swimming or water polo teams in the winter. It is more important that an adolescent learn to be an athlete than that he become an expert in one specific sport.

College, or the few years post–high school, represents a transition time for people's lifestyles. With fewer opportunities to participate in team sports, along with increased freedom and exposure to myriad other activities, a young adult's decisions about nutrition and fitness can influence his or her health for years to come. From my experiences with young adult athletes, I've found that the chances that they will maintain an active lifestyle that promotes personal fitness and the accomplishment of personal goals are directly influenced by the significance athletics held during their high school years. Adolescents who participated in sports only because they were required to, either by parents or school, are more likely to completely drop exercise than are athletes who participated for fun and personal goals.

Adolescents' Focus on Sports

Parents: The #1 Role Models

As parents, our lifestyle choices affect our children's. If they are never encouraged to experience sports and don't see their parents exercising either, they are less likely to pick up sports on their own. With the social, developmental, and fitness benefits of regular exercise, it's in a child's best interest for parents to encourage athletic participation. In order for sports to be a positive, rewarding, and high-priority aspect of a teenager's life, it is important for the focus on sports to be fun first, fitness second, and competition third.

Focus on Fun First

Adolescents yearn for freedom; at the same time, they long for structure and consistency. Sports can satisfy both sides of this paradoxical situation as long as an adolescent has some ownership over his or her sport choices. It's important for parents to steer their children toward sports, but it's equally important that they not force their favorite sport on them. If after-school sports become a requirement, just another assigned task like homework, kids are more likely to quit as a means of exercising some degree of self-determination and autonomy. When adolescents choose their own sport, they are more personally invested in them. They've exercised the freedom they desire because they didn't let Mom and Dad tell them what sport to play.

Of course, letting teenagers make decisions has its drawbacks, especially in the frequency with which they change their minds. A frustrating quandary for parents is often whether to let their kid quit a sport he or she doesn't like anymore, or to use the experience to teach the child character-building concepts like finishing what you start, respecting your team and teammates over your personal desires, and persevering even when you don't like something. As a parent and a coach working with a wide variety of adolescent athletes, I've found that a good compromise is encouraging a high school student to finish out the season in the given sport, then make a decision about choosing another one. This reinforces the character-building concepts mentioned above; but the experience only lasts a few months, and then they can move on to another sport. It's best to make it clear that quitting their current sport isn't a license to lie around and do nothing. Encourage them to try different sports until they find one they look forward to participating in every day.

Fitness Second

In many cases, fitness is a byproduct of participating in school sports throughout the year, rather than the primary reason for playing, and there's nothing wrong with that. Pushing kids to achieve optimal performance often requires more regimen and sacrifice than they're willing to endure, and doing so takes the fun out of participating.

Competition Third

Athletic competition can be very beneficial to adolescents, but it's not the most important aspect of participating in sports. While it is beneficial for student-athletes to strive for excellence in the sports they play, it's also easy for them to lose perspective on the role of sports. A student-athlete's first responsibility is to his or her schoolwork; responsibilities to a team and sport are secondary. No matter how devoted adolescents are to their sports, it is essential that they keep up with their schoolwork. Requiring good grades as a prerequisite for participating in school sports is a good way to teach young people about time management and priori-

Puberty and High School Sports

One challenge adolescent athletes face is that their stage of physical development can influence their success in sports. Teenagers of both genders start puberty at different ages and develop through puberty at different rates. As a result, the strength, speed, and muscular development of adolescent athletes, even those of the same age, is highly variable. The individuals who mature at an earlier age may initially be more successful in high school athletics (due to greater muscular power, height, and weight) than their peers who develop more slowly.

Students who mature quickly and at an early age sometimes struggle later, when other students catch up developmentally. During their freshman and sophomore years of high school, superior strength and speed enabled them to succeed regardless of underdeveloped skills. On the other hand, their smaller peers had to rely on more highly developed skills to be competitive. While the bigger kids were more powerful, the smaller kids had to become more nimble and agile, traits that can be advantageous in sports like soccer, basketball, and even football. As these students mature, they retain their skills and increase their strength and speed, and eventually often surpass the performance of those students who used to be the stars of the team. This can be difficult for former stars to deal with, and it can sometimes lead them to drop out of sports. It is therefore important for coaches to emphasize skill development and good nutrition choices to all student athletes, even the ones who mature through puberty early in their high school years.

ties, and if the time commitment and exertion of sports have a detrimental effect on grades, then parents, coaches, and teachers should withhold an adolescent's privilege to compete.

As long as they keep their grades up and have a healthy social life, adolescents can benefit greatly from competition. It teaches them to work hard in the pursuit of goals, and it allows them the satisfaction of contributing their best individual effort to the success of their team. For students who don't relish competition, there are other ways to learn these important lessons, including the drama club or band, volunteer work, and student government. In many cases, participation in sports or these other activities has a positive effect on students' grades by helping them realize the importance of managing their time.

Training and Nutrition Challenges for Adolescent Athletes

The culture of American high schools and the trends in adolescent eating behaviors lead to substantial challenges to success for teenage athletes. Many high schools have established partnerships with fast-food companies to supply meals for school lunches, and cola companies have contracted with schools to place soda machines in hallways, making it very easy for kids to choose foods that are high in fat and sugar.

Cheyenne Mountain High School, located a few miles from the offices of Carmichael Training Systems in Colorado Springs, is featured in Erik Schlosser's book *Fast Food Nation.* Foods readily available in the school cafeteria include pizza, hamburgers, curly fries, hot pretzels with cheese, Sobe drinks, chocolate milk, nachos, fried chicken, breadsticks with marinara sauce, popcorn, and many varieties of candy. The school has a salad bar, but it also has a slushie machine and Pepsi vending machines. One of the complete meals the school offers includes a deli sandwich with chips, M&Ms, and a drink. Cheyenne Mountain High School's cafeteria selections aren't the exception; rather, they are indicative of food choices in schools around the nation. While it is possible for students to eat healthy, nutrient-dense meals in school cafeterias, it is equally possible, and more likely, that a student's lunch will be high in saturated fat, trans-fat, and empty-carrier carbohydrates.

In One Ear, Out the Other

Studies consistently show that students have limited knowledge of general nutrition and poor knowledge of sports nutrition. In a study by

Peron and Endres, athletes were reasonably knowledgeable about nutrition from a health standpoint, such as how nutrition affects heart-disease risks, but lacked knowledge about sports nutrition. These same studies also suggest that increased knowledge of nutrition doesn't lead to positive changes in students' nutritional choices.

Sometimes the most important nutritional choice an adolescent makes doesn't revolve around which food to eat, but whether to eat at all. In a study by Smalz (1993), 13 percent of the subjects reported skipping breakfast, and another 26 percent reported eating breakfast foods that were high in sugar and fat (yes, doughnuts). Their nutritional choices didn't improve much later in the day, either; Smalz's study indicated only about a quarter of students ate a nutritionally balanced lunch.

Leslie Pearlman, an English teacher and assistant coach of the 2002 Colorado State Champion Cheyenne Mountain High School girls swim team, experienced the consequences of these eating habits firsthand. Girls would routinely come to practice after school having skipped breakfast and only having consumed a soda and candy bar during lunch. During the course of two-hour-long practices, the girls would complain of feeling tired, lethargic, and even nauseated. Miss Pearlman resorted to stocking a drawer in the pool office with peanut butter and crackers, and she skipped one entire day of practice to talk to the girls about sports nutrition.

Nutrition and Overtraining in High School Sports

The seasonal structure of high school sports is problematic for adolescent athletes as well. Students arrive at the first day of practice relatively untrained and have only a few weeks to prepare for their first competitions. The entire season typically lasts about four months, during which time students are asked to go from this relatively untrained state to peak competitive condition in time for league, regional, and state-championship competitions. To prepare them, coaches in some sports hold practices twice a day early in the season. Then, during the entire season, practices are held five days a week, and sometimes at least once during the weekend. Overall, training is characterized by high intensity and high volume with very little emphasis on recovery.

More Isn't Always Better

High school students are advised by coaches, teachers, and parents (and rightly so) that hard work leads to success. When it comes to studying, more is better, especially when a student is struggling. But students often apply this same concept to after-school sports, figuring that if they work harder, such as by running extra laps or training on the weekends, they will improve their performance. Unfortunately, many athletes, including student-athletes, do not fully understand the importance of recovery in training. When you don't allow for enough recovery time, or don't consume proper recovery foods between workouts, training performance suffers, and eventually progress grinds to a halt. While it is possible to structure training to include five days of workouts with two days of recovery, matching the typical school week and weekend schedule, I would rarely institute such a program for an adolescent athlete. Generally speaking, such a schedule would place too high a training stress on an athlete and provide too little time for adequate recovery. However, until there are major reforms in the culture of scholastic sports programs, the best we can do as coaches and parents is guide adolescents to make nutritional choices to better enable them to cope with their training-load demands.

Helping Teenage Athletes Fuel Up for School Sports

There are two issues of primary importance for student athletes: fueling up prior to practice, and eating for recovery during the evening. When athletes begin practice with full fuel stores, they are better prepared to complete the prescribed workouts. However, more commonly, they arrive at practice with partially or completely depleted glycogen stores because they have not consumed enough food throughout the day. Not only does this lead to diminished performance, it also hinders their ability to recover adequately before the next day's practice. Over the span of a few weeks, the effects of this energy deficiency accumulate. Athletes struggle through practice, are constantly tired, suffer small, nagging injuries, and lose motivation to continue participating. Miss Pearlman's swimmers at Cheyenne Mountain High School offer an illustration of this progression.

At the beginning of the season, the girls are eager and excited to get in the water to work on their technique and flip-turns, and they are generally in high spirits. About four to six weeks into the season, they start to skip practice, complain about the length of the workouts, and argue amongst themselves. There is an increase in the number of girls visiting the school's trainer, complaining of real, imagined, or exaggerated injuries so they don't have to get in the water. Though the evidence is anecdotal, girls who consistently maintain higher caloric intakes by eating several times a day tend to see more improvement in performance compared to teammates whose nutritional choices are more suspect. As a result, they tend to retain their enthusiasm for swimming while their teammates struggle to do the same. Speaking with other coaches of high school and youth athletic-league teams, and from my own coaching experience, I've found that Miss Pearlman's swim team's scenario is indicative of many adolescent sports teams.

Breakfast

Breakfast is one of the most important meals for all of us, and maybe even more so for adolescent athletes. During the course of a 10-to-14-hour overnight fast, a large part of their liver glycogen stores are depleted. It is important that they consume a meal that will replenish these stores and provide energy to get through morning classes. Since the reality of a high school student's lifestyle isn't usually conducive to a large, sit-down meal before school, try the following suggestions for quick, nutrient-dense, and in some cases portable breakfasts: All of these options take just two to three minutes to make!

Cereal with Fruit and Yogurt

1 cup low-fat or non-fat yogurt, plain or sugar-free

1 serving fruit of choice

1 cup low-fat or non-fat milk

1–2 handfuls cold cereal

Cereal with Walnuts, Toast, Fruit, and Milk

1 tablespoon unsweetened jelly or jam

1 serving bread of choice

1 tablespoon walnuts (*good for omega-3 fatty acids*)

1 cup low-fat or non-fat milk

1 serving fruit of choice

1 handful cold cereal

Egg Wrap

2 large eggs

1 whole-wheat tortilla (approximately 6 inches in diameter)

1 ounce grated cheese

cooking spray

Spray a small microwaveable bowl with cooking spray, beat egg in bowl, and add cheese. Cook for approximately 2 minutes, until just firm. Place egg on tortilla and fold over. If you don't want to grate the cheese, just put a slice in the tortilla, then put the hot eggs on top of it.

English Muffin or Bagel with Cheese

1 English muffin or bagel

1 ounce low-fat or non-fat cheese of choice

Whole-Grain Waffle with Fruit or Peanut Butter

1–2 frozen waffles

2 tablespoons peanut butter

Toast waffles, then top with fruit or spread with peanut butter.

Peanut Butter Wrap

Wrap together:

1 tortilla (approximately 6 inches in diameter)
1–2 tablspoons low-sodium peanut butter
$^1/_2$ banana

Fruit Shake

$^1/_4$ cup 100% fruit juice of choice
1 cup frozen strawberries or blueberries
4 ice cubes
1 cup low-fat or non-fat milk

In a blender, combine juice, strawberries, ice cubes, and milk. If shake is too thick, add a few tablespoons of water.

Oatmeal with Milk and Fruit

$^1/_3$ cup oats, whole or quick, uncooked
2 tablespoons raisins
3 teaspoons sliced almonds
$^3/_4$ cup low-fat or non-fat milk

In a medium-size bowl, combine oats and milk. Place bowl in a microwave and cook for about 2 to 3 minutes or until milk is absorbed. Stir in raisins and almonds, and serve. NOTE: If desired, an equal amount of water may be substituted for the milk.

Fruit Protein Shake (unsweetened/dairy-free)

1 scoop protein powder, plain (unsweetened)
$^1/_2$ medium banana
3 ice cubes
4 ounces low-fat or non-fat yogurt, dairy-free (soy)

Combine all ingredients in a blender. You can sweeten with sugar or honey, or an artificial sweetener if you prefer.

OTHER ON-THE-GO IDEAS
    Fruit or cereal bars
    Pop-Tarts
    Leftover pizza
    String cheese
    Hard-boiled egg

Lunch

The next challenge for the adolescent athlete is selecting a nutrient-dense lunch from the choices offered at school. Considering that parents have substantial influence over providing quality-carrier foods like whole-grain breads, fresh vegetables, and lean meats at home during breakfast and dinner, I generally don't press adolescents to search the lunch cafeteria for whole grains and fresh vegetables. I've worked with several athletes who have skipped lunch altogether out of frustration over not being able to find foods they felt were nutritious enough. That's totally counterproductive. A deli sandwich on white bread is not bad for you; it would just be better if it was on whole-grain bread. Since consuming enough calories to fuel up for practice is one of the primary concerns for adolescent athletes, it's more important that they eat *something*, preferably something reasonably healthy, as opposed to eating nothing or eating too little.

CAFETERIA CHOICES THAT MAKE THE GRADE:
    Any type of fresh fruit or vegetable
    Low-fat or non-fat (chocolate is okay!)
    Fruit juice or smoothies
    Yogurt (add fruit and/or nuts)
    Hamburger (preferably on a whole-grain bun; go easy on the fries)
    Grilled chicken sandwich
    Bean burritos
    Turkey sandwich
    Soups or chili
    Plain or salted soft pretzels (skip the cheese)
    Vegetable-and-cheese pizza

Brown-Bag Lunch Choices
(don't require refrigeration by lunchtime)

Peanut butter and jelly sandwich

Peanut butter, banana, and honey sandwich

Fruit or fruit cups

Pretzels

Microwaveable container of soup or stew with bread or crackers

Pre-practice Snack

Since students often rotate through the cafeteria for lunch periods be-tween 11 a.m. and 1 p.m., and sports practices begin at around 3:00 to 3:30 p.m., there can potentially be four hours or more between lunch and practice. When students eat an appropriate-sized meal at lunch, the time between lunch and practice actually works to their benefit. Eating a meal about three hours prior to strenuous exercise or competition al-lows enough time for them to absorb most of the energy-containing nutrients in the meal. For those students who have a late lunch, and therefore only two hours between eating and training, a larger breakfast or snack during the morning should give them the ability to eat a smaller, more easily digestible lunch and still have energy for practice.

Regardless of when a student has lunch, a pre-practice snack can be essential to a successful practice. By eating a 200- to 400-calorie food that is high in carbohydrate and contains some protein and fat, they become better able to maintain adequately high blood-sugar levels all the way through practice. This is important because most high school coaches do not make time for athletes to consume food during practice; it's dis-ruptive to the flow and ends up taking much more time than necessary. It's important for athletes to experiment with different snacks, as some foods may settle in the stomach better than others. Energy bars like the PowerBar Performance Bar are a good choice, but they may be hard to come by at school. Some well-prepared students who bring lunch from home can pack an additional sandwich such as peanut butter or turkey, for after school. A piece of fruit, like an apple or a banana, in addition to a candy bar that contains peanuts or almonds, makes a good snack that is both appealing to teenagers' tastes and available on most campuses. See the following table for more pre-practice snack suggestions.

Planning ahead is the best option. You can add these easy-to-carry items to your backpack or gym bag the night before:
PowerBar Performance, Harvest, or Pria bar
Fig Newtons
Nutrigrain bar or other cereal bar
Trail mix (nuts, raisins, dry cereal)
Crackers and cheese/peanut butter
Fruit (apples, oranges, and bananas tend to be the most portable)
Fruit snack cups
Fruit juice in drink boxes or cans
Apple and cheese sticks
Dried fruit
Graham crackers
If you forget and have to make your choice from the vending machine, you can still get a good snack without too much added sugar or fat:
Pretzels
Animal crackers
Cereal bars
Trail mix
Snickers bar (not every day, but once in a while is okay!)

During Practice

Since most after-school sport practices last somewhere between one and three hours, hydration is a big concern. Adolescents have been shown to be less efficient than adults at maintaining their body temperature, and they are therefore at a higher risk of suffering from heat- and dehydration-related illnesses. They start sweating later than adults do and have a slower sweat rate, meaning that at the same level of exercise intensity, an adolescent will have a higher core temperature and a greater degree of dehydration. To make matters even more dangerous, teens are less knowledgeable about the signs and symptoms of dehydration and over-heating, so they don't realize they need to drink more.

Athletes should be encouraged to finish at least one water bottle during practice (two would be much better), but coaches need to be careful about how they emphasize this point. Demanding to see an empty water bottle at the end of practice is not wise because it implies a penalty for drinking too little. In response, kids will deliberately empty water bottles into the grass rather than drink them. Rather, it's better to integrate hy-

Energy Gels: Good, But Not for Replacing Lunch

Some students have discovered energy gels, like PowerBar Power-Gels, and use them for energy during practices. There are a few things you have to remember about these highly concentrated carbohydrate sources:

- A PowerGel only contains 100 calories of energy, and eating one will not make up for skipping lunch. It is designed to provide carbohydrates to maintain your blood-sugar levels so you have energy to supply your brain and keep from bonking.
- An energy gel needs to be consumed with 8 to 16 ounces of water so you can digest it quickly. The water needs to be added to dilute the carbohydrate solution in your stomach and small intestine. Until it's more diluted than it was in the package, you're not going to absorb the carbohydrates quickly.
- Although energy gels taste good and are often sweet, they are not candy. Eating several packets of energy gel is not only expensive, but it can also lead to an upset stomach. You should only consume one or two energy gels per hour of continuous exercise.
- Some energy gels contain caffeine, which can be both beneficial and harmful. Caffeine is a stimulant and promotes fat metabolism, but it is also a diuretic that contributes to dehydration. Considering the adolescent athlete's already-heightened risks of dehydration and heat-related illness, there's really no reason to add caffeine to the equation.

dration into the course of the practice, like sending the athletes to the side-lines to get a drink while explaining the next part of the practice schedule.

Supplying sports drinks like PowerBar Endurance during practices would increase the performance of adolescent athletes. Sports drinks provide carbohydrates and electrolytes and have consistently shown improvement in performance by delaying fatigue and replenishing electrolytes lost through sweating. However, providing sports drinks to student athletes can give rise to logistical problems for coaches and schools. Sports drinks can be expensive, especially in the amounts needed to supply an entire team. The other problem is that if some kids don't like the sports drink provided, they may choose not to drink at all. Ideally, both water and sports drink would be available. I would encourage student athletes to contribute money to a fund that would pay for the team's sports drink if their school is unable to provide it.

Recovery After Practice

Like any other athlete, an adolescent's nutrition choices in the hour directly after practice are critical to the following day's performance. A good recovery meal should include all three macronutrients (carbohydrate, protein, and fat) in order to replenish fuel stores and provide the amino acids needed to repair muscle damage and support the immune system. Student athletes sometimes wait too long to eat following practice, and consequently they fail to take advantage of their bodies' increased readiness to absorb and utilize nutrients for recovery.

Parents who pick their kids up after practice can help their children perform better both in sports and in the classroom by bringing fluids and a mixed-nutrient snack with them. These shouldn't spoil their dinner, but they should keep them alert by preventing their blood sugar from falling too low. A peanut butter sandwich, energy bar, smoothie, or turkey sandwich does the trick. It provides carbohydrates and protein that will be quickly absorbed and used to replenish energy stores and repair damaged tissues, and it also tides them over until they can sit down to a more complete meal at home.

Even after practice, hydration continues to be essential to performance. Athletes should consume at least one bottle of water after practice and continue consuming fluids with dinner and throughout the evening. While water is the obvious choice for rehydration, there are many other beverages that can do the job and may also provide additional benefits. Recovery drinks, orange juice, milk, and tomato or other fruit and vegetable juices provide fluids as well as vitamins, minerals, and electrolytes. Since these drinks also contain calories, it's important not to completely shun water. Drinking a quart of orange juice with dinner adds more than 400 calories to the meal.

Recovery, or lack thereof, may be the primary factor that determines adolescents' success in school sports. They push themselves hard, as do their coaches and parents, to excel on the field and in the classroom; but failing to take the time to focus on recovery establishes a scenario that leads to diminished performance in both areas. With practice, competition, and schoolwork schedules as they are, nutrition is one of the only variables student-athletes can affect in order to improve their recovery from day to day.

Disordered Eating and Adolescents

Body image and social status are heightened concerns for adolescents, so much so that studies have shown that the majority of high school girls would prefer to weigh less than they do and are fearful of becoming fat. Even more interesting, the data from these studies shows that the subjects were primarily of normal or below-normal weights for their heights. Though fewer studies included male subjects, the data shows that boys are every bit as concerned with their weight and appearance. Adolescent athletes often feel pressure to be lean, and studies have shown that the prevalence of weight preoccupation cuts across the entire spectrum of competitive sports. The football and hockey players are just as concerned about body weight as are the swimmers and gymnasts. While disordered eating (fasting, vomiting, and/or using diet pills, laxatives, and diuretics) is dangerous for athletes and nonathletes of all ages, the adolescent athlete is particularly susceptible to developing such problems and is more likely to cause serious and irreversible damage to his or her body.

The Female-Athlete Triad

The Female-Athlete Triad is a cascade of disorders resulting from extreme dieting and/or high levels of athletic activity. (See Chapter 13 for more on special concerns for female athletes.) Dieting to maintain a low body weight restricts caloric intake, and this then contributes to menstrual dysfunction. When an adolescent girl stops menstruating or her cycle becomes erratic, it leads to a decrease in bone density, which then predisposes her to early-onset osteoporosis (a bone disease characterized by reduced bone mass leading to increased susceptibility to fractures). In a study by Drinkwater et al. (1986), young female athletes (an average age of 25) who were amenorrheic (without consistent menstruation) had an average bone-mineral density similar to women of about 51 years of age. Drinkwater's team followed up with the subjects for four years, and though with improved nutrition their menstrual cycles returned to normal and bone density increased, it remained well below average. Since adolescence is such an important period of growth, the female-athlete triad may be even more dangerous for teenage girls. Coaches and parents should inquire as to the menstrual status of adolescent female athletes and direct them to a physician for evaluation.

Disordered Eating Affects Male Athletes, Too

While studies show that fewer male than female athletes suffer from disordered eating, it is a complete misconception to assume that female athletes are the only ones who suffer from disordered eating. It is just as misleading to believe that disordered eating only occurs with male wrestlers attempting to wrestle in lower weight classes. Males in a wide variety of sports are concerned with their body image and the ways their weight affects their performance. Some desire to lose weight, and as a consequence, they restrict their caloric intake, vomit, or take diet pills, laxatives, or diuretics. These athletes are at increased risk for lower-than-normal bone density (although the risk is not as high as it is for women), and for the development of clinical eating disorders like bulimia and anorexia nervosa.

Some male athletes, however, are obsessed with gaining weight, particularly muscle weight. In a misguided attempt to gain muscle mass, some resort to massive oversupplementation with protein, often exceeding two grams of protein per pound (three grams per kilogram) of body weight per day. It has been shown that such high levels of protein intake are not necessary, or effective, for increasing muscle mass. More dangerous than oversupplementation with protein is the increased incidence of drug use among teenage athletes. Anabolic steroids, human growth hormone (HGH), and legal supplements claiming to contain precursors to testosterone have become more easily available, thanks to the Internet, and their use is believed to be on the rise in high school populations. These substances have serious, and even deadly, risks associated with them, including abnormal bone growth and an increased risk of certain cancers. Coaches and parents who suspect that male or female athletes may be using these substances should consult a physician and/or drug counselor immediately.

13

THE ACTIVE WOMAN: WHAT YOU NEED TO KNOW

THOUGH MOST CLINICAL AND SPORTS-NUTRITION INFORMATION applies equally well to both genders, there are some important sports-nutrition considerations that apply specifically to women. Because of the typical smaller size of women in comparison to men, the female athlete generally needs fewer calories to meet the demands of an active lifestyle. I am using the terms "typical" and "general" with caution. Although (in general) most women are smaller and have less muscle mass than men, our CTS coaches work with some recreational and elite female athletes who are bigger and stronger than some of our male athletes. This is why our nutrition recommendations are based on body weight: The bigger you are, the more you need to eat to maintain your energy requirements. It makes sense that smaller athletes need less energy.

Pregnancy

Female athletes often must alter their training and competition schedules during pregnancy. The good news is that athletic women generally have fewer complications with pregnancy and childbirth than do sedentary women. CTS coach Kathy Zawadzki recalled a disappointing revelation during one of her childbirth-preparation classes. The classes are typically held during the seventh month, and most women are pretty big and uncomfortable at that point. During the first class, the instructor asked the class of about 10 couples to raise their hands if they were currently exercising. Kathy was alarmed when only she and one other woman raised their hands. Most of the women continually complained of aches and pains that may have been preventable with a moderate exercise program.

Exercise helps prepare you for childbirth by strengthening your muscles and building endurance, and makes it much easier to get your body

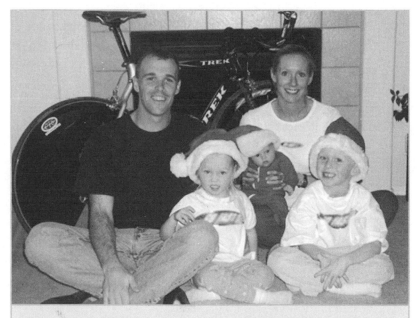

Exercise can be an integral part of your family life, and being active sets a positive example for your children. Photo © by Kevin Dessart

back in shape once the baby's born. Staying active during pregnancy usually means a slight adjustment to an active athlete's training regimen. Since the body releases a hormone called relaxin during pregnancy that loosens joints in preparation for delivery, it may not make sense to exercise as hard as you did before you became pregnant. Ideal exercise gets your heart pumping, keeps you limber, manages weight gain, and prepares your muscles for the hard work of labor and delivery—without causing undue physical stress for you or the baby. Many activities such as running and weight training are fine in the beginning, but your program may need to be modified as you grow bigger. Walking, jogging, swimming, stretching, and yoga all can help maintain muscle tone and keep you flexible. There are many prenatal exercise and yoga classes that are designed to help you through pregnancy and childbirth. You'll be better off avoiding activities that could put you at risk for slips and falls, such as bicycling, rollerblading, horseback riding, and skiing. You should consult your physician regarding your unique situation prior to continuing or starting an exercise program.

Thankfully, the American College of Obstetricians and Gynecologists (ACOG) revised the guidelines for exercise during pregnancy in 2002. Gone are the old guidelines that placed heart-rate and duration restrictions on exercise. The old guideline required women to keep their heart-rate below 140 beats per minute, a continual point of contention between Coach Kathy and her doctor. The following is a summary of the 2002 ACOG guidelines.

1. It is safe to engage in 30 minutes or more of moderate exercise on most, if not all, days of the week.
2. ACOG says that after the first trimester, pregnant women should not exercise in the supine position (flat on your back). This position can make you dizzy and decrease the blood flow to the uterus. However, not all experts consider this a hard-and-fast rule. Many women are comfortable lying on their backs well into their pregnancies. Also, don't stand motionless for long periods.
3. You'll have less oxygen available for aerobic exercise during pregnancy, so modify the intensity of your routine accordingly. Stop exer-

cising when fatigued, and don't exercise to exhaustion. You might be able to continue doing weight-bearing exercises at close to your usual intensity throughout pregnancy, but non-weight-bearing exercise such as swimming is easier to continue and carries less risk of injury.

4. Don't do exercises during which you could lose your balance, especially in the third trimester. Avoid any exercise that risks even mild abdominal trauma.

5. It is recommended that pregnant women eat an additional 300 calories a day during pregnancy, so if you're exercising, be sure to take in enough to meet the energy demands of your fitness routine.

6. During the first trimester, be sure that you stay cool when exercising. Drink 6 to 8 ounces of water every 15 minutes, wear cool clothing, and don't work out in an environment that's too warm.

Obviously, proper nutrition during pregnancy is essential, and when a woman continues to exercise, she needs to pay even more attention to her dietary intake. As we have mentioned again and again, it is important to make sure that energy intake matches energy expenditure. During pregnancy, you need only about 300 extra calories per day, a bit fewer during your first trimester. When exercising, add a few hundred more for your moderate-exercise sessions lasting 30 minutes to one hour. The 300 calories is easy to get—that's about the number of calories found in two and a half cups of low-fat milk or a tuna sandwich. In addition, don't be so concerned about how much you eat, but think more about *what* you eat. You could easily make up those 300 to 500 calories with overly processed foods such as cookies or candy. Making the most of every meal and snack is the best way to ensure that you are getting the best nutrition for yourself and your baby.

Recommendations from some of our current "mothers-to-be" and new moms include the following.

Eat Breakfast Every Day

You'll have more energy and be less susceptible to mid-morning snack attacks. If you have morning sickness, try to eat something—even if ice cream is the only thing you can eat! The calcium, fat, and calories will all be welcomed by your baby. A winning combination: yogurt, fresh fruit, a glass of calcium-fortified orange juice, and a whole-wheat bagel or toast with jam.

Drink Plenty of Water

We recommend 6 to 8 ounces of water every 15 minutes during exercise, but it is just as important to continue to drink water throughout the day. You need the extra fluid to feed your increased blood volume and for amniotic fluid. Water also aids digestion and helps with the constipation that many women face during pregnancy.

Eat Plenty of Fresh Fruits and Vegetables

Not only are these packed with vitamins and minerals, but the high fiber also helps with the constipation and hemorrhoids. You should try to eat seven or more servings of fruits and vegetables a day—three servings of fruit and four of vegetables. Coach Kathy used to prepare a fruit smoothie that included yogurt and frozen strawberries and bananas about an hour before she hit the pool.

Eat Small Meals More Frequently Throughout the Day

To allow the maximum amount of nutrients to be absorbed from the food you eat, digestion and absorption is slowed down during pregnancy. Unfortunately this can lead to heartburn and the dreaded constipation. Eating frequently will help with digestion and keep your energy levels up throughout the day. Be sure to eat a nutritious snack before and after exercise, such as whole-grain breads, granola, string cheese, graham crackers, hard-boiled eggs, or yogurt.

Modify, Modify, Modify

One of our athletes was training for her first marathon when she discovered that she was eight weeks pregnant. With the race only a month away, she was determined to complete her training and finish the marathon. Upon consultation with her doctor, it was decided that the hot climate of the race and the projected four-hour finish time would not be ideal for the baby, so she decided to run the half-marathon instead. By consuming lots of fluids during the race and running at a more moderate pace, she finished in just under two hours.

Take Your Folate Seriously

Folate is a critical B vitamin needed for proper cell division during fetal development. Folic acid taken while trying to conceive and in early pregnancy can help prevent certain birth defects of the brain and spine. Before you conceive, it's best to take a daily multivitamin containing at least 400 micrograms (mcg) of folic acid. Even better, take an over-the-counter prenatal vitamin, which has 800 micrograms. Once you're pregnant, you'll need at least 600 micrograms daily, although many doctors suggest 800 micrograms. Because the fetus's neural tubes close during the first four weeks, you'll want to start taking supplements before then.

Leafy green vegetables are a good source of folate, so try to have a large bowl of salad daily. Other good sources:

- ½ cup chicken liver: 539 mcg
- ½ cup beef liver: 184.5 mcg
- ½ cup lentils: 179 mcg
- ½ cup cereal (fortified): 146–179 mcg
- 1 ounce wheat germ (2 tablespoons): 100 mcg
- 4 spears steamed or boiled asparagus: 88 mcg
- Medium sized papaya: 115 mcg
- ½ cup steamed broccoli: 52 mcg
- 1 cup cantaloupe: 27.2 mcg
- Large hard-boiled egg: 22 mcg
- 3 ounces canned salmon: 17 mcg

Here's an example of a daily menu from the USDA (with a few extra snack suggestions to boost your calcium intake):

Breakfast

¼ cantaloupe

2 whole-wheat pancakes with blueberry sauce

1 cup skim milk

Lunch

Chili-stuffed baked potato topped with low-fat, low-sodium cheddar
  cheese

1 cup spinach-orange salad

6 wheat crackers

1 cup skim milk

Dinner

Apricot-glazed chicken, half of 1 breast

¾ cup rice-pasta pilaf

1 cup tossed salad with reduced-calorie Italian dressing

2 small hard rolls

½ cup vanilla ice milk

Snacks

6 oz non-fat plain yogurt

½ cup fat-free cottage cheese

½ medium apple

1 large soft pretzel

Female Athletes Are Prone to Iron Deficiency

Reduced iron status is a potential problem in all athletes when dietary
intake fails to meet iron requirements; however, female athletes are at a
greater risk because of greater iron loss. Due to menstruation, a woman

may lose an additional 15 to 45 milligrams of iron throughout her cycle. The prevalence of nonanemic iron deficiency is approximately 30 percent for adult women in the U.S. population and 39 percent for adolescent girls. True iron-deficiency anemia is much less common—just under 6 percent for both populations.

Although there is some conflicting scientific evidence that reduced iron status, without anemia, impairs performance, athletes often feel fatigued and unable to recover between training sessions when their iron status falls. In a study published in 2003, it was reported that women with moderate iron deficiency who were then given iron were significantly less fatigued after supplementation, and a 2002 study found that iron supplementation improved aerobic response to exercise in iron-deficient women. These two recent studies strongly suggest that non-anemic iron deficiency *does* impair aerobic and work performance and that correcting it is beneficial.

FACTORS THAT INCREASE THE RISK OF REDUCED IRON STATUS
- Poorly balanced vegetarian diets
- Chronic low-energy diets and other dietary patterns that include infrequent intake of red meat
- Increased iron requirements due to menstruation
- Significant growth spurts during adolescence
- Pregnancy
- Adaptation to high-altitude or high-temperature training

The daily requirement of iron for young girls (ages 9 to 13) is 8 milligrams per day and increases to 15 milligrams per day for premenopausal women. The average American diet typically provides 5 to 7 milligrams of iron for each 1,000 calories consumed. So, in order to get the recommended 15 milligrams, the average female athlete would have to ingest approximately 3,000 calories per day. While this may be a normal caloric intake for some women, it is somewhat high for many as well. Choosing to take a multiple-vitamin-and-mineral pill, which typically contains the RDA of iron—15 milligrams for women, 10 milligrams for men—is safe for those who usually don't meet their iron needs through their diet. Any additional iron supplementation should be supervised by a physician, as some people are susceptible to iron overload.

Female athletes that may be at risk for iron deficiency should have routine checks of their iron status. In addition to hemoglobin, the storage form of iron (plasma ferritin) and the transport iron (transferrin) should be measured.

By choosing the right foods, most women can easily meet their iron needs. Check your diet for iron-rich foods: lean red meat, dark-meat poultry, fish, dried beans, whole grains, dried fruit, enriched grain products, and leafy green vegetables. The body is more efficient at absorbing heme iron, the type found only in red meat, than non-heme iron from vitamin supplements and non-meat sources. Athletes who are vegetarians or eat very few animal products must make a committed effort to consume iron-rich foods, including whole grains, beans, tofu, nuts, dried fruits, and spinach. In addition, it is important to avoid foods that interfere with the absorption of iron into the blood. Caffeine, antacids, vitamin E, and the antibiotic tetracycline all block iron absorption when consumed at the same time as the iron-containing food. On the other hand, vitamin C can enhance iron absorption, so try drinking a glass of orange juice with that iron-fortified breakfast cereal.

Sources of Iron (single servings)

Heme-iron sources		Non-heme-iron sources	
Beef liver (3 oz)	7.5 mg	Fortified cereals such as Wheaties and Smart Start (1 cup)	18 mg
Lean ground beef (3 oz)	3.9 mg	Cream of wheat (1 cup cooked)	12 mg
Pork loin chop (3 oz)	3.5 mg	Soybeans, cooked (1 cup)	9 mg
Chicken breast (3 oz)	0.9 mg	Kidney beans (1/2 cup)	3.0 mg
Dark-meat turkey (3 oz)	2.0 mg	Blackstrap molasses (1 tablespoon)	2.3 mg
White-meat turkey (3 oz)	1.2 mg		
Salmon (3 oz)	0.7 mg	Spinach, cooked (1/2 cup)	2.0 mg

Calcium

Female athletes also have a higher need for calcium in their nutrition programs, and unfortunately, many fall short of meeting their requirements. It has been reported that nearly half of all runners and 40 percent of dancers and gymnasts don't get enough calcium. The primary importance of calcium for women is its function in bone development. Adequate intake of calcium is important in the prevention of osteoporosis, as women are four times more likely to suffer from osteoporosis than men.

Calcium intake is important for female athletes through all stages of life. Adolescents and young adults need to make sure they get enough calcium, as they achieve their peak bone mass during early adulthood. Women continue building bone up until about age 30, so consuming adequate amounts of calcium will help their bones reach optimum density and help protect them from osteoporosis later in life. Mature women need calcium to prevent the breakdown of bone. If untreated, a postmenopausal woman can lose 10 to 40 percent of bone mass between the ages of 50 and 60. Osteoporosis is an irreversible disease; however, you may be able to prevent it by maximizing peak bone mass during the first two to three decades of life in order to sustain bone health during natural periods of bone loss (menopause and aging).

The amount of calcium that a woman should get daily ranges from 1,000 to 1,500 milligrams, depending on her age group and hormonal state. In addition to maintenance of bone, calcium is required for blood clotting, muscle contraction, nerve transmission, and maintenance of normal blood pressure. There is also continuous movement of calcium between the skeleton, the blood, and other parts of the body. Although only about 1 percent of calcium in a woman's body takes care of these additional functions, it is so important to maintain that the body will draw on calcium stores in the bones—even at the expense of causing osteoporosis—to keep blood and cellular-calcium levels within the proper range.

Daily Reference Intakes (DRI) for Calcium According to Age and Gender*

1,300 mg for ages 9–18
1,000 mg for adults aged 19–50
1,200 mg for older adults
1,500 mg for postmenopausal women not taking hormone replacement therapy

*The Upper Intake Level (UL) for calcium is 2,500 mg per day. Intakes above 1,500 mg per day have not been associated with any greater benefits than more moderate intakes in the 1,200-to-1,500-mg-per-day range.

When most of us think of calcium sources, the first things that come to mind are dairy products (milk and milk products). However, if a woman is lactose-intolerant, is a vegan vegetarian, is allergic, has religious or other self-imposed dietary restrictions, or just doesn't like milk, there are many other foods high in calcium that she can choose. (See pages 163–165 in Chapter 9 for more information on calcium).

The Female-Athlete Triad

Consuming adequate calories to meet energy demands is one of the major tenets of the Carmichael Nutrition Program. In order to prevent an energy deficit, vitamin or mineral deficiencies, and/or glycogen depletion, you must consume enough calories to meet your energy demands. This may seem like a simple concept, but it is missed by many and can be a greater problem for female athletes. Inadequate calorie intake can be the first step in the wrong direction for women who participate in endurance sports (distance running, triathlon, cycling, cross-country skiing) or performance sports (figure skating, gymnastics, diving), where low body fat is an advantage. These athletes are at risk for a triad of interrelated disorders known as the "Female-Athlete Triad" syndrome. The Female-Athlete Triad is a serious syndrome that consists of disordered eating, amenorrhea, and decreased bone density; and it can contribute to premature osteoporosis and other medical, as well as psychological, problems. Many mistakenly assume that only elite female athletes that train excessively experience these detrimental effects. The truth is that the syndrome occurs in physically active girls and women participating in a wide range of activities.

Energy Imbalance

While some athletes deliberately restrict caloric intake to maintain a low body weight, others may unintentionally expend more energy than they take in and find themselves in an energy deficit. One situation we typically encounter with our female athletes is that many of them—runners, cyclists, and multisport women—often train with men or women who are stronger than they are. Although this is a great way to push your limits, there are many times when you really need to follow your own individual program. For instance, there are times when you should be training at a heart rate that is reflective of 65 percent of maximum effort, yet you have to ride at 75 percent of maximum in order to keep up with the group. This causes you to burn through your carbohydrate stores faster than your training partners are doing. To make matters worse, we observe that while men often consume massive quantities of food after group rides, the women underestimate the amount of work they did and only consume small meals. I once witnessed one of our elite female riders consuming a green salad after three hours on the bike! There was no way her meal was going to match her energy needs or allow for complete recovery.

Disordered Eating

Disordered eating may cause weakness, dehydration, anemia, lack of concentration, impaired coordination, and delayed recovery from injuries and illness. Studies have revealed that the nutritional intakes of female athletes with eating disorders are low in energy and essential vitamins and minerals, particularly calcium, vitamin D, and iron. In addition, carbohydrate intakes are significantly lower than what is required for optimal performance. Female athletes may diet more aggressively than their sedentary counterparts, with the goal of losing weight in order to improve performance. Unfortunately, consuming insufficient calories hinders performance to a greater extent than their lowered body weight aids it, and a constant energy deficit can alter hormone levels and contribute to menstrual dysfunction, which in turn may lead to a decrease in bone density. In severe cases, this can predispose a woman to early-onset osteoporosis.

Warning Signs of Eating Disorders*

· Excessive leanness or rapid weight loss
· Preoccupation with weight, food, mealtime rituals, and body image
· Wide fluctuations in weight
· Daily vigorous exercise in addition to regular training sessions
· Stress fractures (i.e., microfractures of bones that may progress to complete bone breakage)
· Yellowing of the skin
· Soft "baby hair" on the skin
· Frequent sore throat despite no other signs of respiratory illness (from self-induced vomiting)
· Many dental cavities, foul breath (from self-induced vomiting)
· Fatigue, light-headedness, dizziness
· Depression, low self-esteem

*Reprinted with permission of the American College of Sports Medicine, female athlete brochure, 2001.

Athletic Amenorrhea

When female athletes consume an unbalanced diet or don't eat enough to match their energy needs, they are predisposed to menstrual abnormalities. Amenorrhea is the absence of menstrual cycles and is classified as either *primary* or *secondary.* Primary amenorrhea is the failure to start menstruation at the onset of puberty, while secondary amenorrhea is the discontinuation of normal menstruation for at least three months.

Athletic amenorrhea is a form of secondary amenorrhea, presumed to be the result of poor nutrition and intense training. Although no one factor seems to directly lead to amenorrhea, a combination of low body-fat levels, excessive exercise, and inadequate nutrition may all contribute. Female athletes are strongly encouraged to seek medical advice at the onset of any menstrual irregularity. While the lack of a period is not always a problem in and of itself, disruption of estrogen and progesterone levels ultimately affects other body systems. Research has shown that low estrogen and/or progesterone levels are associated with a multitude of health problems, including higher blood-lipid levels, reduced bone mass, and increased rates of bone loss.

As we mentioned in Chapter 12, a study looked at young (the average age was 25) female athletes who were amenorrheic and found that they had bone-mineral density similar to women of about 51 years of age. When these athletes were tested again four years later, their menstrual cycles had returned to normal, and bone density had increased, but it still remained well below average.

The American College of Sports Medicine considers the Female-Athlete Triad a serious condition and makes the following recommendation: "If an eating disorder or amenorrhea is suspected, the involved individual should be strongly encouraged or required to seek medical attention. If the individual refuses, the concerned coach, friend, or parent should consult with a physician directly. Treatment of the Triad often requires intervention via a team approach. A physician, nutritionist, and psychologist may need to work with the woman or girl, her coach, parents, and close friends. Nutritional monitoring, hormone replacement, and reduced training may be recommended. Early intervention hastens recovery."

In addition to the serious medical conditions we have detailed above, other consequences of a poor nutrition plan include low energy and performance, depleted fuel stores, and deficiencies of iron, calcium, zinc, magnesium, folate (important if the woman plans to one day be pregnant), and other vitamins.

Poor nutrition can also affect your goals and dreams as an athlete. One of the newest members of the CTS management staff, Noriko Moser, was a professional ballet dancer. Like gymnasts, ballet dancers are athletes who begin their professional careers early, often before they hit puberty. The demands of this sport/art are such that you are required to dance several hours a day—more during the performance season—yet also required to maintain a prescribed aesthetic to look waiflike and "sinewy" (otherwise known as "too skinny").

Noriko described to me her own experience of succumbing to the pressures of her professional life, which began at age 15 at a reputable and competitive ballet company. Though she was already thin at 5' 6" and 110 pounds, she began to restrict her eating to get an "edge" on the competition. Here's where a little goes way too far. She lost 20 pounds, her period stopped, and she got injury after injury, including the telltale stress fractures. The worst part was, she sustained this weight loss—and chronic injury pattern—over a period of three years, crucial years in adolescence when her body was still developing.

Needless to say, this affected her goals and dreams as a dancer. Though she received medical attention early on and now eats properly to sustain her high training load, her injuries, and the discouragement they caused, greatly hindered her career. She jokes that she is the poster child for what *not* to do in order to have a long, healthy, injury-free career as a dancer, and since she currently coaches aspiring, adolescent dancers, she is always on the lookout for signs of eating disorders and she keeps tabs on her students' proper fueling during workouts.

WISDOM FOR
OLDER ATHLETES

ONE OF OUR CTS ATHLETES WAS HAVING SOME PROBLEMS with his cycling pedal stroke and he went in to his local bike shop to have his bike fit checked. He had had the same bike setup for over seven years with no problems. However, over those seven years he had gradually become less flexible, and he was advised to raise his handlebars so he wouldn't have to strain to reach them. At first he was bitter about the change because he believed his bike no longer looked like a "racing bike." After he rode several days without any pedaling-related problems, lower-back pain, or numb hands, he accepted the fact that fitting his bike to match the age-related changes in his body was more important than having low handlebars.

The Cold, Hard Truth

- As we age, body composition tends to change due to an increase in body fat and a reduction in muscle mass. It is estimated that you can lose about a half-pound of muscle a year beginning at age 30, but the loss varies according to gender and the level of muscle activity. As you lose muscle, your resting metabolic rate will also fall.
- Less muscle means less strength and less power. Aged skeletal muscle produces less force, and there is a general "slowing" of the mechanical characteristics of muscle. Thus, it takes muscles longer to respond in our fifties than it did in our twenties.
- Flexibility is reduced. Injuries become more likely because the water content of tendons, the cord-like tissues that attach muscles to bones, decreases as we age. This makes the tissues stiffer and less able to tolerate stress.
- Cardiac function is reduced. The heart muscle becomes less able to propel large quantities of blood quickly to the body. The increase in peripheral resistance (higher blood pressure) will also reduce stroke volume (amount of blood ejected with each heartbeat). There may also be a decline in maximum heart rate due to changes in the heart's electrical conduction system and to hormonal changes.
- Metabolically, aerobic enzymes appear to decline with age, lowering aerobic capacity. VO_2 max declines about 10 percent per decade after age 25 in the general population.

The Good News

Neither reduced muscle mass nor the subsequent loss of function is inevitable with aging. Many of the changes in our musculoskeletal and cardiovascular systems result more from lack of use than from simple aging.

- Losses can be minimized or even *reversed* with proper cardiovascular and strength training.

- By exercising and controlling energy intake, older athletes can maintain the same body-fat levels as much younger athletes. Long-term regular exercises may slow the loss of muscle mass and prevent age-associated increases in body fat.
- Exercise also helps maintain the body's response time, as well as its ability to deliver and use oxygen efficiently.
- Muscle strength and size can be improved at any age with proper training. Resistance (strength) training can improve recruitment of muscle and increase muscle mass. One study found that with a 12-week strength-training program, untrained men ages 60 to 72 were able to increase the strength of their quadriceps by over 100 percent and the strength of their hamstring muscles by over 200 percent!
- The bottom line is: Keep moving! Regular endurance and resistance exercise has been proven over and over to slow the hands of Father Time.

Congratulations, You're the Defiant Minority

I have great respect for middle-aged athletes who have made exercise a priority in their lives. I know how hard it can be to juggle the responsibilities of a family, a career, and a social life while also trying to find time to train. But the rewards are worth the effort, as our physical fitness protects us from sliding into old age too quickly. And with proper nutrition, you can help maximize the effectiveness of your limited training time.

Researchers have been relatively slow to look at the changes in sports-nutrition needs that occur as ath-

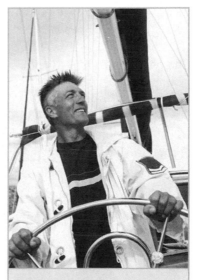

With proper nutrition you can stay active and healthy as you age gracefully.

letes age. As a masters-age athlete, you are definitely part of a minority group, and the most sedentary group is over age 50. Much of the research that looks at the nutritional status of older adults looks at their decreased mobility and their subsequent decrease in activity levels as they age. As these older adults become more sedentary, they eat less and become more susceptible to diseases linked with nutritional deficiencies. Keep in mind, most of these recommendations are based on populations that are less active than you are. Since you exercise more, your caloric requirement is higher, and by meeting this requirement through eating high-quality, nutrient-dense foods, you increase your chance of obtaining all of the essential vitamins and minerals.

Dietary needs for active older athletes are not significantly different from those of younger adult athletes. The biggest nutrition concern should be to routinely eat quality calories from nutrient-dense, health-protective foods that provide clean-burning energy, promote long-term health, and enhance recovery from hard workouts. Overall, masters athletes should follow the same recommendations as everyone else for carbohydrates, fat, and protein across all the phases of periodization, but there are a few points to consider.

Carbohydrates

To get the most out of your selection of carbohydrate foods, focus on the quality-carrier foods that bring the highest amount of vitamins and minerals, fiber, and phytochemicals. Since 33 percent of all cancers are related to poor nutrition choices, you want to spend a little more time making the best choices. And since recovery can take a bit longer as we get older, it is important to take advantage of the rapid glycogen-resynthesis window immediately after exercise. (See the recovery section in Chapter 11).

Protein

Protein intake needs to increase *slightly* as we get older, so be sure to consume high-quality protein-rich foods. Be sure to have some protein as part of at least two meals per day to build, repair, and protect your muscles. Breakfast is usually an easy place to get protein, with milk, yogurt, or eggs. A midday turkey or tuna sandwich on multigrain bread will do the job as well.

Fats

Since heart disease is the number-one killer of adults over age 65, you want to do everything in your power to decrease your risk. The heart-healthy effects of the "good" fats (see Chapter 8) should be essential to an older athlete's diet. Obviously, being and staying active is the best preventive measure, but you may consider replacing as much saturated fat as possible with monounsaturated fats. You also need to be sure to get some omega-3 and omega-6 fatty acids—the essential fatty acids found in many foods, including fish, flaxseed, walnuts, and wheat germ. Use nuts such as almonds and walnuts as a topping in your cereal or add them to salads. Substitute monounsaturated oils (olive oil and canola) and polyunsaturated oils (safflower oil and sunflower oil) for saturated oils and trans-fatty acids (lard, margarine, butter).

Calcium

Calcium absorption begins to decline beginning at age 60 for women and age 70 for men. Often seen as a "normal" effect of aging, this can eventually lead to osteoporosis and increased likelihood of bone fractures. Research strongly supports strength training and weight-bearing exercise as great ways to increase bone mass and reverse the loss of skeletal calcium. See Chapter 9 for ways to increase calcium intake and absorption.

Fiber

Consuming a diet high in whole grains, fruits, and vegetables is not only a good diet to support the demands of an active lifestyle; it also provides a ton of fiber, which is critical in helping to maintain a healthy heart and colon. A minimum recommendation is approximately 25 to 30 grams of fiber a day.

Antioxidant Vitamins

In Chapter 9 we discussed mitochondrial oxidative stress and the effect that antioxidants can have on your well-being. As you grow older, you don't necessarily have to increase your intake of nutrients like vitamin E, vitamin C, beta-carotene, vitamin A, selenium, and zinc, but you should definitely make sure you're not deficient in them.

Vitamin B12

Older adults may have difficulty with vitamin B12 absorption from food, so B12-fortified foods or supplements should be used—they are usually well-absorbed. Many cereals and breads are fortified with this vitamin.

One final thought is that as we get older, we may have to take more medications. Since they may interact with foods, it's critical that you make careful food choices when you are taking medications. Be sure to ask your pharmacist or doctor if or how your medications can interact with or detract from your nutritious diet.

15

EATING ON THE GO

AS THE PACE OF MODERN LIVING KEEPS ACCELERATING, THE majority of Americans are eating more and more meals away from home. There is an astonishing number of choices available to us, from fast-food joints to sit-down restaurants and convenience stores. Athletes sometimes feel challenges to find healthy, fuel-packed meals on restaurant menus, but with a little patience and forethought, you can find foods that will enhance your training.

As with most purchases you make, you need to become an educated consumer when it comes to eating out. If your quest for food starts with a solid knowledge base, then you'll be able to make choices that support your lifestyle. The combination of knowledge with patience will allow you to find foods that complement your training rather than hinder it. A little bit of knowledge goes a long way toward weeding through the myriad of marketing ploys and convenience scams to find foods that are right for you.

Portion Size: More Is Not Always Better

One of the first concerns you need to address when eating out is portion size. Over the past twenty years, restaurants have increased the average serving size in nearly every area of the menu. This includes fast-food restaurants as well as sit-down dining establishments. This means you have to be aware of how much you are eating. You don't need to order the largest size to get enough calories or nutrients. With many foods and even soft drinks, increasing the order size drastically increases the fat and sodium content of your meal without adding much beneficial nutrition.

Statistics on Portion Size

	Portion Sizes of 10–15 years ago	Calories	Current Portion Sizes	Calories
Bagel	3" diameter	140	5–6" bagel	350–400
Beer	7-oz bottle	85	12-oz bottle	150
			20-oz bottle	243
Chips	1-oz bag	150	1.75-oz "grab bag"	260
French fries	Large (McDonald's) 3.5 oz	305	Large (McDonald's) 6.2 oz	540
Hamburger (fast food)	5.7 oz	420	8.4 oz	600
Portion size spaghetti and meatballs	1 cup cooked spaghetti + 3 meatballs	500	2 cups spaghetti + 3 large meatballs	1025
Snickers bar	Regular bar (1.25 oz, *estimated*)	170	Regular bar— 2.07 oz	280
			KING size bar— 4 oz	540
Soft Drinks at 7-Eleven	Small: 12-oz cup	135	Big Gulp— 32-oz cup	360
	Large: 20-oz cup	225	Double Gulp— 64-oz cup	720
Soda Machine	12-oz can	140	20-oz bottle	230

Brown-Bagging It

The best option for eating on the go is to "brown-bag" it. This guarantees that you will have high-quality, wholesome foods for meals and snacks. This way you can ensure that you have healthy food choices at your fingertips. Successful brown-bagging starts in the grocery store. One of the main reasons people end up going out for lunch or stopping by a convenience store is that they didn't have anything in their cupboards or refrigerator that they could easily take with them. The next time you go to the grocery store, stock up on some of the following:

- Fresh fruits and vegetables
- Whole-grain breads for sandwiches
- Cold cuts (sliced roast beef, turkey, cheese)
- Nuts
- Energy bars
- Granola and cereal bars
- Bagels
- Bottled water
- Raisins or other dried fruit
- Lean beef jerky or turkey jerky

It is also important to have the means to carry and eat your food with you. You want to be able to keep your food fresh, safe, and clean. Ecologically, it would be better to carry your food in reusable containers. Some of the employees at CTS keep sets of silverware in their desk drawers rather than use disposable plastic utensils. To start brown-bagging your lunch, consider purchasing some of the following:

- Resealable storage bags (Ziploc)
- Reusable plastic containers (Gladware, Tupperware)
- Plastic flatware (forks, knives, spoons)
- Reusable water bottles (Nalgene)
- Personal cooler (Igloo, Coleman)

Going Out to Eat

Sometimes our schedules are too hectic and unpredictable to take a brown-bag lunch to work, and we end up going out for lunch or grabbing something to eat between appointments. These meals and snacks can fit quite well into your athletic nutrition program; it just takes a few minutes to think about your choices.

Many restaurants are addressing the public's demands for healthier meals and offering better choices on their menus. They are now adding items that are "heart smart," which means that these menu choices are lower in saturated fats, calories, and sodium. Try to select items from this list, but keep in mind that these choices may only be low in fat compared to the other menu items, and they may still be very high in calories. This is another instance when you need to be an informed consumer. Remember that you're looking at the number of calories in a meal as well as where they are coming from.

Fast-Food Burger Joints

The average fast-food menu is full of fried items, which are typically high-fat and high-calorie foods. Frying can make a gut bomb out of a potentially beneficial food, adding enough fat to outweigh the good nutrients a food, such as chicken, originally had. Try to substitute grilled, roasted, or broiled chicken rather than the breaded or fried options. This way, you'll still have the benefits of chicken without all the added fat and calories. Another option is a grilled veggie burger, which is lower in fat and provides a good source of protein.

When you order a hamburger, stick to the smaller sizes and avoid the "special" sauce and mayonnaise, as they are often fat- and calorie-laden. A better choice is to ask for extra toppings such as tomatoes, pickles, lettuce, or onions, and to use ketchup or mustard.

Sometimes there's nothing more satisfying than a pile of french fries, which may be one reason I can't advocate completely avoiding them. On the other hand, they contain a whole lot of fat and sodium. If you're dining with someone else, consider buying one order of fries and splitting them, or order yourself a small size. Also, stick to the normal french fries as opposed to curly or waffle fries; believe it or not, the regular, straight fries have less fat per serving.

Calories and Fat in French Fries

Restaurant	Calories in Medium-Sized Fries	% French Fry Calories from Fat	Grams of Fat in Medium-Sized Fries
McDonald's	450	44%	22
Wendy's	390	38%	17
Burger King	320	44%	16
Arby's (curly fries)	400	45%	20

Source: All tables on pages 259-263 compiled from information on packaging, menus, and corporate websites, 2003.

As we were looking over fast-food menus and nutritional information for this book, I was really impressed with the good choices you can make at Wendy's. While it is possible to put together some meals there that are terribly high in fat and sodium, these restaurants also have several low-fat, nutrient-dense options on their menu. What's more, these good options are easy to find and easy to order. You don't have to request specially configured items; they're already right there on the menu:

Good Choices at Wendy's

Food	Calories	Fat	% Calories from Fat
Baked potato (plain)	270	0	0
Baked potato (broccoli & cheese)	440	15	29
Chili (large)	300	7	23
Grilled chicken sandwich	300	6	20
Mandarin chicken salad (no dressing)	190	3	13
Mandarin chicken salad (fat-free French dressing)	270	3	10
Frosty (Small)	330	8	22
How Bad Can You Get at Wendy's?			
Classic Triple with everything, made with 3 slices of cheese (14.5 oz)	1,030	65	57

To help you make good choices at fast-food burger joints, we reviewed the nutrition information found on their websites and assigned "medals" (gold, silver, bronze) to their top three menu items as well as to their worst combined meal choice (the lead medal). It's important to note that even the best choices at fast-food joints are relatively high in fat, relatively low in nutrient content (lower-quality ingredients), and high in sodium. However, late at night or in the middle of nowhere on a highway, your choices may be pretty limited, and it's better to eat fast food than to eat nothing at all.

Burger King

		Calories	Total Fat (g)	% Calories from Fat	Sodium (mg)
GOLD	BK Veggie burger (6 oz)	330	10	27	760
SILVER	Chicken Whopper with reduced-fat mayo (10 oz)	490	14	25	1,420
BRONZE	Chicken Whopper Jr. (6 oz)	350	14	36	1,050
LEAD	*Double Whopper with cheese, king fries, and king Coca-Cola Classic	2,050	95	41	2,600

Kentucky Fried Chicken

		Calories	Total Fat (g)	% Calories from Fat	Sodium (mg)
GOLD	Tender roast chicken sandwich without sauce (6 oz)	270	5	17	690
SILVER	Tender roast chicken sandwich with sauce, with corn on the cob	500	17	31	900
BRONZE	Tender roast chicken sandwich with sauce (7.5 oz)	350	15	39	880
LEAD	*Extra-crispy chicken (drumstick and 2 thighs), potato wedges, and biscuit	1,420	89	56	3,230

McDonald's

		Calories	Total Fat (g)	% Calories from Fat	Sodium (mg)
GOLD	Grilled chicken caesar salad (5.5 oz)	100	3	27	240
SILVER	Chicken McGrill without mayo (7.5 oz)	340	7	19	890
BRONZE	Hamburger (4 oz)	280	10	32	590
LEAD	*Double Quarter Pounder with cheese, large fries, and a 16-oz Nestle Crunch McFlurry	2,230	108	44	2,130

Sub Shops

Subs or wraps make an excellent fast-food choice because they often include lean meats, whole-grain breads, and plenty of vegetable toppings. Choose options like lean roast beef, turkey, or grilled chicken, and then top them off with plenty of vegetables. Again, be wary of the heavy sauces and opt for mustard or oil and vinegar to garnish your sandwich. Cheese can be a good protein source, especially for vegetarian sandwiches, but use it sparingly.

The Subway Diet gained popularity a few years ago after the company launched a marketing campaign based on the weight-loss success of one of the chain's patrons. A little while later, CTS hired a new employee who religiously ate the same Subway sandwich every day for lunch. While he could have definitely chosen a worse place to eat every day, the coaches in the office suggested that he would benefit from some more variety in his nutrition program. There's nothing wrong with eating sandwiches for lunch, but you should take advantage of the variety of meats, cheeses, and vegetables that your local sub shop offers. See Chapter 6 for information regarding the Subway low-carb wraps.

Italian

Traditional Italian food can provide excellent, well-balanced meals for active, healthy people. This is especially true of the cuisine that is based on the traditions of Southern Italy. These foods tend to rely on fresh vegetables, pasta, olive oil, and fresh herbs. Meat and cheese are used sparingly in these dishes. Some of the larger, chain Italian restaurants have deviated from these traditions, however, and serving sizes can be larger than anticipated, with extra breading and more cheese and meat added to the meals.

Focus on the traditional ingredients when ordering Italian food. Start with a salad full of fresh, dark, green leafy lettuce and top it with a variety of vegetables and a small side of low-fat dressing. It's okay to include a few croutons, but go light on them as many times they are fried, so they are high in fat and calories. For your entrée, stick with pasta and marinara sauce or meat sauce, but avoid the heavy cream-based sauces. Small portions of fettucini Alfredo and manicotti are nice, rich treats, but they're almost always extremely high in fat, so they're not your best choice for either heart hearth or athletic performance. The final piece to your Italian meal would be a slice of fresh bread with a drizzle of olive oil.

Family-style and sit-down Italian restaurants often get around listing their nutritional information by saying the seasonality of their dishes and the fact they make them to each customer's tastes means they can't accurately tell you what's in it. The Olive Garden publishes some information, but only on the "Garden Fare," healthier portion of their menu. Then there's Fazoli's, where it is difficult to find any main dish that's low in fat or sodium. Overall, wherever you go for Italian food, stick with tomato-based sauces (marinara) rather than cream sauces (Alfredo), and you can reduce calories, fat, and sodium by asking the restaurant to go light on the cheese.

Mexican

Mexican food may seem like a healthy choice, but you need to be careful here as well. The taco salad is probably the biggest pitfall. The contents may be healthy, but the "shell" that forms the bowl is where the danger lies. This is typically a deep-fried tortilla and will turn this option into a nutritional nightmare. If you do order this item, eat the salad contents and leave the bowl behind.

Try to choose healthy alternatives such as whole-wheat tortillas, grilled chicken or seafood, and brown rice. Some restaurants may allow you to build your own burrito or taco, so you can pick the ingredients you like and build a healthy, flavorful meal for yourself. Of the fast-food burrito chains, Chipotle appears to be one of the best choices. Their steak and chicken are grilled as opposed to being cooked on a griddle, and their black and pinto beans are low in fat and vegetarian (they're not prepared with lard). In addition, their guacamole is not prepared with sour cream or mayonnaise. To reduce the fat content of your burrito, go light on the sour cream and cheese or skip them altogether. Tortillas can be relatively high in fat as well, so ordering a burrito in a bowl is also a good option.

Of course, Taco Bell is the most pervasive of the drive-through Mexican-food restaurants, and their menu has some pretty good choices for athletes as well.

Taco Bell

		Calories	Total Fat (g)	% Calories from Fat	Sodium (mg)
GOLD	Chicken Fiesta burrito (6.5 oz)	370	12	29	1,000
SILVER	Bean burrito (7 oz)	370	12	29	1,080
BRONZE	Chicken Gordita nacho cheese (5.5 oz)	290	13	40	690
LEAD	*Mucho Grande nachos (18 oz)	1,320	82	56	2,670

At many sit-down Mexican restaurants, chips and salsa are brought to the table right when you arrive. Although you may be hungry, don't go crazy with the chips and salsa before your meal arrives. The salsa can be fresh and relatively healthy for you, but it's the chips that will sink your ship and fill you up. Substitute salsa for the sour cream and cheese that typically come with tacos and burritos; this will add excellent flavor to your meal and let you avoid the fat and calories that come with the former options.

Pizza

Pizza can be a very good choice for you if you make sound topping selections. The two biggest unhealthy factors in pizza are cheese and the high sodium content that is usually associated with pizza (880 to 2,200 milligrams per slice).* You can request a cheeseless pizza as a healthier option. Although this may go against conventional pizza wisdom, this tomato pie is a great choice. Have the kitchen add a little extra sauce so it doesn't dry out too much in the oven, and then top it with your favorite veggies, chicken, or ham. As a general rule, avoid the combination pizzas (except the veggie one), as they typically have an abundance of toppings and extra cheese that make them heavy in the calorie department.

Chinese

Most Chinese restaurants can provide quick meals, and many of them will even deliver to your home or office. As with all choices, there are good and bad options; here are a few things for you to look for on the menu. "Crispy" is another way to describe fried foods, so keep an eye out for that word as you're scanning the menu and try to avoid it if possible. You will frequently see tofu as an option, too. Although this can be a good choice, be careful to ask whether or not it will be served "crispy." Hold the fried noodles, too.

You may find that your local Chinese restaurant has added a selection of "light" items to the menu. These choices may not be the most healthy, but they are typically lower in fat and calories than the rest of the menu options. You can also request that the kitchen use less oil when preparing your dish, or you can ask them to steam your vegetables rather than fry or sauté them. In addition, ask for brown rice rather than white rice. The brown rice is higher in fiber, vitamin B6, and magnesium, and contains vitamin E as well. Opt for steamed rice instead of fried rice, once again keeping the fat calories to a minimum.

*Information from *Restaurant Confidential,* by Michael F. Jacobsen, Jayne Hurley, Workman Publishing, 2002, p. 137.

Convenience Stores

Travel through almost any American town and you will undoubtedly see several convenience stores. They have become a cornerstone of our economy and something that many Americans have learned to rely on. Most of the shelves are stocked with ready-to-eat packaged foods, many of which are not exactly healthy choices: chips, cookies, candy bars, soft drinks, doughnuts, hot dogs, etc. While this may not appear to be the best place to find food that could contribute to health, let alone athletic performance, it can be done. Next time you enter one of these neon-lit, open-24-hours-a-day smorgasbords, take a moment to look around, and with a keen eye, you'll be able to put together a reasonable selection of snacks and the makings of a meal.

Since they're called "convenience stores," it makes sense that most of them are conveniently laid out in the same way. There's the aisle of candy bars, the aisle of bagged chips (which usually also contains the pretzels and nuts), the aisle of boxed cookies and crackers, and the walls lined with refrigerator cases and, hopefully, a deli case. Of course there are also the aisles of household cleaners, car parts, and magazines, but we're not concerned with those right now.

Remember that "fat-free" does not necessarily mean low-calorie, although it often does mean more carbohydrate. In order to make low-fat foods taste good, many companies add sugar, enough to almost completely make up for the eliminated calories from fat. The table on page 266 shows some comparisons between low-fat foods and their regular counterparts.

The Aisle of Chips

If you're looking for a snack, this should be one of the first aisles you walk down, not because potato chips or Doritos are good for you, but because this is usually the aisle that also contains pretzels, nuts, and seeds. While pretzels are an empty-carrier carbohydrate source, they provide energy and sodium without added fat. If you go for the nuts, skip the honey-roasted varieties and go with the dry-roasted ones. They are lower in total calories, and you still get the protein, vitamins, and

Fat-Free or Reduced Fat		Regular	
	Calories		Calories
Reduced-fat peanut butter, 2 tablespoons	187	Regular peanut butter, 2 tablespoon	191
Reduced-fat chocolate-chip cookies, 3 cookies (30 g)	118	Regular chocolate-chip cookies, 3 cookies (30 g)	142
Fat-free fig cookies, 2 cookies (30 g)	102	Regular fig cookies, 2 cookies (30 g)	111
Non-fat vanilla frozen yogurt (<1% fat), 1/2 cup	100	Regular whole milk vanilla frozen yogurt (3–4% fat), 1/2 cup	104
Low-fat blueberry muffin, 1 small (2 1/2 inch)	131	Regular blueberry muffin, 1 small (2 1/2 inch)	138
Low-fat cereal bar, 1 bar (1.3 oz)	130	Regular cereal bar, 1 bar (1.3 oz)	140
Low-fat granola cereal, approximately 1/2 cup (55 g)	213	Regular granola cereal, approximately 1/2 cup (55 g)	257

Source: National Heart, Lung, and Blood Institute. Nutrient data taken from Nutrient Data System for Research, Nutrition Coordinating Center, University of Minnesota. *http://www.nhlbi.nih.gov/health/public/heart/obesity/lose_wt/fat_free.htm.*

minerals. Sunflower seeds are also a good choice, and many traveling athletes like passing the time in the car by cracking sunflower seeds.

The Aisle of Boxed Cookies and Crackers

This aisle contains a mixture of good and bad choices. Almost all pre-packaged baked goods contain trans-fat, but some are not so bad for you. Your best choices include cereal bars and Fig Newtons, but you should avoid most of the other cookies. If you're in the mood for crackers, try to find Triscuits or crackers made of stoned wheat, and generally avoid varieties that have "cheese taste baked right in!" Crackers of that type are almost always higher in calories, trans-fat, and artificial ingredients.

The Candy Aisle

Before you dismiss the candy aisle, consider what it has to offer. Many candies are neither good nor bad for you; they're just energy. There are no beneficial nutrients with the sugar, which is why they're empty-carrier carbohydrate sources, but as a snack or a treat, they're fair game. Fruit candies are the lowest in fat, and varieties like Skittles, jelly beans, and Gummy Bears contain no fat at all. If you're craving chocolate, eat some; just don't get the king-sized bar. The regular bar will most likely satisfy your craving just as well as the bigger bar, but with far fewer calories and much less fat. Some other decent choices for chocolate lovers include chocolate-covered raisins or peanuts, due to the additional nutrients in the fruit or nuts.

Most convenience stores now stock a selection of energy bars. These are a great meal substitute or mid-workout fuel source, and they will get you through the afternoon until you can get home for a complete meal. As mentioned in Chapter 6, make sure you don't inadvertently grab a low-carb "energy" bar, as most are high in indigestible sugar alcohols. Their protein content will fill you up, but it won't provide you with the clean-burning energy you're looking for. In addition, there are fat-free pretzels, fig bars, juices, carbohydrate drinks, fresh fruit, raisins, dried apricots, nuts, and lean beef jerky aplenty in these stores. These are great, healthy snacks that will allow you to maintain your training and nutritional goals and can be wonderful on-the-go snacks to throw in your backpack or your car's glove compartment. Some of these stores may even have full deli services, so you can get a fresh sandwich made right before your eyes.

Emergency Foods

Try as you might, there will come a day when you experience a training fuel emergency. You'll be far from home, trying to finish a workout that has unexpectedly taken much longer than you thought it would, and you'll have that disheartening feeling of emptiness in your stomach. Your ability to focus will disappear; you'll feel lethargic and hazy. You've already eaten all your food, you're hypoglycemic (low in blood sugar), and you need to find food quickly so you can make it home. As we discussed in Chapter 11, endurance athletes refer to this scenario as "bonking," and it's not only unpleasant; it can become dangerous. Your body is running out of the carbohydrate it needs to fuel the central nervous system, so as an act of self-preservation, your brain takes action to stop you from exercising. You become dizzy, disoriented, and nauseated, and athletes who don't eat something to raise their blood sugar sometimes faint or crash their bikes.

During a food emergency, nutrition is not a concern. The key is to quickly get sugar into the bloodstream, and convenience stores have shelves brimming with sugar. Grab your favorite candy bar and either a sports drink, cola, or fruit juice, and then go outside and sit down for a while as you eat. You don't need massive amounts of food, and eating a lot may exacerbate your nausea. One energy bar or candy bar and 12 to 20 ounces of sports drink or cola should get you home. Cola has caffeine in it, and this stimulant can help keep you alert as you continue on toward home. While caffeine also increases fat oxidation, the amount you get in a cola won't increase fat metabolism much, and it won't fuel your brain or central nervous system, which still need carbohydrate.

Every athlete and coach I have ever worked with has had a training fuel emergency at least once. The following table provides a list of emergency foods we have all used to get home.

Convenience-Store Emergency Foods That Will Get You Home

Snickers or Baby Ruth bar and a Mountain Dew or Coca-Cola	Little Debbie's Oatmeal Creme Pies (just 25 cents each!)
PowerBar Performance Bar	Fig Newtons
Grandma's Chocolate Cookies	Peanut M&Ms
Little Debbie's Swiss Cake Rolls	PowerBar PowerGel
Honey Buns	Slim-Fast shake
Microwave burritos (especially on winter rides)	Milky Way bar

PART

Recipes, Training Programs, Meal Plans, and More

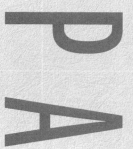

4

16

HIGH-OCTANE COOKING

AN ATHLETE'S LIFE REVOLVES AROUND FOOD, BUT IN A DIFferent way than most people's do. It's easy to consume well over 2,000 calories in a day—you can even accomplish it in one meal at a fast-food joint—but consuming that much high-octane fuel for athletic performance takes some more planning. Many athletes become interested in cooking because it puts us in complete control over our nutrition. Instead of wondering what is really in a take-out meal, you can ensure you're eating quality ingredients by preparing your meals at home.

Of course, the reality of modern living is that we don't have time to spend hours in the grocery store and kitchen purchasing and preparing elaborate meals. Working with CTS coach and head chef Greg Brown, I've compiled a wide variety of unique and easy-to-prepare recipes that will provide the fuel you need for optimal performance and recovery. The majority of the recipes found in the following sections take 15 to

20 minutes from start to finish, time well spent in the pursuit of optimal nutrition.

I first became interested in cooking as a matter of necessity; having moved out of my mother's house, I had to figure out how to feed myself well enough to continue racing. The meals I prepared in the early days were terrible, but they were effective. As I mentioned in the beginning of this book, I didn't necessarily care what it tasted like or looked like, as long as it got the job done. As I matured, so did my tastes, and I realized I deserved to enjoy my meals.

One of the privileges of being an athlete is the ability to cook with high-calorie ingredients. When you are consuming well over 2,000 calories a day, you can include foods that sedentary dieters conspicuously avoid, including olive oil, butter, and sour cream. These ingredients are high in fat, but when used appropriately in recipes, they add flavor and richness without really adding that many additional calories.

That said, there are times when reducing the fat content of a recipe is desirable. Chef Brown provided me with a great—albeit unconventional—way to reduce the fat content of recipes that normally contain sour cream and/or mayonnaise: substitute with yogurt. I have to admit, when I first saw some of his recipes on paper, I thought he had made a mistake. The concept of combining yogurt with cayenne pepper, as in the Fettucini with Sweet Pepper-Cayenne Sauce (page 281), sounded ludicrous and mildly revolting. He just laughed and showed up the next day with a container of the fettuccini for me to try. I loved it. As he explained, when you cook with yogurt, it contributes a rich and creamy taste that is completely different (i.e., less sweet) from the way it tastes when you eat it cold out of a container. In the particular case of the spicy fettuccini, he uses vanilla yogurt because the sugar and vanilla are a nice contrast to the heat of the cayenne pepper. As you will see in recipes for less-spicy recipes, he recommends using plain yogurt because there is less need for sweetness. I've been using yogurt in recipes for some time now, and even though it still looks strange on paper, I strongly recommend trying it. You will be surprised and pleased with the results.

An Athlete's Guide to Preparing Food

Your primary goal is to preserve the nutritional quality of the foods you are cooking. Depending on the food, this can mean eating it raw, steamed, or fully cooked in a variety of ways. In general, overcooking any food reduces its nutritional quality.

The way you cook a food can significantly influence its nutritional quality. Boiling, for instance, can completely destroy some foods, but is also a great way to make the carbohydrates in potatoes available for digestion. When you boil broccoli and similar vegetables, most of their vitamins, minerals, and phytochemicals end up in the water instead of in your body. However, in the case of starchy vegetables, grains, and legumes, like potatoes, barley, rice, and beans, boiling makes it easier for your body to get to carbohydrates trapped inside stiff cell walls.

Preparing Vegetables

Most fresh vegetables are best eaten raw or steamed. Sautéing them with cooking spray, butter, or olive oil is also good, as long as they still have some of their crunch afterward. A soft, mushy pepper or limp stalk of asparagus is overcooked and less nutritious. Soups and stews offer exceptions to this rule because you are consuming the liquid the vegetables were cooked in, and therefore obtaining their vitamins and minerals. I've included several soup recipes in this book because you can prepare a lot of food at one time, soups freeze well, and they're a great way to increase your fluid intake.

Preparing Pasta

One of Lance Armstrong's pet peeves in his early years as a professional cyclist in Europe was the terrible pasta he and his teammates were served in France. While it is definitely possible to find good pasta in France, bike racers from my era all the way to the present day have all had the same experiences with overcooked pasta in France. That was part of the reason I loved racing in Italy; they knew how to make a good plate of pasta.

Good food is such an important component of winning the Tour de France that Lance hired a chef to travel with the team during his first attempt at winning the race. One of the things he was looking for was a person who would cook pasta *al dente,* meaning it is firm, instead of mushy, when bitten. Of course, another major reason for hiring a team chef was ensuring the safety of the team's food. The extreme exertion of the Tour de France strains riders' immune systems, and they are incredibly susceptible to stomach illnesses. Having a team chef means having a person specifically in charge of making sure everything is clean and fresh, from the vegetables to the meat, and even the pots, pans, and knives.

Tips for Cooking Pasta

- Use a pot big enough to allow the pasta to move freely; this prevents it from clumping together.
- To make 1 pound of pasta, bring 4 quarts of water to a rapid boil.
- Adding a little salt to the water makes it boil faster and heightens the flavor a bit.
- Adding a little olive oil to the water helps prevent the pasta from sticking to itself.
- Rinsing cooked pasta helps prevent it from sticking together, but is generally only necessary if you're making a cold dish like pasta salad.

Portion Sizes

- A typical portion of pasta is 1 cup, which alone accounts for about 210 calories. It takes 2 ounces of dried pasta to make 1 cup of cooked pasta.
- A typical serving of spaghetti in an Italian restaurant is usually 3–3½ cups.
- As you progress through the four periods of the year, your portion sizes may increase.
- Standard serving size: 1 cup (may be enough for a side dish for an athlete)
- Realistic serving size for an 150-pound athlete:
  - Foundation Period: 2 to 2½ cups
  - Preparation Period: 2½ to 3 cups

- Specialization Period: 3 to 4 cups
- Transition Period: 2 cups (and include more low-calorie side dishes, such as a large green salad or steamed veggies)

Preparing Rice

You can use rice as the base of an entire meal or as a side dish, and you can add it to soups and stews to make a thicker, higher-carbohydrate meal. Brown rice has more fiber than white rice does because it still has its high-fiber bran. When this is removed to make white rice, plenty of nutrients come off with it. While brown rice is preferred over white rice, it takes considerably longer to cook. I recommend cooking a large pot of brown rice and storing it in your refrigerator so you can easily use it in a variety of meals for the next several days.

While brown rice has some advantages, there's nothing wrong with white rice. And don't be afraid to use instant rice—it has the same nutritional quality as regular white rice; it just takes less time to prepare.

TIPS FOR COOKING RICE
- Boil 2 cups of water for each cup of rice you want to prepare.
- Cooking times: brown rice, about 45 to 50 minutes; white rice, about 20 to 30 minutes; instant rice, about 5 to 10 minutes.
- Unlike with pasta, you don't want to use excess water. If you cook rice in too much water, you have to pour it through a colander, and a lot of the nutrients in the rice go down the drain. You want the rice to absorb all the water in the pot.
- Using an inexpensive rice cooker is another great way to prepare your rice. You just add the rice and water, turn it on, and 45 minutes later it is done.
- Cooking rice in broth or soup instead of plain water adds flavor.

PORTION SIZES
- 1 cup of dry white rice yields 3 cups of cooked rice, about 700 calories.

- 1 cup of dry brown rice yields between 3–4 cups of cooked rice, but still about 700 calories. The brown rice has a higher content of B-vitamins and slightly more fiber.
- Standard serving size: ½ cup of cooked rice
- Realistic serving size for an athlete: 1–2 cups
  - Foundation Period: 1 cup
  - Preparation Period: 1–1½ cups
  - Specialization Period: 1½ to 2 cups
  - Transition Period: 1 cup

Preparing Potatoes

Potatoes are a major source of carbohydrates for athletes: They're easy to prepare, they're packed with fuel, vitamins, and minerals, and they're really cheap. If you're looking to reduce your grocery bill, start using more potato recipes. Cooking potatoes makes their carbohydrates more readily available, and there are almost countless ways to use this versatile tuber.

During the Tour de France, Lance and his U.S. Postal Service teammates grab cotton bags full of food on the fly in designated "feed zones" along the racecourse. Cold baked potatoes are found among the sandwiches, PowerBars, PowerGels, cakes, and fruit in the bags. The riders unwrap the potatoes and eat them like apples.

TIPS FOR COOKING POTATOES
- Leave the skin on, even when boiling potatoes for mashed potatoes. The vitamin, mineral, and fiber content of potatoes decreases when you peel them.
- Baking a medium-sized brown potato takes about 40 to 50 minutes in a 400-degree-Fahrenheit oven, or about 6 to 10 minutes in a microwave. In either case, prick the skin several times with a fork prior to cooking.
- A properly cooked potato will be tender but firm when you squeeze it, and you can easily stick a fork all the way into it. An overdone potato will feel dense and rubbery when you squeeze it.

- Baked potatoes keep well in the refrigerator. You can reheat them in the microwave in 1 to 3 minutes. Baked sweet potatoes are great cold, right out of the fridge.
- Red potatoes, new potatoes, russet potatoes, etc. are all equivalent choices in terms of nutritional value.

Portion Sizes
- Standard serving size: ½ medium-sized potato
- Realistic serving size for an athlete: 1 medium-sized potato
  - Foundation: 1 medium-sized potato topped with 1 cup steamed veggies
  - Preparation: 1 medium-sized potato topped with low-fat chili and cheese
  - Specialization: 1 large potato topped with veggies, low-fat yogurt
  - Transition: 1 med potato topped with ½ cup steamed veggies

Preparing Poultry

Many athletes prefer chicken and turkey to red meat because they are lower in saturated fat. It is important to fully cook poultry to kill any salmonella bacteria that may be present.

Tips for Cooking Poultry
- While you can cook it with the skin on, discard the skin rather than eat it because it is almost entirely fat.
- You know your chicken is done when you cut into it and its juices run clear.
- If you're cooking an entire bird, place it breast-*down* in a pan instead of legs-down. This makes the chicken breasts moister as the juices flow downward from the rest of the bird. It will slightly increase the fat content of the breast meat, but the difference is not very big and it tastes great.
- You can roast a whole chicken or turkey a few different ways:
  - Breast-down in a brown paper bag—moist and golden

- Breast-down uncovered in a nonstick pan—more golden-brown in color
- Breast-down in ½ inch of water in a covered pan—moist and tender
- When marinating, don't bother piercing the chicken breasts. According to Chef Greg, it doesn't significantly increase the absorption of the marinade.

Portion Sizes
- Standard serving size: 4 ounces (meat only, no skin), about 140 calories. Size of a normal chicken breast: 4–6 ounces, about 140–200 calories.

Preparing Beef and Pork

The earliest writings about sports nutrition included recommendations for eating meat, specifically that eating the muscles of strong and fast animals made athletes strong and fast. While the logic wasn't perfect, it was and still is true that beef and pork are wonderful sources of protein, iron, and zinc—nutrients athletes need for optimal performance. By selecting lean cuts, beef and pork can be an integral part of your nutritional program.

Tips for Cooking Meat
- To select lean cuts, look for the words "loin" or "round" in the name, such as tenderloin, sirloin, eye of round, or top round.
- If you choose to marinate meat, first prick it in several places with a fork.
- Grilling meat gets rid of some of the fat because the fat melts and drips into the coals.
- Roasting and broiling meat in the oven often means the meat is sitting in a pan of its own melted fat. If you serve the meat by itself, the process of broiling or roasting will reduce the fat content. If, however, you use the fat in the pan to make gravy, you may actually consume more saturated fat than was originally in the portion of meat on your plate.

- Boiling meat is just a bad idea. It doesn't taste good afterward, and its nutritional value is significantly diminished. Adding meat to soups and stews is an exception. By consuming the liquid the meat was boiled in, you're receiving many of the nutrients it originally contained.
- If you pan-fry meat, you can drain the fat from the pan after the meat has cooked. Please note: Do not pour hot grease from beef, bacon, pork, etc. directly down the drain, and if you do, run hot water down the drain at the same time. Otherwise, the hot, liquid saturated fat will congeal and solidify to sides of your plumbing as it cools, which contributes to clogged drains. I mention this after spending one too many hours unclogging my own kitchen sink.

Preparing Fish

Purchasing fish can be intimidating to those of us living in landlocked areas of the country, like Colorado. However, many modern fishing boats are equipped to flash-freeze fish very soon after they are caught, and they are delivered to grocery stores around the world frozen solid. This advancement in packaging and delivery makes fresh fish safe and available to people far away from the nearest ocean. When purchasing fish, make sure it is firm and nearly odorless. If it has a strong, fishy smell, don't buy it. Fish fillets should be firm to the touch, not slimy or mushy, and should be somewhat translucent. The color of fish gives an indication of its fat content; white or light-colored fish are lower in fat, while fish with more fat, such as salmon and tuna fillets and steaks, are more colorful.

Artichoke and Sun-Dried Tomato Pasta

A versatile pasta dish with a wine-based sauce. Shrimp and chicken are excellent additions to this recipe.

READY IN: APPROX. 25 MINUTES
MAKES 4 SERVINGS

1 (8-ounce) package fresh fettuccine pasta
4 tablespoons butter
½ medium onion, chopped
1 (8-ounce) package sliced mushrooms
3 cloves garlic, crushed
⅔ (8-ounce) jar sun-dried tomatoes, packed in oil
1 (2-ounce) can sliced black olives, drained
10 ounces marinated artichoke hearts
1 cup dry white wine
2 tablespoons lemon juice
1 ripe tomato, chopped
1 cup Parmesan cheese
salt and pepper to taste

1. Bring a large pot of lightly salted water to a boil. Add psta and cook for 8 to 10 minutes or until al dente; drain.

2. Melt butter over medium heat in a large saucepan. Saute onions, mushrooms, and garlic until tender. Stir in sun-dried tomatoes, olives, artichoke hearts, wine, and lemon juice. Bring to a boil; cook until liquid is reduced by a third, about 5 minutes.

3. Toss pasta with sauce. Top with tomatoes and dust with Parmesan cheese. Add salt and pepper to taste, and serve.

CPF RATIO: 48-15-37

Calories (kcal)	Carbohydrate (g)	Protein (g)	Fat (g)
555	67	20	23

Fettuccine with Sweet Pepper-Cayenne Sauce

This recipe has a lot of flavor and packs quite a kick. Be careful with the cayenne pepper, though. One of our coaches misread the recipe and added ¾ of a tablespoon of cayenne instead of ¾ of a teaspoon. He didn't realize anything was wrong until everyone at the table was sweating. Grilled chicken is a great addition to this meal.

READY IN: APPROX. 15 MINUTES
MAKES 4 SERVINGS

12 ounces dry fettuccine pasta
2 red bell peppers, julienned
3 cloves garlic, minced
¾ teaspoon cayenne pepper
1 cup reduced-fat vanilla yogurt
¾ cup chicken broth
¾ cup grated Parmesan cheese
salt and pepper to taste

1 | Bring a large pot of lightly salted water to a boil. Add pasta and cook for 8 to 10 minutes or until *al dente;* drain.

2 | Meanwhile, spray cooking oil in a large skillet and sauté red bell peppers, garlic, and cayenne pepper over medium heat for 3 to 5 minutes.

3 | Stir in sour cream and broth; simmer uncovered for 5 minutes. Remove from heat and stir in cheese.

4 | Toss hot pasta with sauce and season with salt and pepper to taste; serve.

CPF RATIO: 50-23-27

Calories (kcal)	Carbohydrate (g)	Protein (g)	Fat (g)
532	66	31	16

Olive Blast Pasta

The distinct flavors of black olives and sun-dried tomatoes intermin-gled with chicken make this a wonderful recipe for all pasta lovers! Try it topped with Parmesan cheese.

READY IN: APPROX. 20 MINUTES
MAKES 2 SERVINGS

4 ounces fettuccini pasta

2 skinless, boneless chicken-breast halves—cut into bite-sized pieces

2 green onions, chopped

½ teaspoon dried basil

½ cup sliced black olives

2 tablespoons olive oil

½ teaspoon minced garlic

2 tablespoons grated Parmesan cheese

10 sun-dried tomatoes, softened

1 tablespoon minced fresh parsley

1 | Bring a large pot of lightly salted water to a boil. Add pasta and cook for 8 to 10 minutes or until *al dente;* drain.

2 | In a large skillet over medium-high heat, heat olive oil and cook chicken until brown and juices run clear, 5 to 10 minutes. Stir in green onions, basil, olives, olive oil, garlic, Parmesan, sun-dried tomatoes, and parsley; cook 5 minutes or until garlic is golden and whites of onions are translucent. Toss chicken mixture with pasta; serve.

CPF RATIO: 39-25-36

Calories (kcal)	Carbohydrate (g)	Protein (g)	Fat (g)
521	50	33	21

Broccoli Pesto Angel Hair

This recipe can be made with either fresh or frozen broccoli and served with tomato slices and warm garlic bread. Chef Greg uses bouillon cubes instead of canned chicken stock to lower the saturated-fat content.

READY IN: APPROX. 20 MINUTES
MAKES 4 SERVINGS

1 (9-ounce) package angel hair pasta
1 cup hot water
2 chicken bouillon cubes
1 (16-ounce) package frozen chopped broccoli,
    prepared according to package directions
¼ cup grated Romano or Parmesan cheese
¼ cup fresh basil leaves
2 tablespoons olive oil
1 large clove garlic, peeled
coarsely ground black pepper to taste

1   Bring a large pot of lightly salted water to a boil. Add pasta and cook for 8 to 10 minutes or until *al dente;* drain.

2   Combine water and bouillon in small bowl; stir to dissolve.

3   Place broccoli, broth, cheese, basil, oil, and garlic in food processor or blender; cover. Process until smooth.

4   Toss broccoli pesto with pasta. Season with coarsely ground black pepper.

CPF RATIO: 53-22-25

Calories (kcal)	Carbohydrate (g)	Protein (g)	Fat (g)
367	49	20	10

Rigatoni and Broccoli Florets

A light and quick meal! As written it will work for most vegetarians, and some non-vegetarians like to substitute chicken broth for the vegetable broth. To complete the meal, serve with a side salad and garlic bread.

READY IN: APPROX. 15 MINUTES
MAKES 4 TO 6 SERVINGS

1 pound rigatoni pasta

8 tablespoons olive oil

2 tablespoons butter

4 cloves garlic, minced

1 pound fresh broccoli florets

1 cup vegetable broth

1 cup chopped fresh basil

2 tablespoons grated Parmesan cheese

1 | Bring a large pot of lightly salted water to a boil. Add pasta and cook for 8 to 10 minutes or until *al dente;* drain.

2 | In large skillet, heat oil and butter. Gently brown garlic, add broccoli, and sauté gently for 2 to 3 minutes. Add broth; cover and simmer until broccoli is tender.

3 | Toss the broccoli mixture with the basil and cooked pasta. Serve with grated Parmesan cheese on top.

CPF RATIO: 48-18-34

Calories (kcal)	Carbohydrate (g)	Protein (g)	Fat (g)
682	82	30	26

Penne Pasta with Tomatoes and White Beans

This is a nice medley of tomatoes, beans, feta cheese, and spinach, which stand out individually and meld together. Even though it doesn't take long to prepare, this dish has a great, complex flavor that will make your guests or family think you were in the kitchen for hours.

READY IN: APPROX. 25 MINUTES
MAKES 4 SERVINGS

8 ounces penne pasta

2 (14.5-ounce) cans Italian-style diced tomatoes with basil

1 (19-ounce) can cannellini beans, drained and rinsed

10 ounces fresh spinach, washed and chopped

½ cup crumbled feta cheese

1 | Bring a large pot of lightly salted water to a boil. Add pasta and cook for 8 to 10 minutes or until *al dente;* drain.

2 | Meanwhile, combine tomatoes and beans in a large non-stick skillet. Bring to a boil over medium-high heat. Reduce heat and simmer 10 minutes.

3 | Remove skillet from heat and add spinach to the sauce, letting the spinach wilt; stirring constantly.

4 | Serve sauce over pasta and sprinkle with feta.

CPF RATIO: 63-23-14

Calories (kcal)	Carbohydrate (g)	Protein (g)	Fat (g)
451	71	26	7

Pasta with Yogurt Sauce

This is a revised version of a traditional Middle Eastern dish. While you can make it using any pasta—fusilli, elbow macaroni, penne, shells—it is traditionally made with couscous. It is just as tasty eaten cold or warm, and it's a quick fix for a hurry-up meal. For added texture and nutrition, throw in some toasted pine nuts. Sahtain!—To your health!

READY IN: 15 MINUTES
MAKES 6 SERVINGS

1 (16-ounce) package pasta
1 teaspoon salt
4 cloves garlic, minced
2 cups plain yogurt
1 tablespoon butter or olive oil
2 tablespoons chopped fresh parsley

1 | Bring a large pot of lightly salted water to a boil. Add pasta and cook for 8 to 10 minutes or until *al dente;* drain.

2 | Using a mortar and pestle, mash the salt and garlic cloves together into a paste. Warm the yogurt slightly in a saucepan. Be careful not to overheat, as the yogurt will separate. Remove a small amount of warmed yogurt from the pan and stir it together with the garlic paste. Stir this mixture into the remaining yogurt.

3 | Drain the pasta and rinse in cold water. Place in a casserole or deep serving dish, toss with butter or olive oil. Toss with half of the garlic-yogurt sauce. Spread the remaining sauce over the pasta. Garnish with the parsley.

CPF RATIO: 59-22-19

Calories (kcal)	Carbohydrate (g)	Protein (g)	Fat (g)
372	55	20	8

Bow-Tie Pasta with Eggplant, Mushrooms, and Goat Cheese

A delicious and hearty bowl of bow-tie pasta, eggplant, mushrooms, and goat cheese. If goat cheese isn't your thing, this recipe also tastes great with Parmesan cheese.

READY IN: APPROX. 55 MINUTES
MAKES 6 SERVINGS

1 (16-ounce) package rigatoni pasta

3 tablespoons olive oil

1 large onion, chopped

2 cloves garlic, sliced

1 (8-ounce) package fresh mushrooms,
    coarsely chopped

1 eggplant, cut into ½-inch cubes

1 (28-ounce) can crushed tomatoes in puree

½ cup chicken broth

15 Kalamata olives, pitted and chopped

1 teaspoon dried thyme

1½ teaspoons salt

¼ teaspoon crushed red-pepper flakes

8 ounces goat cheese,
    cut into large chunks

1 | Bring a large pot of lightly salted water to a boil. Add pasta and cook for 8 to 10 minutes or until *al dente;* drain.

2 | Heat olive oil in a large saucepan over medium low heat. Sauté onion and garlic until soft and translucent, about 5 minutes.

3 | Increase heat to medium high. Stir in mushrooms and cook until lightly browned, about 5 minutes. Stir in the eggplant and cook 5 minutes.

4 | Stir in the tomatoes, chicken broth, and olives. Season with thyme, salt, and red-pepper flakes.

5 | Bring to a boil. Reduce heat, cover, and simmer 30 minutes or until eggplant is tender. Toss with pasta and goat cheese.

CPF RATIO: 43-19-38

Calories (kcal)	Carbohydrate (g)	Protein (g)	Fat (g)
426	46	20	18

Couscous with Roasted Vegetables

Just to prove that yams are for more than Thanksgiving, here's a great Middle Eastern recipe that combines roasted yams, crunchy cashews, and rich olives for a balanced and tasty meal.

READY IN: APPROX. 45 MINUTES
MAKES 6 SERVINGS

1 (8-ounce) yam, peeled and diced (½-inch)

1 (8-ounce) red onion, peeled and diced (½-inch)

8 ounces zucchini, halved and sliced (½-inch thick)

2 tablespoons olive oil

½ teaspoon kosher salt

¼ teaspoon coarsely ground black pepper

2½ cups low-sodium chicken broth

12 ounces couscous

½ cup scallions, chopped

1 cup Kalamata olives, pitted and halved

¾ cup cooked garbanzo beans

⅓ cup toasted cashews, coarsely chopped

¼ cup parsley, chopped

¼ cup orange juice

¼ teaspoon ground cinnamon

Cayenne pepper to taste

1 | Preheat oven to 450 degrees F (230 degrees C).

2 | In a large mixing bowl, toss yams, onions, and zucchini with olive oil, salt, and pepper. Spread onto a baking sheet and roast for 30 minutes until lightly browned and tender.

3 | While vegetables are cooking, heat broth to a boil in a medium-sized saucepan. Stir in couscous and scallions, cover, and cook for 1 more minute. Remove from heat and set aside for 5 minutes, then uncover and fluff with a fork.

4 | Mix in Kalamata olives, garbanzo beans, cashews, parsley, orange juice, and cinnamon. Season with a dash of cayenne pepper to taste.

5 | Top couscous with roasted vegetables and toss together just before serving.

CPF RATIO: 62-12-26

Calories (kcal)	Carbohydrate (g)	Protein (g)	Fat (g)
441	68	13	13

Spinach and Salmon Fettuccine

You can spend a little or a lot to make this dish, but any way you do it, it tastes great. Smoked salmon is a wonderful substitution, albeit a little costly. And if you don't have the time or desire to bake your own salmon filet, this dish tastes good with canned salmon as well.

READY IN: APPROX. 40 MINUTES
MAKES 4 SERVINGS

8 ounces dry fettuccine pasta
¼ cup butter
1 cup milk
1 tablespoon all-purpose flour
1 cup freshly grated Parmesan cheese
½ pound baked salmon, cooked and chopped
1 cup chopped fresh spinach
2 tablespoons capers
¼ cup chopped sun-dried tomatoes
½ cup chopped fresh oregano

1 | Bring a large pot of lightly salted water to a boil. Add fettuccine, and cook for 11 to 13 minutes or until *al dente;* drain.

2 In a medium saucepan over medium heat, melt the butter and blend with milk. Mix in the flour to thicken. Gradually stir in the Parmesan cheese until melted.

3 Crumble salmon into the butter mixture. Stir in the spinach, capers, sun-dried tomatoes, and oregano. Cook and stir about 3 minutes, until heated through. Serve over the cooked pasta.

CPF RATIO: 35-28-37

Calories (kcal)	Carbohydrate (g)	Protein (g)	Fat (g)
713	63	50	29

Leafy Spinach Lasagna

You can make this recipe with fresh or frozen spinach. You can make plenty of fresh vegetable additions to the recipe as well, including zucchini, squash, mushrooms, and broccoli.

READY IN: APPROX. 1 HOUR 40 MINUTES
MAKES 8 SERVINGS

1 tablespoon extra-virgin olive oil

20 ounces chopped spinach

½ onion, chopped

½ teaspoon dried oregano

½ teaspoon dried basil

2 cloves garlic, crushed

1 (32-ounce) jar spaghetti sauce

1½ cups water

2 cups non-fat cottage cheese

1 (8-ounce) package part-skim mozzarella cheese, shredded

¼ cup grated Parmesan cheese

½ cup chopped fresh parsley

1 teaspoon salt

⅛ teaspoon black pepper

1 egg

8 ounces lasagna noodles

1 | Preheat oven to 350 degrees F (175 degrees C).

2 | In a large pot over medium heat, sauté spinach, onion, oregano, basil, and garlic in the olive oil. Pour in spaghetti sauce and water; simmer 20 minutes.

3 | In a large bowl, mix cottage cheese, mozzarella cheese, Parmesan cheese, parsley, salt, pepper, and egg.

4 | Place a small amount of sauce in the bottom of a lasagna pan. Place four uncooked noodles on top of sauce and top with layer of sauce. Add four more noodles and layer with half-sauce-and-half-cheese mixture, then noodles, and repeat until all is layered, finishing with sauce.

5 | Cover with foil and bake in a preheated oven for 55 minutes. Remove foil and bake another 15 minutes. Let sit 10 minutes before serving.

CPF RATIO: 39-27-34

Calories (kcal)	Carbohydrate (g)	Protein (g)	Fat (g)
316	31	21	12

Spinach and Black Bean Pasta

This is a recipe that combines two of athletes' favorite vegetables: spinach and black beans. It's a great dish for getting your carbohydrates and your protein, as well as a big dose of vitamins. This can also be served over brown rice, especially since brown rice takes 45 to 50 minutes to prepare. The rice will be ready just as the rest of the recipe is ready.

READY IN: APPROX. 45 MINUTES
MAKES 8 SERVINGS

1 (16-ounce) package rotini pasta
1½ cups vegetable broth
2½ cups chopped fresh spinach
½ cup chopped red onion
1 clove garlic, chopped
½ teaspoon cayenne pepper
salt and pepper to taste
1 (15-ounce) can black beans, drained and rinsed
1 cup frozen chopped broccoli
1 cup diced tomatoes
2 ounces freshly grated Parmesan cheese

1   Bring a large pot of lightly salted water to a boil. Add rotini, and cook for 8 to 10 minutes, or until *al dente;* drain.

2   In a large saucepan over medium heat, bring the vegetable broth to a boil. Reduce heat and mix in spinach, onion, garlic, cayenne pepper, salt, and pepper. Stir in the black beans and broccoli. Continue to cook and stir 5 to 10 minutes.

3   Stir in the tomatoes, and continue cooking 10 minutes, or until all vegetables are tender. Serve over the cooked pasta. Garnish with Parmesan cheese.

CPF RATIO: 71-21-8

Calories (kcal)	Carbohydrate (g)	Protein (g)	Fat (g)
452	80	24	4

Pasta in a Hurry

This recipe is so easy to prepare, you can make it in the morning and take it with you for lunch. If you have a little extra time, go for fresh herbs instead of dried ones. When you cut up your basil and oregano, Chef Greg advises that you cut them into long, matchstick-sized strips rather than finely chopping them. This puts more of their flavor into the dish rather than the cutting board.

READY IN: 15 MINUTES
MAKES 8 SERVINGS

16 ounces rotini pasta

4 tablespoons olive oil

4 skinless, boneless chicken-breast halves, cut into bite-sized pieces

3 cloves garlic, minced

1¼ teaspoons salt

1¼ teaspoons garlic powder

1¼ teaspoons dried basil

1¼ teaspoons dried oregano

1 cup chopped sun-dried tomatoes

¼ cup grated Parmesan cheese

1 Cook and drain pasta as directed.

2 While pasta is cooking, in a 5-quart pot, heat olive oil and sauté chicken, garlic, salt, garlic powder, basil, and oregano until chicken is cooked. Add sun-dried tomatoes and cook for 2 more minutes.

3 Remove from heat and toss with pasta. Serve with grated Parmesan cheese if desired.

CPF RATIO: 48-26-26

Calories (kcal)	Carbohydrate (g)	Protein (g)	Fat (g)
350	42	23	10

Yogurt Shrimp Fettuccini

Here's an exotic shrimp pasta recipe with a creamy yogurt sauce that you can use to impress your spouse or significant other while still getting the nutrients you need for recovery and great performance. What's more, you don't have to be a trained chef to make it; it's really very easy.

READY IN: 25 MINUTES
MAKES 7 SERVINGS

16 ounces dry fettuccini pasta

2 tablespoons butter or margarine

1½ pounds medium shrimp—peeled and deveined

salt and pepper to taste

2 teaspoons paprika

1 red bell pepper, chopped

1 green bell pepper, sliced

1 tablespoon minced shallots

1 teaspoon chopped garlic

½ cup sour cream

1 cup plain yogurt

4 tablespoons chopped fresh cilantro

1 | Bring a large pot of lightly salted water to a boil. Add pasta and cook for 8 to 10 minutes or until *al dente.* Drain and set aside.

2 | Heat butter or margarine in a large skillet. Add the shrimp, salt, and pepper to taste, and paprika. Stir with a wooden spatula. When the shrimp become pink (it should take 2 to 3 minutes), remove them with a slotted spoon, leaving the cooking liquid in the skillet.

3 | Add red and green bell peppers, shallots, garlic, and salt and pepper to taste. Cook, stirring, about 3 to 4 minutes over medium-high heat. Add shrimp. Cook over medium heat for 2 more minutes.

4 | Add sour cream and yogurt and blend all together. Add cilantro and bring to a simmer for about 30 seconds. Do not boil or sauce will separate. Serve over cooked fettuccini.

CPF RATIO: 46-34-20

Calories (kcal)	Carbohydrate (g)	Protein (g)	Fat (g)
438	50	37	10

Speedy Gnocchi

Gnocchi means "potato pasta" in Italian. This is a much easier version of an Italian favorite, using instant mashed potatoes. You can make a few batches at once and freeze what you don't immediately use. To freeze, put on wax paper until frozen (or they will stick together), and then put into plastic bags. Serve with your favorite pasta sauce.

READY IN: APPROX. 15 MINUTES
MAKES 2 SERVINGS

1 cup dry potato flakes

1 egg, beaten

1 cup boiling water

1 teaspoon salt

⅛ teaspoon ground black pepper

3 tablespoons of basil

1½ cups all-purpose flour

salt and pepper to taste

1 | Place potato flakes, egg, and water in a medium-sized bowl and mix together. Stir in salt, pepper, and basil. Blend in flour to make a fairly stiff dough. Turn dough out on a well-floured board. Knead lightly.

2 | Shape dough into a long, thin roll the thickness of a breadstick. With a knife dipped in flour, cut into bite-sized pieces.

3 | Place a few gnocchi at a time into pot of boiling water. As the gnocchi rise to the top of the pot, remove them with a slotted spoon. Repeat until all are cooked.

4 | Top with your favorite pasta sauce, add salt and pepper to taste.

CPF RATIO: 85-13-2

Calories (kcal)	Carbohydrate (g)	Protein (g)	Fat (g)
437	93	14	1

CHICKEN

Garlic Chicken Delight

Simple to make, just dip and bake! If you like garlic, this is the recipe for you. Much of the oil in this recipe stays in the bowl you use to dip the chicken in, so the actual fat content of the prepared chicken is lower than what's in the recipe.

READY IN: APPROX. 55 MINUTES
MAKES 4 SERVINGS

2 teaspoons crushed garlic
¼ cup olive oil
¼ cup dry bread crumbs
¼ cup grated Parmesan cheese
4 skinless, boneless chicken-breast halves

1 | Preheat oven to 425 degrees F (220 degrees C).

2 | Mix the garlic and olive oil in a shallow dish, and warm to blend the flavors. In a separate dish, combine the bread crumbs and Parmesan cheese. Dip the chicken breasts in the olive-oil-and-garlic mixture, then into the bread-crumb mixture. Place in a shallow baking dish.

3 | Bake for 30 to 35 minutes, until no longer pink and juices run clear.

CPF RATIO: 14-42-44

Calories (kcal)	Carbohydrate (g)	Protein (g)	Fat (g)
202	7	21	10

Apple and Orange Chicken

This is another recipe that looked like a mistake the first time I read it. I have to admit, I'd never added apple and orange juice to a cream sauce. With Chef Greg's urging, I made this recipe at home and loved it. It's great—full of flavor, high in protein, and wonderful over rice.

READY IN: APPROX. 1 HOUR 30 MINUTES
MAKES 4 SERVINGS

4 bone-in chicken-breast halves, skinless

1 (1-ounce) package dry onion soup mix

1 (.6-ounce) package cream-of-chicken soup mix

2 tablespoons soy sauce

2 cloves crushed garlic

1 cup apple juice

1 cup orange juice

salt and pepper to taste

1 Preheat oven to 350 degrees F (175 degrees C).

2 Place the chicken pieces in a lightly greased 9×13-inch baking dish.

3 In a medium bowl, combine the onion soup mix, cream-of-chicken soup mix, soy sauce, garlic, apple and orange juice, salt, and pepper. Mix together and pour mixture over chicken.

4 Cover and bake for 1 hour, then remove cover/lid and bake for another ½ hour to brown the chicken.

CPF RATIO: 46-40-14

Calories (kcal)	Carbohydrate (g)	Protein (g)	Fat (g)
191	22	19	3

Mediterranean Lemon Chicken

This goes nicely with roasted potatoes!

READY IN: 1 HOUR
MAKES 6 SERVINGS

1 lemon

2 teaspoons dried oregano

3 cloves garlic, minced

1 tablespoon olive oil

¼ teaspoon salt

¼ teaspoon ground black pepper

6 skinless, boneless chicken-breast halves

1 | Preheat oven to 425 degrees F (220 degrees C).

2 | Grate the peel from half the lemon, squeeze out the juice (about ¼ cup) and add to peel with the oregano, garlic, oil, salt, and pepper in a 9×13-inch baking dish. Stir until mixed.

3 | Coat chicken pieces with the lemon mixture and arrange, bone-side up, in the baking dish. Cover dish and bake for 20 minutes. Turn and baste chicken.

4 | Reduce heat to 400 degrees F (205 degrees C) and bake uncovered, basting every 10 minutes, for about 30 more minutes. Serve chicken with pan juices.

CPF RATIO: 16-48-36

Calories (kcal)	Carbohydrate (g)	Protein (g)	Fat (g)
75	3	9	3

Baked Honey-Mustard Chicken

This is a good post-workout meal because the honey provides simple sugar and the chicken provides a lot of protein. Together, you consume everything you need to replenish your energy stores and build and maintain your muscles. It doesn't hurt that the recipe tastes great as well.

READY IN: APPROX. 1 HOUR
MAKES 6 SERVINGS

6 skinless, boneless chicken-breast halves

salt and pepper to taste

½ cup honey

½ cup prepared mustard

1 teaspoon dried basil

1 teaspoon paprika

½ teaspoon dried parsley

1   Preheat oven to 350 degrees F (175 degrees C).

2   Sprinkle chicken breasts with salt and pepper to taste, and place in a lightly greased 9×13 inch baking dish. In a small bowl, combine the honey, mustard, basil, paprika, and parsley. Mix well. Pour half of this mixture over the chicken, and brush to cover.

3   Bake for 30 minutes. Turn chicken pieces over and brush with the remaining half of the honey-mustard mixture.

4   Bake for an additional 10 to 15 minutes, or until chicken is no longer pink and juices run clear. Let cool 10 minutes before serving.

CPF RATIO: 54-36-10

Calories (kcal)	Carbohydrate (g)	Protein (g)	Fat (g)
186	25	17	2

Cashew Crusted Chicken

Chicken breasts dipped in an apricot/mustard sauce, then rolled in chopped cashew nuts for a wonderfully tangy, crunchy, and easy baked-chicken dish. Try this with either raw or dry-roasted cashews, especially if you normally eat a bit more salt.

READY IN: APPROX. 40 MINUTES
MAKES 4 SERVINGS

1 (12-ounce) jar apricot preserves
¼ cup prepared Dijon-style mustard
1 teaspoon curry powder
1 cup coarsely chopped cashews
4 skinless, boneless chicken-breast halves

1 | Preheat oven to 375 degrees F (190 degrees C).

2 | Combine the preserves, mustard, and curry powder in a large skillet and heat over low heat, stirring constantly, until preserves are completely melted and smooth.

3 | Place cashews in a shallow dish or bowl. Dip chicken breasts in skillet sauce, then roll in nuts to coat and place in a lightly greased 9×13 inch baking dish.

4 | Bake at 375 degrees F (190 degrees C) for 20 to 30 minutes. Boil any remaining sauce and serve on the side with the baked chicken.

CPF RATIO: 18-52-30

Calories (kcal)	Carbohydrate (g)	Protein (g)	Fat (g)
513	23	67	17

Italian Crumb-Topping Cod

This is a variation on the traditional crab cake. Personally, I like dishes like this a little spicier, so when I make them at home I add chili powder or cayenne pepper. As is, this recipe is a good, low-fat, and quick cod recipe, and you can also substitute salmon or any other cold-water fish instead of cod. This works well served over Couscous with Roasted Vegetables (page 288).

READY IN: APPROX. 25 MINUTES
MAKES 4 SERVINGS

¼ cup fine dry Panco bread crumbs

2 tablespoons grated Parmesan cheese

1 tablespoon cornmeal

1 teaspoon olive oil

½ teaspoon Italian seasoning

⅛ teaspoon garlic powder

⅛ teaspoon ground black pepper

4 (3-ounce) cod fillets

1 egg white, lightly beaten

1 | Preheat oven to 450 degrees F (230 degrees C).

2 | In a small, shallow bowl, stir together the bread crumbs, cheese, cornmeal, oil, Italian seasoning, garlic powder, and pepper; set aside.

3 | Coat the rack of a broiling pan with cooking spray. Place the cod on the rack, folding under any thin edges of the fillets. Brush with the egg white, then spoon the crumb mixture evenly on top.

4 | Bake for 10 to 12 minutes or until the fish flakes easily when tested with a fork and is opaque all the way through.

CPF RATIO: 16-70-14

Calories (kcal)	Carbohydrate (g)	Protein (g)	Fat (g)
256	10	45	4

Tuna Burgers

These tuna burgers are an economical way to utilize almost your entire spice rack. Chef Greg discovered this recipe one night when he was all set to make hamburgers but had forgotten to buy ground beef. With people on their way over to his house, he improvised and came up with this simple yet tasty alternative.

READY IN: 25 MINUTES
MAKES 4 SERVINGS

1 (6-ounce) can tuna, packed in water,
    drained
1 egg
½ cup Italian seasoned bread crumbs
⅓ cup minced onion
¼ cup minced celery
¼ cup minced red bell pepper
¼ cup mayonnaise
2 tablespoons chili sauce
½ teaspoon dried dill weed
¼ teaspoon salt
⅛ teaspoon ground black pepper
1 dash hot pepper sauce
1 dash Worcestershire sauce
4 hamburger buns
1 tomato, sliced
4 leaves of lettuce (optional)

1 | Combine tuna, egg, bread crumbs, onion, celery, red bell pepper, mayonnaise, chili sauce, dill weed, salt, pepper, hot pepper sauce, and Worcestershire sauce. Mix well.

2 | Shape into 4 patties (mixture will be very soft and delicate). Refrigerate for 30 minutes to make the patties easier to handle, if desired.

3 | Coat a non-stick skillet with cooking spray; fry tuna patties for about 3 to 4 minutes per side, or until cooked through. These are fragile, so be careful when turning them.

4 | Serve on buns with tomato slices and lettuce leaves, if desired.

CPF RATIO: 43-20-37 (WITH BUN)

Calories (kcal)	Carbohydrate (g)	Protein (g)	Fat (g)
363	39	18	15

Blackened Tuna

This is a very simple way to prepare tuna, and it also works well with salmon and other fish. The fat content may seem high, but most of it is in the oil and butter you're using to cook the fish in. A lot of it stays in the pan when you're done, so you're actually consuming less fat than is in the recipe itself.

READY IN: APPROX. 20 MINUTES
MAKES 6 SERVINGS

1½ pounds fresh tuna steaks, 1 inch thick
3 tablespoons Cajun seasoning
2 tablespoons olive oil
2 tablespoons butter

1 | Generously coat tuna with Cajun seasoning.

2 | Heat oil and butter in a large skillet over high heat. When oil is very hot (flows more like water than thick oil), place steaks in pan. Cook on one side for 3 to 4 minutes or until blackened. Turn steaks, and cook for 3 to 4 minutes or to desired doneness.

CPF RATIO: 0-57-43

Calories (kcal)	Carbohydrate (g)	Protein (g)	Fat (g)
189	0	27	9

Stuffed Flank Steak

This is a delicious flank steak. The stuffing makes it much more fill-ing, but there's never any left over! Although the sauce from the pan contains fat, ladling some over the meat tastes really good.

READY IN: APPROX. 1 HOUR 10 MINUTES
MAKES 4 SERVINGS

2 cups dry stuffing mix

1 cup boiling water

2 tablespoons butter or margarine

1½ pounds flank steak, pounded thin for easy rolling

2 green onions, chopped

1 red bell pepper, chopped

1 (10.5-ounce) can mushroom gravy

¼ cup red wine or apple juice

1 clove garlic, minced

2 tablespoons grated Parmesan cheese

1 | Preheat oven to 350 degrees F (175 degrees C).

2 | In a medium bowl, combine the stuffing mix, water, and butter or margarine. Mix well and let stand for 5 minutes. Spoon the stuffing onto the steak, leaving a 1-inch border. Add the green onions and the red bell pepper.

3 | Roll from the long edge of the steak and secure with wooden tooth-picks. Place steak seam-side down in a 9×13 inch baking dish.

4 | In a separate small bowl, combine the gravy, wine or apple juice, garlic, and cheese. Mix well and pour over the steak.

5 | Bake for 1 hour, remove from oven, and let stand before slicing.

CPF RATIO: 55-28-17

Calories (kcal)	Carbohydrate (g)	Protein (g)	Fat (g)
697	95	50	13

Tomato Orzo Soup

Delicious hearty soup perfect for cold winter days. I sometimes combine all the ingredients in a crock pot on medium heat before long outdoor workouts. When I return hours later, all I have to do is heat it up a little more and I have a nice treat waiting for me. Orzo pasta and vegetables make this soup absolutely wonderful. I love combining this soup with a turkey or roast-beef sandwich to add some protein after training.

READY IN: APPROX. 40 MINUTES
MAKES 8 SERVINGS

7½ cups water
2 (10.5-ounce) cans vegetable broth
2 (10.75-ounce) cans condensed tomato soup
5 teaspoons chicken bouillon powder
1½ cups diced carrots
1½ cups diced celery
1 cup green peas
1½ cups uncooked orzo pasta
½ cup fresh parsley
salt and pepper to taste

1 | Place water, vegetable broth, tomato soup, chicken bouillon, carrots, celery, peas, and orzo pasta in large stock pot and bring to a boil.

2 | Reduce heat and simmer for 30 minutes, or until vegetables are tender. Sprinkle with parsley just before serving. Add salt and pepper to taste.

CPF RATIO: 73-20-7

Calories (kcal)	Carbohydrate (g)	Protein (g)	Fat (g)
258	47	13	2

Cabbage Soup

Although Chef Greg really doesn't like cabbage, this has been one of the most popular soups he's made in restaurants. I have to admit, I agree with Greg's opinion of cabbage, but even I really liked this soup. You can make it a vegetarian soup very easily by substituting vegetable broth for beef broth.

READY IN: APPROX. 45 MINUTES
MAKES 15 SERVINGS

5 carrots, chopped

3 onions, chopped

2 (16-ounce) cans whole peeled tomatoes, with liquid

1 large head cabbage, chopped

1 (15-ounce) can cut green beans, drained

2 green bell peppers, diced

10 stalks celery, chopped

1 (1-ounce) envelope dry onion soup mix

2 quarts tomato juice

1 (14-ounce) can beef broth

1 | Place carrots, onions, tomatoes, cabbage, green beans, peppers, and celery in a large pot. Add onion-soup mix, tomato juice, beef broth, and enough water to cover vegetables. Simmer until vegetables are tender. May be stored in the refrigerator for several days.

CPF RATIO: 77-15-8

Calories (kcal)	Carbohydrate (g)	Protein (g)	Fat (g)
109	21	4	1

Tomato Florentine Recovery Soup

This was a new recipe to me, but it has made this past winter much more pleasant. I live in the mountains above Colorado Springs, and it's great to come home from hiking, mountain biking, or snowshoeing in the cold to a hot bowl of this soup. I'd recommend cooking large pots of it because it keeps well, freezes well, and tastes even better in the days after it's originally cooked.

READY IN: APPROX. 45 MINUTES
MAKES 6 SERVINGS

2 (14.5-ounce) cans chicken broth

1 (14.5-ounce) can chopped stewed tomatoes

1 (12-fluid-ounce) can tomato-vegetable juice cocktail

1 (10.75-ounce) can condensed tomato-bisque soup

1 tablespoon white sugar

1 pinch ground nutmeg

salt and pepper to taste

½ cup cooked macaroni

10 ounces of loose leaf spinach

1   Combine broth, tomatoes, juice, and soup in a saucepan with a wire whisk over medium heat. Add sugar and nutmeg, then add salt and pepper to taste. Allow to heat gently 20 minutes on medium-low heat. Keep hot without letting it boil.

2   Add cooked pasta and cook for 10 minutes more.

3   Take off heat and add loose-leaf spinach and serve.

CPF RATIO: 58-24-18

Calories (kcal)	Carbohydrate (g)	Protein (g)	Fat (g)
204	30	12	4

A Spicy Chicken Soup

This an updated, twenty-first-century version of an old standard. There are plenty of ways to adjust the spices in this to suit your tastes, but no matter what you add, the longer it simmers, the better it gets. Top with crushed tortilla chips and shredded cheese.

READY IN: APPROX. 1 HOUR 45 MINUTES
MAKES 8 SERVINGS

2 quarts water

8 skinless, boneless chicken-breast halves

½ teaspoon salt

1 teaspoon ground black pepper

1 teaspoon garlic powder

2 tablespoons dried parsley

1 tablespoon onion powder

5 cubes chicken bouillon

1 onion, chopped

3 cloves garlic, chopped

3 tablespoons olive oil

1 (16-ounce) jar chunky salsa

2 (14.5-ounce) cans peeled and diced tomatoes

1 (14.5-ounce) can whole peeled tomatoes

1 (10.75-ounce) can condensed tomato soup

3 tablespoons chili powder

1 (15-ounce) can whole-kernel corn, drained

2 (16-ounce) cans chili beans, undrained

1 (8-ounce) container sour cream

1 | In a large pot over medium heat, combine water, chicken, salt, pepper, garlic powder, parsley, onion powder, and bouillon cubes. Bring to a boil, then reduce heat and simmer 1 hour, or until chicken juices run clear.

2 | Remove chicken and shred it; reserve broth.

3 | In a large pot over medium heat, cook onion and garlic in olive oil until slightly browned.

4 | Stir in salsa, diced tomatoes, whole tomatoes, tomato soup, chili powder, corn, chili beans, sour cream, shredded chicken, and 5 cups broth. Simmer 30 minutes.

CPF RATIO: 44-27-29

Calories (kcal)	Carbohydrate (g)	Protein (g)	Fat (g)
442	49	30	14

Grandma's Chicken Soup

Chef Greg's grandmother used to make a soup similar to this when he didn't feel well. As he learned to cook, he doctored her original recipe. I know better than to offer an opinion as to which version tastes better.

READY IN: APPROX. 2 HOURS
MAKES 8 SERVINGS

1 (2- to 3-pound) whole chicken

3 stalks celery with leaves, chopped

1 pound baby carrots

2 onions, chopped

2 cubes beef bouillon, crumbled

1 packet chicken-noodle soup mix

2 (14.5-ounce) cans low-sodium chicken broth

1 pinch dried thyme

1 pinch poultry seasoning

1 pinch dried basil

5 black peppercorns

2 bay leaves

1 pinch dried parsley

1 (8-ounce) package farfalle (bow-tie) pasta

1 | Place chicken in a large pot and cover with water. Place celery leaves in pot and bring to a boil, then reduce heat and simmer until chicken is cooked through, 30 to 40 minutes. Remove chicken from pot and place in a bowl until cool enough to handle.

2 | Meanwhile, place celery, carrots, onion, bouillon, soup mix, and chicken broth in pot and let simmer. Season with thyme, poultry seasoning, basil, peppercorns, bay leaves, and parsley.

3 | Bone chicken and cut up meat into bite-sized pieces. Return meat to pot. Cook until vegetables are tender and flavors are well blended, up to 90 minutes.

4 | Stir in pasta and cook 10 to 15 minutes more, until noodles are *al dente*. Serve hot.

CPF RATIO: 57-34-9

Calories (kcal)	Carbohydrate (g)	Protein (g)	Fat (g)
190	27	16	2

Fresh Asparagus Soup

A yogurt-based asparagus soup, thickened with new red potatoes and accented with lemon and Parmesan cheese. This used to be a great soup after long spring rides, but now that asparagus is available year-round, so is this soup. You can also substitute soy products to make this recipe vegan.

READY IN: APPROX. 30 MINUTES
MAKES 4 SERVINGS

1 pound fresh asparagus
2½ cup of new red potatoes
¾ cup chopped onion
2¾ cups vegetable broth
½ cup vanilla yogurt
1 cup vanilla soy milk
1 teaspoon lemon juice
1 teaspoon salt
1 pinch ground black pepper

1 | Place asparagus, potato, and onion in a saucepan with 1½ cups of vegetable broth. Bring the broth to a boil, reduce heat and let simmer until the vegetables are tender.

2 After vegetables are cooked, place a few asparagus tips aside for garnish. Place remaining vegetable and broth mixture in an electric blender and puree until smooth.

3 Add 1¼ cups vegetable broth, yogurt, soy milk, lemon juice, and salt and pepper to mixture and blend into pureed vegetables. Pour mixture into pot over medium heat. Continue stirring until the soup comes to a boil, and then simmer and serve.

4 Garnish with reserved asparagus tips. Sprinkle with Parmesan cheese if desired.

CPF RATIO: 63-1-16

Calories (kcal)	Carbohydrate (g)	Protein (g)	Fat (g)
230	36	12	4

SMOOTHIES

Seriously Filling Strawberry Oatmeal Breakfast Smoothie

This smoothie is perfect in the morning or after a long workout, but it's so filling you might not want to drink it prior to exercise. As written, it is suitable for vegans, but you can make it with skim milk instead.

READY IN: APPROX. 5 MINUTES
MAKES 2 SERVINGS

1 cup soy milk
½ cup raw rolled oats
½ cup ice
1 banana, broken into chunks
14 frozen strawberries
½ teaspoon vanilla extract (optional)
1½ teaspoons white sugar (optional)

1 | In a blender, combine soy milk, oats, ice, banana, and strawberries. Add vanilla and sugar if desired. Blend until smooth and serve.

CPF RATIO: 71-13-16

Calories (kcal)	Carbohydrate (g)	Protein (g)	Fat (g)
224	40	7	4

Quick Start Breakfast Drink

This is a very quick and easy way to start your morning off right. It will keep in the fridge for a while as well, and one CTS member who fancies this smoothie doubles the recipe and pours the rest in a tall travel cup for her son, Robert, who wakes up an hour after she leaves in the morning. He used to skip breakfast before school, but now he grabs the smoothie and a bagel as he rushes to make it to the bus. Robert's first-period teacher recently called his mother to tell her that Robert was much more alert in his class; he hadn't fallen asleep in weeks.

READY IN: APPROX. 5 MINUTES
MAKES 4 SERVINGS

2 cups pineapple juice

2 bananas

2 cups vanilla yogurt

1 cup strawberries

¼ cup wheat germ

1 teaspoon vanilla extract

1 | In a blender, combine pineapple juice, bananas, yogurt, strawberries, wheat germ, and vanilla extract. Blend until smooth.

CPF RATIO: 77-13-10

Calories (kcal)	Carbohydrate (g)	Protein (g)	Fat (g)
271	52	9	3

Bananerberry Smoothie

It's great on a hot summer day and easy to prepare.

READY IN: APPROX. 10 MINUTES
MAKES 2 SERVINGS

1 cup fresh strawberries

1 banana, sliced

1 cup fresh peaches

1 cup apples

1½ cups vanilla yogurt

1½ cups ice cubes

½ cup milk

1 | In a blender combine strawberries, banana, peaches, apples, and yogurt. Blend until smooth. Add ice, pour in milk, and blend again until smooth. Serve immediately.

CPF RATIO: 75-15-10

Calories (kcal)	Carbohydrate (g)	Protein (g)	Fat (g)
352	66	13	4

BEANS AND VEGETABLES

Sweet Lentil Soup with Asparagus Tips

READY IN: 1 HOUR (WITH PRECOOKED LENTILS), 1 HOUR 30 MINUTES
(INCLUDING COOKING TIME FOR LENTILS)
MAKES 9 SERVINGS

1 medium head garlic

3 tablespoons olive oil

¼ teaspoon dried basil

1 red bell pepper

2½ cups dry lentils

2 (32-ounce) containers chicken broth

1½ large carrot, shredded

1 large onion, grated

1 cup asparagus tips

1 cup sweet peas

¼ cup white sugar

2 tablespoons orange marmalade

2 tablespoons curry powder

1 pinch saffron

1 teaspoon kosher salt

ground black pepper to taste

1 | Preheat oven to 450 degrees F (230 degrees C).

2 | Cut the top off of the head of garlic and place in a shallow dish in 1 inch of water. Drizzle with 2 tablespoons olive oil, sprinkle with basil, cover, and place on a baking sheet. Halve and seed the bell pepper, drizzle with remaining 1 tablespoon olive oil, and place on the baking sheet.

3 | Bake garlic and pepper until pepper is browned and garlic is soft, 20 to 40 minutes.

4 | While garlic and pepper are baking, combine lentils and chicken broth in a large pot over medium heat. Bring to a boil, then reduce heat and simmer 40 minutes, until lentils are just tender.

5 | Remove garlic and pepper from oven and, when cool enough to handle, remove and discard pepper skin, and chop the flesh of the pepper. Squeeze out garlic cloves and mash in a bowl to form a paste.

6 | Stir garlic paste, bell pepper, carrots, onion, asparagus, and peas into lentil mixture, adding more broth to thin, if necessary. Season with sugar, marmalade, curry powder, saffron, salt, and pepper. Simmer 30 minutes more, until vegetables are soft.

CPF RATIO: 57-25-18

Calories (kcal)	Carbohydrate (g)	Protein (g)	Fat (g)
350	50	22	7

Loaf of Lentil

This vegetarian staple features a crunchy bread-crumb topping. Make it the centerpiece of your meal, and serve with a vegetarian gravy, mashed potatoes, and peas.

READY IN: 30 MINUTES (WITH PRECOOKED LENTILS), OR 1 HOUR (INCLUDING COOKING TIME FOR LENTILS)
MAKES 5 SERVINGS

1⅛ cups green lentils

2¼ cups water

6 slices white bread, torn into small pieces

2 eggs

1 cup vegetable broth

2 tablespoons tomato paste

½ teaspoon dried basil

¼ teaspoon garlic powder

½ teaspoon ground black pepper

1 teaspoon dried parsley

1 tablespoon olive oil

1 packet dry vegetable soup mix

⅓ cup dried bread crumbs

1 Combine lentils and water in a small saucepan. Bring to a boil. Reduce heat, and simmer until tender, about 40 minutes.

2 Preheat oven to 400 degrees F. Grease a 9 × 5-inch loaf pan.

3 In a large bowl, mix together 2 cups cooked lentils, bread, eggs, broth, tomato paste, basil, garlic powder, black pepper, parsley, olive oil, and dry soup mix. Spread into prepared pan.

4 Bake for 40 minutes. Sprinkle top with dry bread crumbs, and continue baking another 10 minutes. Let sit for 10 minutes before serving.

CPF RATIO: 62-23-15

Calories (kcal)	Carbohydrate (g)	Protein (g)	Fat (g)
290	45	17	5

Cuban Black Beans

Serve these flavorful beans over rice, as a sauce for pasta, or with a good loaf of bread.

READY IN: APPROX. 2 TO 3 HOURS IF YOU USE THE BEANS SHORTCUT ON PAGE 118, FOURTEEN HOURS IF YOU SOAK THE BEANS OVERNIGHT.
MAKES 6 SERVINGS

1 pound black beans, washed

1 onion, chopped

1 red bell pepper, chopped

1 green bell pepper, chopped

2 bay leaves

1½ teaspoons paprika

1½ teaspoons ground cumin

1 tablespoon dried oregano

2 minced hot green chili peppers

3 cloves garlic, minced

¼ cup balsamic vinegar

salt and pepper to taste

1 | In a large bowl, soak beans in water to cover overnight. You can also use the shortcut on page 118.

2 | Rinse beans and transfer to a large stock pot. Add onion, bell peppers, bay leaves, paprika, cumin, oregano, and chili peppers, along with water to cover. Bring to a boil, reduce heat, and simmer for 1½ hours.

3 | Test beans for tenderness, and when tender, add garlic and balsamic vinegar. Add salt and pepper to taste.

CPF RATIO: 72-22-6

Calories (kcal)	Carbohydrate (g)	Protein (g)	Fat (g)
145	26	8	1

Black-Bean Hummus

Greg Brown started making this recipe when he worked in a café in At-
lanta, Georgia, and he continues to make it because it's so good. It goes
great with some toasted pita bread. Greg recommends adding a bit
more lemon juice if this hummus tastes like it needs a little extra kick.

READY IN: APPROX. 5 MINUTES
MAKES 8 SERVINGS

1 clove garlic
1 (15-ounce) can black beans; drain and reserve liquid
2 tablespoons lemon juice
1½ tablespoons tahini
¾ teaspoon ground cumin
½ teaspoon salt
¼ teaspoon cayenne pepper
¼ teaspoon paprika
10 Greek olives

1 | Mince garlic in the bowl of a food processor. Add black beans, 2 ta-
blespoons reserved liquid, 2 tablespoons lemon juice, tahini, ½
teaspoon cumin, ½ teaspoon salt, and ⅛ teaspoon cayenne pepper; process until smooth, scraping down the sides as needed. Add
additional seasoning and liquid to taste. Garnish with paprika and
Greek olives.

CPF RATIO: 62-20-18

Calories (kcal)	Carbohydrates (g)	Protein (g)	Fat (g)
98	15	5	2

Black Bean and Rice Salad

This is a simple dish to prepare, and it can be used as a side dish or a main meal. You can add steamed vegetables, sautéed chicken, and even baked salmon to this recipe for variety and some additional carbohydrate or protein.

READY IN: 15 MINUTES
MAKES 8 SERVINGS

2 tomatoes, chopped

1 large red bell pepper, chopped

2 jalapeño peppers, minced

¾ cup lemon juice

1¼ teaspoons dried cilantro

½ teaspoon dried basil

⅛ teaspoon red pepper flakes

1 (15-ounce) can whole-kernel corn;
    drain and reserve liquid

1 (15-ounce) can black beans;
    drain and reserve liquid

1 tablespoon olive oil

½ cup chopped onion

½ teaspoon minced garlic

1½ cups instant or brown rice

salt and pepper to taste

1 | In a large bowl, combine tomatoes, red bell pepper, jalapeño pepper, lemon juice, cilantro, basil, red pepper flakes, corn, and beans. Stir to combine the vegetables, and then set aside.

2 | In a medium saucepan, heat olive oil at a medium-low heat. Add onions and sauté until they are translucent. Add garlic and sauté for another minute. Pour in rice and toss to coat. Add reserved liquid from the corn and beans, along with any additional liquid, to equal the amount of water directed on the rice box.

3 | Cook the rice to package specifications. Let it cool slightly.

4 | Combine the rice and vegetable mixtures. Add salt and pepper to taste and serve.

CPF RATIO: 73-18-9

Calories (kcal)	Carbohydrate (g)	Protein (g)	Fat (g)
315	58	14	3

Butter-Bean Burgers

While there are a lot of veggie burgers in the freezer case of your local grocery store, they're also easy to make at home and much cheaper than the frozen variety. They are great with your favorite toppings. This recipe contains an egg, which helps hold the patties together as they cook but also means it is only appropriate for vegetarians who eat eggs. These burgers are pan-seared in a bit of oil, and it's important to place them on paper towels when you take them from the pan. Patting both sides with paper towels will help remove a lot of excess oil before you place the burger on a bun.

READY IN: APPROX. 25 MINUTES
MAKES 4 SERVINGS

1 (15-ounce) can butter beans, drained

1 small onion, chopped

1 tablespoon finely chopped jalapeño pepper

6 saltine crackers, crushed

1 egg, beaten

½ cup shredded cheddar cheese

¼ teaspoon garlic powder

salt and pepper to taste

¼ cup vegetable oil

1 | In a medium bowl, mash butter beans. Mix in onion, jalapeño pepper, crushed crackers, egg, cheese, garlic powder, salt, and pepper. Divide into 4 equal parts and shape into patties.

2 | Heat oil in a large skillet over medium-high heat; use more or less oil to reach ¼ inch in depth. Fry patties until golden, about 5 minutes on each side.

CPF RATIO: 34-27-39 (WITHOUT BUN)

Calories (kcal)	Carbohydrate (g)	Protein (g)	Fat (g)
117	10	8	5

Easy Stuffed Peppers

This microwave recipe is quick and very simple—a good meal for a busy work week.

READY IN: APPROX. 30 MINUTES
MAKES 4 SERVINGS

2 large red bell peppers, halved and seeded

1 (8-ounce) can stewed tomatoes, with liquid

⅓ cup quick-cooking brown rice

2 tablespoons hot water

2 green onions, thinly sliced

½ cup frozen corn, thawed and drained

½ (15-ounce) can kidney beans, drained and rinsed

¼ teaspoon crushed red pepper flakes

½ cup shredded mozzarella cheese

1 tablespoon grated Parmesan cheese

1 | Arrange pepper halves in a 9-inch-square glass baking dish. Cover dish with plastic wrap. Poke a few holes in the plastic wrap for vents, and heat 4 minutes in the microwave or until tender.

2 | In a medium bowl, mix tomatoes and their liquid, rice, and water. Cover with plastic, and cook in the microwave for 4 minutes or until rice is cooked.

3 | Stir green onions, corn, kidney beans, and red pepper flakes into the tomato mixture. Heat in the microwave for 3 minutes or until heated through.

4 | Spoon hot tomato mixture evenly into pepper halves, and cover again with plastic wrap. Poke a few holes in the plastic to vent steam, and heat in the microwave 4 minutes. Remove plastic, sprinkle with mozzarella cheese and Parmesan cheese, and allow to stand 1 to 2 minutes before serving.

CPF RATIO: 70-19-11

Calories (kcal)	Carbohydrate (g)	Protein (g)	Fat (g)
247	43	12	3

SNACKS AND DESSERTS

Creamy Rice Pudding

READY IN: 50 MINUTES
MAKES 6 SERVINGS

¾ cup uncooked white rice
2 cups milk
⅓ cup white sugar
¼ teaspoon salt
1 egg, beaten
⅔ cup golden raisins
1 tablespoon butter
½ teaspoon vanilla extract

1 | In a medium saucepan, bring 1½ cups water to a boil. Add rice and stir. Reduce heat, cover and simmer for 20 minutes.

2 | In another saucepan, combine 1½ cups cooked rice, 1½ cups milk, sugar, and salt. Cook over medium heat until thick and creamy, 15 to 20 minutes. Stir in remaining ½ cup milk, beaten egg, and raisins. Cook 2 minutes more, stirring constantly. Remove from heat, and stir in butter and vanilla. Serve warm.

CPF RATIO: 81-9-10

Calories (kcal)	Carbohydrate (g)	Protein (g)	Fat (g)
259	52	6	3

Road Trip Cookie

This was one of Chef Greg's first recipes, discovered by virtue of using what was left in his college cupboards. This high-energy snack has been a staple for his road trips ever since.

READY IN: 20 MINUTES
MAKES 5 DOZEN (30 SERVINGS).

3 bananas, mashed
¾ cup butter
1 egg
1 cup white sugar
¼ cup packed brown sugar
1 teaspoon baking soda
2½ cups all-purpose flour
¼ teaspoon ground nutmeg
½ teaspoon ground cinnamon
1½ cups rolled oats
¾ cup chopped walnuts
½ cup raisins (optional)

1 | Preheat oven to 350 degrees F (175 degrees C).

2 | Mix together all ingredients in order given, making sure that butter is well beaten in. You can add up to ½ teaspoon more cinnamon if you like spice. More flour may be added if batter is runny.

3 | Drop by tablespoonfuls on greased baking sheet. Bake for 10 minutes or until edges are slightly brown. Cookies will be soft. Put them in a plastic bag and hit the road.

CPF RATIO: 63-6-31

Calories (kcal)	Carbohydrate (g)	Protein (g)	Fat (g)
203	32	3	7

17

SAMPLE PERFORMANCE
MEAL PLANS

MEAL PLANS ARE AS PERSONAL AS TRAINING PLANS AND MUST be tailored to your individual needs and tastes in order to be effective. By providing meal plans in this book, I only hope to give you an idea of what an effective nutrition program looks like in practice. I've tried to show examples across different sports and different periods of training, as well as across varying body weights, and hopefully one of the following examples will provide some insight into your own nutrition program. As I've done before, I'll encourage you to take advantage of the nutrition-coaching offer on the back page of this book; let the CTS coaches help you apply these concepts directly to your training-and-nutrition program.

Sample Meal Plans

Sample Meal Plan #1

Athlete: 135-pound female cyclist

Training Period: Foundation

Training load: 11 hours/week

Recommended grams/pound body weight:
CARBOHYDRATE: 2.5–3.0 g/lb
PROTEIN: 0.5–0.6 g/lb

	Monday	Tuesday	Wednesday
Sample Training	Rest day	2 hrs cycling with 7 × 10 sec PowerStarts™	1.5 hrs cycling
% CPF	65-13-22	72-12-17	66-15-18
Calories	2,315	2,321	2,194
Carbohydrate (g)	387	421	380
Protein (g)	77	70	88
Fat (g)	59	43	46
Saturated Fat (g)	10	13	12
Fiber (g)	40	31	30

Average Daily CPF Ratio: 65-14-21

Energy (kcal)	2,282
Carbohydrate (g)	385
% Calories from Carbohydrate	65
Protein (g)	823
% Calories from Protein	14
Total Fat (g)	54
% Calories from Fat	21
Saturated Fat (g)	13
Fiber (g)	33

Thursday	Friday	Saturday	Sunday
2 hrs cycling 6 × 12 Stomps™	Rest day	3 hrs group ride	2.5 hrs cycling
59-16-25	66-15-20	66-11-23	63-17-21
2,263	2,072	2,511	2,300
342	359	424	377
90	80	72	102
64	47	64	55
20	6	19	11
30	41	27	30

MONDAY

TOTAL CALORIES: 2,315   CPF RATIO: 65-13-22

Breakfast
1 cup of oatmeal (regular or instant), 1 apple, 1½ cups of orange juice, and ½ cup of skim milk

Morning Snack
1 orange-juice muffin with honey spread, 1 cup of mixed fruit or vegetable juice

Lunch
Cheese ravioli with marinara sauce, 1 medium-sized roll, and 2 cups of mixed-greens-and-vegetable salad (low-fat dressing of your choice)

Afternoon Snack
1 medium-sized bowl of yogurt (plain or flavored) with granola, raisins, and nuts

Dinner
Mediterranean Lemon Chicken (page 298), 1 cup of long-grain brown rice, 2 cups of steamed broccoli, and 2 whole-wheat rolls

TUESDAY

TOTAL CALORIES: 2,321   CPF RATIO: 72-12-17

Breakfast
1 honey-wheat bagel, 2 teaspoons of butter or cream cheese, 1 banana, and 1 cup of fruit or vegetable juice

Morning Snack
1 6-ounce container of low-fat yogurt, any flavor

Lunch

Peanut-butter-and-jelly sandwich (up to 2 tablespoons of each) on whole-wheat bread, 1 piece of fresh fruit, and 1 cup of cow or soy milk

Afternoon Snack/Training Food

1 PowerBar Performance Bar, 20 ounces of PowerBar Endurance drink, and at least an equal amount of water

Dinner

Black-bean-and-roasted-pepper burrito with black-bean salsa and 1 cup of long-grain brown rice

WEDNESDAY

TOTAL CALORIES: 2,194   CPF RATIO: 66-15-18

Breakfast

1 bran muffin with 2 tablespoons of fruit preserves and 1½ cups of orange juice

Morning Snack

1 whole-wheat English muffin with 2 tablespoons of hummus and 1 cup of fruit or vegetable juice

Lunch

Tuna salad with vegetables on whole-grain bread or pita, with 2 handfuls of pretzels, 1 piece of fruit, and water

Afternoon Snack/Training Food

20 ounces of sports drink, at least that much water, and a PowerBar PowerGel

Dinner

Barbecue chicken (4–6 ounces), 1 cup of tomato soup with 1 buttered whole-grain roll, 1 piece of fresh fruit, and 1 ice cream sandwich

THURSDAY

TOTAL CALORIES: 2,263   CPF RATIO: 59-16-25

Breakfast
1 cup of oatmeal (regular or instant) made with a handful of raisins and ½ cup of skim milk; 1 cup of orange juice

Morning Snack
1 banana with 1–2 tablespoons of peanut butter

Lunch
Turkey sandwich with Swiss cheese on whole-grain bread or pita, topped with lettuce, tomato, carrot, and cucumber; a handful of pretzels, and 1–2 cups of fruit or vegetable juice

Afternoon Snack/Training Food
PowerBar Harvest Bar

Dinner
Garlic Chicken Delight (page 296), 1 cup of grilled potatoes, 1½ cups of mixed-greens salad with low-fat Caesar dressing, 1 whole-grain roll

Evening Snack
Bananerberry Smoothie (page 313)

FRIDAY

TOTAL CALORIES: 2,072   CPF RATIO: 66-15-20

Breakfast
1 medium bowl of yogurt with a handful of whole-grain cereal and fruit, 1½ cups of fruit juice

Morning Snack
A handful of wheat crackers and ¼ cup of hummus, 1 piece of fresh fruit

Lunch

Pasta salad with honey-mustard chicken, spinach, and almonds

Afternoon Snack

1 6-ounce container of low-fat yogurt, any flavor

Dinner

2 cups of angel-hair pasta, tossed with olive oil; 1 cup of steamed vegetables, 2 cups of mixed-greens salad with 2 tablespoons of low-fat dressing, and 1 slice of garlic bread

Evening Snack

1 medium-sized piece of strawberry shortcake (angel food cake, 1 cup of strawberries, and 2 tablespoons of whipped cream)

SATURDAY

TOTAL CALORIES: 2,511   CPF RATIO: 66-11-23

Breakfast

1 cup of oatmeal made with ½ cup of skim milk, 1 piece of fruit, 1–2 slices of buttered toast, and 1 cup of orange juice

Training Food

During training, you may need about 36 ounces of sports drink, at least an equal amount of water, two PowerBar PowerGels, and either an energy bar or a fig bar.

Post-Training Food

16 ounces of PowerBar Recovery drink and at least an equal amount of water

Lunch

2 cups of cheese ravioli with marinara sauce, 2 cups of mixed-greens salad with low-fat dressing, 1 buttered whole-grain roll, and more water

Dinner

Grilled beef tenderloin (4–6 ounces), one medium-sized baked potato (topped with a tablespoon of low-fat yogurt), and 1½ cups of mixed vegetables

SUNDAY

TOTAL CALORIES: 2,300   CPF RATIO: 63-17-21

Breakfast

1 medium bowl of yogurt (any flavor) with ½ cup of granola cereal, 1 large banana, and 1½ cups of orange juice

Morning Snack/Training Food

1 energy bar, about 24 ounces of PowerBar Endurance drink, and at least an equal amount of water

Post-Training Food

16 ounces of PowerBar Recovery drink and at least an equal amount of water

Lunch

Tuna-salad sandwich (topped with vegetables) on whole-wheat bread or pita, 1 cup of fruit salad, and water

Afternoon Snack

Peanut butter (2 tablespoons) and honey (1–2 tablespoons) sandwich on whole-grain bread

Dinner

Poached salmon (4 ounces) with cucumber sauce, a whole-grain roll, and 1½ cups of angel-hair pasta tossed with a drizzle of olive oil, spinach, and almonds

Sample Meal Plan #2

Athlete: 135-pound female cyclist

Training Period: Specialization

Training load: 11 hours/week

Recommended grams/pound body weight:
CARBOHYDRATE: 4.0–4.5 g/lb
PROTEIN: 0.8–0.9 g/lb

Average Daily CPF Ratio: 69-13-17

7-DAY AVERAGES

Energy (kcal)	3,152
Carbohydrate (g)	567
% Calories from Carbohydrate	69
Protein (g)	109
% Calories from Protein	13
Total Fat (g)	62
% Calories from Fat	17
Saturated Fat (g)	16
Cholesterol (mg)	117
Fiber (g)	46

	Monday	Tuesday	Wednesday
Sample Training	Rest day	2 hrs cycling with 3 × 3 min PowerIntervals™	1.5 hrs cycling
% CPF	72-12-16	68-14-18	69-14-16
Calories (g)	2,869	3,148	3,173
Carbohydrate (g)	535	555	574
Protein (g)	87	111	117
Fat (g)	52	66	58
Saturated Fat (g)	11	17	17
Fiber (g)	42	38	42

MONDAY

TOTAL CALORIES: 2,869   CPF RATIO: 72-12-16

Breakfast
1 cup of oatmeal (regular or instant) made with ½ cup of skim milk, 2 slices of whole-grain toast with 2 teaspoons of fruit preserves, 1 piece of fresh fruit, and 1½ cups of fruit juice

Morning Snack
1 oat-bran muffin and 1½ cups of fruit or vegetable juice

Lunch
Cheese ravioli with marinara sauce and 2 whole-grain rolls

Afternoon Snack
1 medium-sized bowl of yogurt (plain or flavored) with granola, raisins, and nuts

Dinner
2 cups of chicken-spinach-and-rice casserole, 1 medium baked potato (with skin) topped with low-fat yogurt, and 2 dinner rolls

Thursday	Friday	Saturday	Sunday
2 hrs cycling with 3 × 3 min PowerIntervals™	Rest day	3 hrs cycling	2.5 hrs cycling with 6 × 10 sec HighSpeedSprints™
70-13-18	66-15-20	70-13-16	71-13-16
3,227	3,025	3,171	3,447
585	507	585	628
106	114	111	113
66	68	60	63
8	21	15	21
65	46	48	40

Evening Snack

A handful of graham crackers (approximately 8) and 1 cup of chocolate-raspberry pudding (or flavor of your choice)

TUESDAY

TOTAL CALORIES: 3,148   CPF RATIO 68-14-18

Breakfast

2 cups of whole-grain cereal, 1 cup of skim milk, and 1½ cups of orange juice

Morning Snack/Training Food

24 ounces of sports drink, at least that much water, and a PowerBar PowerGel

Lunch

Chicken-salad sandwich, topped with spinach, on whole-grain bread or pita; 2 pieces (2 x 2-inch squares) of corn bread, ¼ cantaloupe, and 1½ cups of grapes

Afternoon Snack
Bananerberry Smoothie (page 313)

Dinner
Bow-Tie Pasta with Eggplant, Mushrooms, and Goat Cheese (page 287), 2 slices of garlic bread, 1½ cups of low-fat Caesar salad, and 1 cup of skim milk

Evening Snack
1 6-ounce container of yogurt (any flavor) with a handful of almonds and 1 cup of fresh fruit

WEDNESDAY

TOTAL CALORIES: 3,173   CPF RATIO: 69-14-16

Breakfast
Quick Start Breakfast Drink (page 312) and 1 oat-bran muffin

Morning Snack
Peanut butter (2 tablespoons), honey (1 tablespoon), and banana sandwich on a multigrain bagel, and 1½ cups of orange juice

Lunch
Baked Honey-Mustard Chicken (4–6 ounces) (page 299) with 1½ cups of brown rice, 1 cup of mixed vegetables, and 1 cup of fruit or vegetable juice

Afternoon Snack
1 energy bar (or cereal bar), 30 ounces of PowerBar Endurance drink, and at least an equal amount of water

Dinner
Artichoke and Sun-Dried Tomato Pasta (page 280) with 3 ounces of boiled or sautéed shrimp added, and 2 cups of mixed-greens salad with low-fat dressing

Evening Snack
2 cups of fruit or vegetable juice and up to 1 bag (4 cups) of microwave popcorn

THURSDAY

TOTAL CALORIES: 3,227   CPF RATIO: 70-13-18

Breakfast
1 cup of oatmeal with 1 cup of blueberries, 1–2 slices of toast with 2–3 tablespoons of fruit preserves, and 1½ cups of fruit juice

Morning Snack
1 oat-bran muffin and 1 piece of fresh fruit

Lunch
Chicken sandwich with American cheese, ½–1 cup of Black Bean and Rice Salad (page 318), 1 piece of fresh fruit, 1 handful of pretzels, and 1 can of cola

Afternoon Snack/Training Food
1 handful of almonds, 1 piece of fresh fruit, 1 PowerBar PowerGel, 20 ounces of sports drink, and at least an equal amount of water

Post-Training Food
16 ounces of PowerBar Recovery drink

Dinner
Couscous with Roasted Vegetables (page 288), 1 cup of baked sweet potato, 1 large pita, and 1½ cups of soy milk

Evening Snack
16 ounces of fruit smoothie

FRIDAY

TOTAL CALORIES: 3,025   CPF RATIO: 66-15-20

Breakfast

1½ cups of fruit smoothie, 2 slices of whole-grain toast with 2–3 tablespoons of fruit preserves, and 1 cup of cantaloupe

Morning Snack

1 cinnamon-raisin bagel with 2 ounces of Neufchâtel cheese (a lighter version of cream cheese) and 1½ cups of fruit or vegetable juice

Lunch

Tomato Florentine Recovery Soup (page 307) with a slice of whole-grain bread, and 2 cups of mixed-greens salad with low-fat dressing

Afternoon Snack

1 6-ounce container of yogurt (any flavor) with a handful of granola in it, and 1½ cups of fruit juice

Dinner

Baked Atlantic salmon (3 ounces) over 1½ cups of pasta and sautéed spinach; 1 slice of garlic bread

Evening Snack

2 scoops of ice cream (your favorite flavor) with 1 cup of fresh fruit and 1 banana

SATURDAY

TOTAL CALORIES: 3,171   CPF RATIO: 70-13-16

Breakfast

1 toasted cinnamon-raisin bagel with 2 tablespoons of fruit preserves; 1 cup of honeydew melon, 1 6-ounce container of low-fat yogurt (any flavor), 1 cup of green tea

Morning Snack/Training Food

During training, you may need about 36 ounces of sports drink, at least an equal amount of water, two PowerBar PowerGels, and either an energy bar or a fig bar.

Post-Training Food

16 ounces of PowerBar Recovery drink and at least an equal amount of water

Lunch

Black-bean-and-roasted-pepper burrito with black-bean salsa, 1 tablespoon of sour cream, 1½ cups of brown rice, a handful of tortilla chips, 1 piece of fresh fruit, plenty of water, and 1 cup of green tea

Afternoon Snack

1 muffin and 1 piece of fruit

Dinner

Broiled herbed chicken, 1½ cups of brown rice, 1 cup of mixed vegetables, 1½ cups of garden salad, and 1 whole-grain roll

Evening Snack

1 6-ounce container of yogurt (any flavor)

SUNDAY

TOTAL CALORIES: 3,447   CPF RATIO: 71-13-16

Breakfast

Seriously Filling Strawberry Oatmeal Breakfast Smoothie (page 311) and 1 honey-wheat bagel with 1–2 tablespoons of butter or cream cheese

Morning Snack/Training Food

About 30 ounces of sports drink, at least an equal amount of water, 2 energy gels, and 1 PowerBar Performance Bar

Post-Training Food
16 ounces of PowerBar Recovery drink and at least an equal amount of water

Lunch
Chicken-salad sandwich on whole-grain bread, 1 cup of sweet potato salad, and 1 piece of fruit

Afternoon Snack
1 6-ounce container of yogurt (any flavor) with a handful of granola and raisins in it

Dinner
Pasta in a Hurry (page 293) and 1 cup of Tomato Florentine Recovery Soup (page 307), and a large handful of whole-grain crackers

Evening Snack
½ cup of low-fat cottage cheese (any flavor)

Sample Meal Plan #3

Athlete: 135-pound general-fitness athlete

Training Period: Preparation

Training load: 9–10 hours/week

Recommended grams/pound body weight:
 CARBOHYDRATE: 3.0–3.5 g/lb
 PROTEIN: 0.6–0.7 g/lb

Average Daily CPF Ratio: 66-14-20

7-DAY AVERAGES

Energy (kcal)	2,611
Carbohydrate (g)	446
% Calories from Carbohydrate	66
Protein (g)	94
% Calories from Protein	14
Total Fat (g)	60
% Calories from Fat	20
Saturated Fat (g)	13
Cholesterol (mg)	102
Fiber (g)	43

	Monday	Tuesday	Wednesday
Sample Training	Rest day	75 min cardio 40 min strength training, core strengthening, and stretching	80 min outdoor cardio
% CPF	62-13-25	63-15-23	64-14-20
Calories	2,545	2,803	2,726
Carbohydrate (g)	402	454	454
Protein (g)	82	105	102
Fat (g)	73	73	64
Saturated Fat (g)	15	20	19
Fiber (g)	36	35	35

MONDAY

TOTAL CALORIES: 2,545   CPF RATIO: 62-13-25

Breakfast
1 cup of oatmeal (regular or instant) made with ½ cup of skim milk; 2 slices of whole-grain toast with 2 teaspoons of fruit preserves, 1 piece of fresh fruit, and 1½ cups of fruit juice

Morning Snack
1 orange-juice muffin with honey spread, and 1 cup of mixed fruit or vegetable juice

Lunch
Spaghetti with marinara sauce, broccoli, and red peppers, 1 whole-grain roll, and 1½ cups of fruit or vegetable juice

Afternoon Snack
A handful of crackers and 2 tablespoons of peanut butter

Thursday	Friday	Saturday	Sunday
75 min cardio 40 min strength training, core strengthening, and stretching	Rest day	75 min cardio 40 min strength training	120 min outdoor activity and core-strengthening work
63-13-24	72-14-14	69-14-16	69-14-17
2,666	2,439	2,581	2,518
443	451	470	450
93	84	98	93
73	39	50	50
9	9	11	9
51	59	41	40

Dinner

Grilled beef sirloin steak (3 ounces); 1 medium-sized baked potato topped with yogurt; 2 cups of garden salad with low-fat dressing, and 2 dinner rolls

TUESDAY

TOTAL CALORIES: 2,803   CPF RATIO: 63-15-23

Breakfast

1½ cups of whole-grain cereal and 1 cup of skim milk; 1 oat-muffin with 2 teaspoons of fruit preserves

Morning Snack/Training Food

16 ounces of sports drink, at least that much water, and 1 PowerBar PowerGel

Lunch
Chicken-salad sandwich topped with spinach, on whole-grain bread or pita; ¼ cantaloupe, 1 Bananerberry Smoothie (page 313)

Afternoon Snack
1 cup of grapes

Dinner
Bow-Tie Pasta with Eggplant, Mushrooms, and Goat Cheese (page 287), 2 slices of garlic bread, 1½ cups of low-fat Caesar salad, and 1 cup of skim milk

Evening Snack
1 6-ounce container of yogurt (any flavor) with a handful of almonds and 1 cup of fresh fruit

WEDNESDAY
TOTAL CALORIES: 2,726   CPF RATIO: 64-14-20

Breakfast
Bananerberry Smoothie (page 313)

Morning Snack
Peanut butter (2 tablespoons) and honey (1 tablespoon) sandwich on whole-grain bread

Lunch
Baked Honey-Mustard Chicken (4–6 ounces) (page 299) with 1 cup of brown rice, ¾ cup of whole-kernel corn, and 1 cup of fruit or vegetable juice

Afternoon Snack
Energy bar (or cereal bar), 30 ounces of PowerBar Endurance drink, and at least an equal amount of water

Dinner
Artichoke and Sun-Dried Tomato Pasta (page 280) with 3 ounces of boiled or sautéed shrimp added, and 2 cups of Greek salad (greens, olives, feta cheese, oil-and-vinegar dressing)

Evening Snack
1 cup of skim milk and 1 chocolate-covered graham cracker

THURSDAY
TOTAL CALORIES: 2,666   CPF RATIO: 63-13-24

Breakfast
1 cup of oatmeal with 1 cup of blueberries, and 1½ cups of fruit juice

Morning Snack
1 oat-bran muffin and 1 piece of fresh fruit

Lunch
Chicken sandwich with American cheese, ½–1 cup boiled green soybeans, 1 piece of fresh fruit, and 1 can of cola

Afternoon Snack/Training Food
1 handful of mixed nuts, 1 piece of fresh fruit, 1 PowerBar PowerGel, 20 ounces of sports drink, and at least an equal amount of water

Post-Training Food
16 ounces of PowerBar Recovery drink

Dinner
Couscous with Roasted Vegetables (page 288) with 1 cup of baked sweet potato, 2 cups of Greek salad (greens, olives, feta cheese, oil-and-vinegar dressing) and 1½ cups of soy milk

Evening Snack
1 6-ounce container of low-fat yogurt with 1 banana and 1 cup of raspberries

FRIDAY

TOTAL CALORIES: 2,439   CPF RATIO: 72-14-14

Breakfast
2 slices of whole-grain toast with 2 tablespoons of fruit preserves, 1 cup of cantaloupe, and 1½ cups of fruit juice

Morning Snack
1 multigrain bagel and 1 6-ounce container of low-fat yogurt with ½ cup of sliced peaches mixed in

Lunch
Sweet Lentil Soup with Asparagus Tips (page 313), 1 slice of French bread, 2 cups of garden salad with 2 tablespoons of low-fat dressing

Afternoon Snack
A handful of whole-wheat crackers and 1½ cups of fruit or vegetable juice

Dinner
Speedy Gnocchi (page 295) with marinara sauce and 2 slices of garlic bread

Evening Snack
16 ounces of fruit smoothie

SATURDAY

TOTAL CALORIES: 2,581   CPF RATIO: 69-14-16

Breakfast
Seriously Filling Strawberry Oatmeal Breakfast Smoothie (page 311)
and a bagel with 1–2 tablespoons of butter or cream cheese

Morning Snack
During training, you may need around 24 ounces of PowerBar
Endurance sports drink, at least an equal amount of water, and either
an energy bar or a fig bar.

Post-Training Food
16 ounces of PowerBar Recovery drink and at least an equal amount of
water

Lunch
Black-bean-and-roasted-pepper burrito with black-bean salsa, 1 cup of
brown rice, a handful of tortilla chips, 1 piece of fresh fruit, plenty of
water, and 1 cup of green tea

Afternoon Snack
1 oat-bran muffin and 1 large banana

Dinner
Broiled herbed chicken, 1½ cups of pineapple rice, 1 cup of mixed
vegetables, 1½ cups of garden salad, and 1 whole-grain roll

Evening Snack
1 scoop of premium ice cream (any flavor)

SUNDAY

TOTAL CALORIES: 2,518   CPF RATIO: 69-14-17

Breakfast
1 toasted cinnamon-raisin bagel with 2 tablespoons of fruit preserves, 1 cup of honeydew melon, 1 6-ounce container of low-fat yogurt (any flavor), 1 cup of green tea

Morning Snack/Training Food
About 32 ounces of sports drink, at least an equal amount of water, 1 energy gel, and 1 PowerBar Performance Bar

Post-Training Food
16 ounces of PowerBar Recovery drink and at least an equal amount of water

Lunch
Tuna-salad sandwich on whole-grain bread, 1 small baked potato, 1 piece of fruit, and water

Afternoon Snack
1 6-ounce container of yogurt (any flavor) with a handful of granola in it, and 1½ cups of fruit juice

Dinner
Pasta in a Hurry (page 293) and 1 cup of Tomato Florentine Recovery Soup (page 307), 1 large handful of whole-grain crackers

Evening Snack
½ cup of whole-grain cereal, 1 small handful of almonds, ½ cup of strawberries, and ½ cup of skim milk

Sample Meal Plan #4

Athlete: 135-pound general-fitness athlete

Training Period: Transition

Training load: 4–6 hours/week

Recommended grams/pound body weight:
CARBOHYDRATE: 2.0–2.5 g/lb
PROTEIN: 0.6–0.7 g/lb

Average Daily CPF Ratio: 56-17-27

7-DAY AVERAGES

Energy (kcal)	2,029
Carbohydrate (g)	294
% Calories from Carbohydrate	56
Protein (g)	89
% Calories from Protein	17
Total Fat (g)	62
% Calories from Fat	27
Saturated Fat (g)	14
Cholesterol (mg)	88
Fiber (g)	29

	Monday	Tuesday	Wednesday
Sample Training	Rest day	20 min cardio 30 min strength training, core strengthening, and stretching	30 min active recovery
% CPF	56-16-28	54-15-30	58-18-22
Calories	2,057	2,073	2,080
Carbohydrate (g)	294	292	310
Protein (g)	81	83	97
Fat (g)	66	73	52
Saturated Fat (g)	17	15	10
Fiber (g)	32	35	27

MONDAY

TOTAL CALORIES: 2,057   CPF RATIO: 56-16-28

Breakfast
2 slices of whole-grain toast with 1 tablespoon of chunky peanut butter and 1 tablespoon of fruit preserves, 1½ cups of orange juice and 1 cup of skim milk

Lunch
Veggie burger with tomato and Swiss cheese, small portion of french fries, a side Caesar salad, and water

Dinner
Black-bean stew, 2 whole-grain rolls, and 2 cups of garden salad with non-fat dressing

Thursday	Friday	Saturday	Sunday
30 min cardio, core strengthening, and stretching	Rest day	60 min outdoor activity— core strengthening work	Yoga class
61-18-21	57-14-29	53-17-30	54-21-25
1,898	2,050	2,054	1,986
295	304	281	280
84	74	92	108
45	70	70	56
15	10	15	17
23	28	34	25

TUESDAY

TOTAL CALORIES: 2,073   CPF RATIO: 54-15-30

Breakfast
1 cup of oatmeal made with ½ cup of skim milk, 1 medium-sized piece of fruit

Lunch
2 slices of veggie pizza, a side garden salad with non-fat dressing, and 2 wedges of cantaloupe (about ⅛–¼ of the melon)

Afternoon Snack/Training Food
1 piece of fruit, 16 ounces of PowerBar Endurance sports drink, and at least an equal amount of water

Dinner
Chicken enchiladas, dirty rice, 1–2 handfuls of baked tortilla chips, and ¼ cup of fresh guacamole

WEDNESDAY

TOTAL CALORIES: 2,080   CPF RATIO: 58-18-22

Breakfast
1 medium-sized bowl (1¼ cups) multigrain cereal with 1 cup of skim milk and 1 banana

Lunch
Grandma's Chicken Soup (page 309), 1 whole-grain roll with 1 pat of butter, and 1 piece of fruit

Afternoon Snack
1 fresh-fruit tart with about ½ cup of fruit

Dinner
Stuffed Flank Steak (page 304) with 1 small baked potato, 1 cup of spinach salad with non-fat dressing, and 1 cup of fruit juice

Evening Snack
1 medium-sized bowl of yogurt (plain or flavored) with granola, raisins, and nuts

THURSDAY

TOTAL CALORIES: 1,898   CPF RATIO: 61-18-21

Breakfast
1 multigrain bagel with 1 tablespoon of Neufchâtel cheese (a lighter version of cream cheese), ½ grapefruit, and 1 cup of skim milk

Morning Snack
1 cup of orange juice

Lunch
Ham sandwich on multigrain bread with mustard, tomato, and Swiss cheese; 2 cups of hearty tomato soup

Afternoon Snack
1 6-ounce container of low-fat yogurt and ½ cup each of strawberries and blueberries

Dinner
Vegetarian quiche lorraine, 1 slice of bran bread with 1 pat of butter, and a cup of brewed tea

Evening Snack
1 fruit popsicle

FRIDAY

TOTAL CALORIES: 2,050   CPF RATIO: 57-14-29

Breakfast
1 medium-sized bowl of yogurt with 1 handful each of whole-grain cereal, raisins, and nuts; 1 cup of orange juice

Morning Snack
1 piece of fruit (e.g., an apple or a banana) with 2 tablespoons of peanut butter

Lunch
Baked, marinated chicken over long-grain brown rice, sautéed spinach and almonds, 1 cup of fruit or vegetable juice

Dinner
Angel-hair pasta (1½ cups) tossed with olive oil and roasted vegetables, 1½ cups of mixed-greens salad with honey-mustard dressing, 1 or 2 breadsticks

Evening Snack
1 piece of strawberry shortcake with whipped cream

SATURDAY

TOTAL CALORIES: 2,054   CPF RATIO: 53-17-30

Breakfast
1½ cups of whole-grain cereal with 1 cup of skim milk and ½ cup of blueberries

Training Food
16 ounces of sports drink, an equal amount of water, and a PowerBar PowerGel if the workout is hard

Lunch
Chicken-salad sandwich with spinach on whole-grain bread, 2 pieces (2 x 2-inch squares) of corn bread, ¼ cantaloupe

Dinner
Bow-Tie Pasta with Eggplant, Mushrooms, and Goat Cheese (page 287), 2 slices of garlic bread, 1½ cups of low-fat Caesar salad, and 1 cup of grapes

Evening Snack
1 6-ounce container of low-fat yogurt or cottage cheese, 1 handful of almonds and ½ cup of berries, all mixed together

SUNDAY

TOTAL CALORIES: 1,986   CPF RATIO: 54-21-25

Breakfast
1 bran muffin with 1 tablespoon of fruit preserves and 1 tablespoon of apple butter, 1 cup of orange juice

Morning Snack
2 ounces of low-fat cheese

Lunch
Tuna salad in a pita pocket with lettuce and tomato, 1 cup of hearty tomato soup, 1 handful of pretzels, 1 piece of fruit and 1 cup of skim milk

Afternoon Snack
1 apple and 1 handful of mixed nuts or trail mix

Dinner
Spinach and Salmon Fettuccini (page 289)

Sample Meal Plan #5

Athlete: 165-pound runner

Training Period: Preparation

Training load: 5–8 hours/week

Recommended grams/pound body weight:
CARBOHYDRATE: 3.0–3.5 g/lb
PROTEIN: 0.6–0.7 g/lb

	Monday	Tuesday	Wednesday
Sample Training	Rest day	45 min running (moderate pace) 4 strides	60 min running 15 min warm-up, 45 min TempoRun™ (faster pace), 15 min cool down
% CPF	61-17-23	63-14-23	65-14-22
Calories	3,169	3,262	3,454
Carbohydrate (g)	504	524	570
Protein (g)	139	115	121
Fat (g)	83	86	84
Saturated Fat (g)	20	29	30
Fiber (g)	42	48	43

Average Daily CPF Ratio: 65-14-21

Energy (kcal)	3,217
Carbohydrate (g)	540
% Calories from Carbohydrate	65
Protein (g)	113
% Calories from Protein	14
Total Fat (g)	76
% Calories from Fat	21
Saturated Fat (g)	24
Cholesterol (mg)	126
Fiber (g)	44

Thursday	Friday	Saturday	Sunday
45 min running (moderate pace) 4 strides	Rest day	60 min running 15 min warm-up 6 strides, fartlek intervals (5 x [3 min fast, 3 min slow]) 15 min cool down	70 min running (moderate pace)
67-13-20	68-13-19	65-12-20	68-13-19
3,237	2,918	3,285	3,190
543	521	555	560
105	98	100	110
74	64	74	68
22	17	30	17
36	54	41	45

MONDAY

TOTAL CALORIES: 3,169   CPF RATIO: 61-17-23

Breakfast
2 cups of whole-grain cereal, 1 banana, 1 cup of skim milk, and 2 cups of orange juice

Morning Snack
1 cinnamon-raisin bagel with 2 tablespoons of cream cheese

Lunch
Pasta in a Hurry (page 293), 2 whole-grain rolls, and 1 piece of fresh fruit

Afternoon Snack
2 handfuls of mixed nuts and 1½ cups of fruit or vegetable juice

Dinner
Apple and Orange Chicken (page 297), 1½ cups of mixed vegetables, 1 cup of skim milk

TUESDAY

TOTAL CALORIES: 3,262   CPF RATIO: 63-14-23

Breakfast
2 packets of instant oatmeal, 1 cup of blueberries, 1 cup of soy milk

Morning Snack
1 banana (or other fruit) with 1 tablespoon of chunky peanut butter and 1½ cups of orange juice

Lunch
Tuna Burger (page 302), 1 cup of pasta salad, 1 piece of fruit, water

Afternoon Snack/Training Food
16 ounces of PowerBar Endurance sports drink, at least an equal amount of water, 1 energy gel (if necessary)

Dinner
Black-bean-and-roasted-pepper burrito, 1½ cups of long-grain brown rice, ⅓ cup of shredded cheese, ¼ cup each of picante salsa and fresh guacamole

WEDNESDAY
TOTAL CALORIES: 3,454   CPF RATIO: 65-14-22

Breakfast
1 muffin (any flavor) with 2 tablespoons of fruit preserves, 1 6-ounce container of low-fat yogurt, 1 piece of fruit, and 1½ cups of orange juice

Morning Snack
1 multigrain bagel or cereal bar and 1 cup of skim milk

Lunch
Peanut-butter-and-jelly sandwich on whole-grain bread, 1 large banana, 1 cup of fruit or vegetable juice, and 1–2 handfuls of pretzels

Afternoon Snack/Training Food
16 ounces of sports drink, at least an equal amount of water, 1 PowerBar PowerGel

Post-Training Food
16 ounces of PowerBar Recovery drink, cereal bar

Dinner
Spinach and Salmon Fettuccini (page 289), 2 cups of non-fat Caesar salad, 2 slices of whole-grain bread, plenty of water

Evening Snack
1 fruit popsicle

THURSDAY
TOTAL CALORIES: 3,237   CPF RATIO: 67-13-20

Breakfast
Egg sandwich on whole-grain bread, with 2 eggs (cooked as you prefer), Swiss cheese, tomato, 1 teaspoon of butter (for cooking the eggs), and 1½ cups of orange juice

Morning Snack
1 medium-sized slice of banana nut bread and 1½ cups of fruit or vegetable juice

Lunch
Butter-Bean Burger (page 319) on a whole-wheat bun with spinach and tomato, 1 small bag of barbecue potato chips, and water

Afternoon Snack/Training Food
16 ounces of PowerBar Endurance sports drink and at least an equal amount of water, 1 energy gel packet (if necessary)

Dinner
Cashew Crusted Chicken (page 300) over 1 cup of brown rice, 2 cups of steamed broccoli, and 1 cup of mixed-greens salad with low-fat Caesar dressing.

Evening Snack
A handful of graham crackers and 1 piece of fresh fruit

FRIDAY

TOTAL CALORIES: 2,918   CPF RATIO: 68-13-19

Breakfast
1½ cups of bran cereal with raisins, 1 large banana, 1 cup of skim milk (or soy milk), and 1½ cups of orange juice

Morning Snack
1 carrot muffin with 1 tablespoon of blackstrap molasses

Lunch
Black-Bean Hummus (page 317) in a pita pocket with cucumber, romaine lettuce, tomato slices, and 2 ounces of feta cheese; 1 handful of pretzels, 1 cup of fruit salad

Afternoon Snack
16 ounces of fruit-and-yogurt smoothie

Dinner
Speedy Gnocchi (page 295) with marinara sauce, tossed with sautéed spinach and almonds

Evening Snack
6-ounce container of low-fat yogurt with a handful each of granola and blueberries

SATURDAY

TOTAL CALORIES: 3,285   CPF RATIO: 65-12-20

Breakfast
Quick Start Breakfast Drink (page 312), 2 cups whole-grain cereal, 1 cup skim milk and 1 banana

Morning Snack
1 whole-grain bagel with 2 tablespoons of peanut butter

Lunch
Turkey sandwich with cheddar cheese and a bowl of Tomato Orzo Soup (page 305); 1 piece of fresh fruit

Afternoon Snack/Training Food
24 ounces of PowerBar Endurance sports drink, at least an equal amount of water, and either an energy bar or an energy gel, depending on how you tolerate food during harder workouts

Dinner
Artichoke and Sun-Dried Tomato Pasta (page 280), 1½ cups of honey-ginger carrots, and 1 glass of red wine (optional)

Evening Snack
2 scoops of premium ice cream, ½ cup of fresh strawberries, and 1 banana

SUNDAY
TOTAL CALORIES: 3,190   CPF RATIO: 68-13-19

Breakfast
Seriously Filling Strawberry Oatmeal Breakfast Smoothie (page 311) and 2 packets of instant oatmeal (This might be a little heavy if you're going to train within an hour after breakfast.)

Morning Snack/Training Food
20 ounces of PowerBar Endurance sports drink and 1 energy bar (carry an energy gel in case the run is longer than planned)

Post-Training Food
16 ounces of PowerBar Recovery drink

Lunch
Chicken-salad sandwich in a pita pocket or on whole-grain bread, a side of ½–1 cup of Black Bean and Rice Salad (page 318), 1 piece of fresh fruit, and 1 can of cola

Afternoon Snack
16 ounces of sports drink and 1–2 handfuls of mixed nuts

Dinner
Leafy Spinach Lasagna (page 290), 2 slices of garlic bread, 1½ cups of Caesar salad with low-fat dressing

Evening Snack
A handful of graham crackers and 1 cup chocolate-raspberry pudding (or flavor of your choice)

Sample Meal Plan #6

Athlete: 165-pound runner

Training Period: Specialization

Training load: 5–8 hours/week

Recommended grams/pound body weight:
CARBOHYDRATE: 4.0–4.5 g/lb
PROTEIN: 0.8–0.9 g/lb

	Monday	Tuesday	Wednesday
Sample Training	Rest day	50 min running (steady pace) 4 strides	15 min warm-up 6 strides 8 x 400 meters w/2 min rest 15 min cool down
% CPF	69-14-17	72-14-14	68-13-19
Calories	3,769	3,783	3,871
Carbohydrate (g)	674	696	672
Protein (g)	135	139	133
Fat (g)	75	61	81
Saturated Fat (g)	20	18	15
Fiber (g)	54	39	49

Average Daily CPF Ratio: 69-13-17

Energy (kcal)	3,738
Carbohydrate (g)	668
% Calories from Carbohydrate	69
Protein (g)	130
% Calories from Protein	13
Total Fat (g)	73
% Calories from Fat	17
Saturated Fat (g)	19
Cholesterol (mg)	119
Fiber (g)	50

Thursday	Friday	Saturday	Sunday
50 min running (steady pace) 4 strides	Rest day	15 min warm-up 6 strides 10 x 200 meters w/ 1 min rest 15 min cool down	75 min running (steady pace)
68-13-19	72-12-16	68-14-16	68-13-19
3,806	3,445	3,895	3,598
675	644	675	640
127	108	141	120
82	61	69	78
22	13	22	22
56	55	48	51

MONDAY

TOTAL CALORIES: 3,769   CPF RATIO: 69-14-17

Breakfast

2 cups of whole-grain cereal with 1 banana and 1 cup of skim milk, 1½ cups of orange juice

Morning Snack

1 cinnamon-raisin bagel with 2 tablespoons of cream cheese, Bananer-berry Smoothie (page 313)

Lunch

Fresh Asparagus Soup (page 310), peanut-butter-and-jelly (2 table-spoons of each) sandwich on whole-grain bread, 1 piece of fresh fruit, and 1 handful of corn chips

Afternoon Snack

1 cup of grapes and 1½ cups of fruit or vegetable juice

Dinner

Baked Honey-Mustard Chicken (page 299) over 2 cups of long-grain brown rice; 1½ cups of mixed vegetables, and 2 dinner rolls

Evening Snack

3 chocolate-chip cookies (approximately 3-inch diameter)

TUESDAY

TOTAL CALORIES: 3,783   CPF RATIO: 72-14-14

Breakfast

Quick Start Breakfast Drink (page 312), 1 oat-bran muffin with 1 tablespoon of fruit preserves

Morning Snack
1 6-ounce container of low-fat yogurt with 1 handful of granola and raisins, 1½ cups of fruit or vegetable juice

Lunch
Chicken-breast sandwich on a whole-wheat bun, 2 cups of pasta salad, 1 piece of fruit, and water

Afternoon Snack/Training Food
12–20 ounces of PowerBar Endurance sports drink, and at least an equal amount of water. Carry an energy gel in case the workout takes longer than planned.

Post-Training Food
16 ounces of PowerBar Recovery drink

Dinner
Leafy Spinach Lasagna (page 290), 2 slices of garlic bread, and 2 cups of mixed-greens salad with 2 tablespoons of non-fat dressing

WEDNESDAY

TOTAL CALORIES: 3,871   CPF RATIO: 68-13-19

Breakfast
1 cup of oatmeal made with ½ cup of skim milk; 2 slices of whole-grain toast with 2 tablespoons of fruit preserves, and 1½ cups of orange juice

Morning Snack
1 large banana

Lunch
Black-bean-and-roasted-pepper burrito with 2 tablespoons of plain yogurt instead of sour cream, ½ avocado, 2 cups of brown rice; 1 handful of tortilla chips and ¼ cup of picante salsa, and 1 piece of fresh fruit

Afternoon Snack/Training Food

16 ounces of sports drink, at least an equal amount of water, 1 PowerBar PowerGel

Post-Training Food

16 ounces of PowerBar Recovery drink

Dinner

Vegetarian lasagna and a cup of Tomato Orzo Soup (page 305), 1 slice of whole-grain bread, and 2 cups of mixed-greens salad with non-fat dressing

Evening Snack

1 fruit popsicle

THURSDAY

TOTAL CALORIES: 3,806   CPF RATIO: 68-13-19

Breakfast

2 cups of multigrain cereal with ½ cup of blueberries and 1 cup of skim or low-fat milk (1% milkfat), ½ bagel or English muffin, and 1½ cups of orange juice

Morning Snack

1 oat-bran muffin and 1½ cups of fruit or vegetable juice

Lunch

2 butter-bean burgers on whole-wheat buns with spinach and tomato, 1 cup of Tomato Florentine Recovery Soup (page 307) with a handful of crackers; 1 small bag of barbecue potato chips, and water.

Afternoon Snack/Training Food

12–20 ounces of PowerBar Endurance sports drink and at least an equal amount of water. Carry an energy gel in case the workout takes longer than planned.

Post-Training Food
16 ounces of PowerBar Recovery drink, 1 cereal bar

Dinner
Bow-Tie Pasta with Eggplant, Mushrooms, and Goat Cheese (page 287) with 1½ cups of steamed broccoli, 2 dinner rolls, and 2 cups spinach Caesar salad (2 tablespoons low-fat dressing)

Evening Snack
A handful of graham crackers (approximately 8)

FRIDAY

TOTAL CALORIES: 3,445   CPF RATIO: 72-12-16

Breakfast
1½ cups of bran cereal with raisins, 1 banana, 1 cup of skim milk (or soy milk), and 1½ cups of orange juice

Morning Snack
1 6-ounce container of low-fat yogurt and a muffin of your choosing

Lunch
Black-Bean Hummus (page 317) in a pita pocket with cucumber, romaine lettuce, tomato slices, and carrot slices; 1 handful of pretzels, 1 cup of fruit salad

Afternoon Snack
16 ounces of banana smoothie

Dinner
Speedy Gnocchi (page 295) with marinara sauce, honey-glazed carrots and 2 cups of mixed-greens-and-vegetable salad (2 tablespoons of low-fat dressing)

Evening Snack
2 chocolate-chip cookies (approximately 3-inch diameter) and 1 cup of soy milk

SATURDAY

TOTAL CALORIES: 3,895   CPF RATIO: 68-14-16

Breakfast
Quick Start Breakfast Drink (page 312), 1 cup of oatmeal with 1 table-spoon of brown sugar and ¼ cup of raisins; 1½ cups of fruit juice

Morning Snack
1 multigrain bagel, 2 teaspoons of peanut butter and 1 banana

Lunch
Smoked-turkey-breast sandwich on whole-grain bread, ¾ cup of Cous-cous with Roasted Vegetables (see page 288), a handful of tortilla chips, 1 piece of fresh fruit

Afternoon Snack/Training Food
16–24 ounces of PowerBar Endurance sports drink and at least an equal amount of water. 1 energy gel or a few bites of an energy bar. Carry an energy gel in case the workout takes longer than planned.

Post-Training Food
16 ounces of PowerBar Recovery drink, ½ turkey sandwich

Dinner
Cuban Black Beans (page 316) with 1 roasted chicken breast (4–6 ounces), and 2 dinner rolls.

Evening Snack
1 cup of fresh strawberries and blueberries with ¼ cup cream

SUNDAY

TOTAL CALORIES: 3,598   CPF RATIO: 68-13-19

Breakfast
16 ounces of berry-banana-peach smoothie, 1 whole-grain bagel, 1½ cups orange juice

Morning Snack/Training Food
20–30 ounces of PowerBar Endurance sports drink and at least an equal amount of water. 1 energy bar or cereal bar. Carry an energy gel in case the workout takes longer than planned.

Post-Training Food
16 ounces of PowerBar Recovery drink

Lunch
Veggie burger on whole-wheat bun with tomato and provolone cheese slices; medium-sized baked potato or sweet potato, 1 piece of fresh fruit and 1 can of cola

Afternoon Snack
2 cups of fruit or vegetable juice, 2–3 ounces of fig bar cookies

Dinner
Cabbage Soup (page 306), grilled Atlantic salmon (four ounces) over long-grain and wild rice, lightly cooked spinach and toasted almonds, 1 slice of Italian bread, and 1 glass of white wine (optional)

Evening Snack
A handful of graham crackers (approximately 8) and 1 cup of chocolate-raspberry pudding (or flavor of your choice)

Sample Meal Plan #7

Athlete: 180-pound triathlete

Training Period: Specialization

Training load: 9–10 hours/week

Recommended grams/pound body weight:
CARBOHYDRATE: 4.0–4.5 g/lb
PROTEIN: 0.8–0.9 g/lb

	Monday	Tuesday	Wednesday
Sample Training	Rest day	Endurance swim 45 min	Endurance running 80 min
		Endurance cycling 75 min 7 × 3 min Power Intervals™ (These workouts can be done separately)	Recovery bike 1 hr (These workouts can be done separately)
% CPF	67-16-17	70-13-17	68-14-18
Calories	4,146	4,131	4,005
Carbohydrate (g)	717	740	708
Protein (g)	166	139	145
Fat (g)	80	80	80
Saturated Fat (g)	19	15	24
Fiber (g)	64	41	57

Average Daily CPF Ratio: 69-14-17

Energy (kcal)	4,028
Carbohydrate (g)	720
% Calories from Carbohydrate	69
Protein (g)	140
% Calories from Protein	14
Total Fat (g)	79
% Calories from Fat	17
Saturated Fat (g)	21
Cholesterol (mg)	155
Fiber (g)	52

Thursday	Friday	Saturday	Sunday
Rest day	Endurance swim 60 min	Bike/run brick: cycling 90 min w/4 × 5 min ClimbingRepeats™ Endurance run 30 min	Endurance swim 45 min
			Run 40 min 4 × 3 min RunIntervals™ (These workouts can be done separately)
70-12-18	72-14-14	70-13-17	67-13-20
4,054	3,764	3,964	4,130
741	692	720	720
125	140	134	134
86	59	75	94
26	17	23	23
60	41	40	65

MONDAY

TOTAL CALORIES: 4,146   CPF RATIO: 67-16-17

Breakfast

3 eggs (prepared as you prefer: scrambled, poached, hard-boiled, etc.),
2 slices of whole-grain toast topped with 2 teaspoons of fruit preserves,
1 piece of fruit

Morning Snack

1 oat-bran muffin with honey spread and 1 6-ounce container of low-
fat yogurt

Lunch

2½ cups of macaroni, ½ cup of tomato sauce, 1 cup of potato soup, and
2 bran muffins, each with 1 pat of butter

Afternoon Snack

16 ounces of berry-banana-peach smoothie

Dinner

Beef tenderloin (4 ounces), 1 large baked russet or sweet potato topped
with 3 tablespoons of low-fat plain yogurt; 2 dinner rolls, 2 cups of
steamed broccoli, and 1 cup of fruit juice

Evening Snack

1 cup of chocolate ice cream with 1 cup of strawberries and chocolate
syrup

TUESDAY

TOTAL CALORIES: 4,131   CPF RATIO: 70-13-17

Breakfast

1 cup of oatmeal, 1 cup of skim milk, 1 cup of blueberries, ½ cup of raspberries, and 1 cinnamon-raisin bagel with 2 tablespoons of cream cheese

Morning Snack/Training Food

1 banana with 2 tablespoons of peanut butter. If you do part of your training in the morning, you may want to drink about 20 ounces of sports drink and at least an equal amount of water during your workout.

Lunch

Chicken-salad sandwich on whole-grain bread or pita, 1 cup of mixed vegetables, 2 pieces (2 x 2-inch squares) of corn bread, 1–2 pieces of fresh fruit, 1 cup of fruit or vegetable juice, and water.

Afternoon Snack/Training Food

20–24 ounces of PowerBar Endurance sports drink, at least an equal amount of water, and 1 PowerBar or cereal bar

Post-Training Food

16 ounces of PowerBar Recovery drink

Dinner

3 cups of spaghetti with marinara sauce, 2 slices of garlic bread, and 2 cups of mixed-greens salad with 2 teaspoons of low-fat dressing

Evening Snack

1 medium-sized slice of carrot cake with 1 cup of soy milk

WEDNESDAY

TOTAL CALORIES: 4,005   CPF RATIO: 68-14-18

Breakfast

3 blueberry pancakes with maple syrup, 3 strips of vegetarian bacon, 1 banana, and 1½ cups of orange juice

Morning Snack

1 cranberry-orange muffin with honey spread and 1 6-ounce container of low-fat yogurt

Lunch

Tuna-salad sandwich on whole-grain bread or in a pita pocket, with 2 cups of fruit salad, 2 handfuls of pretzels, and 1 cup of fruit or vegetable juice

Afternoon Snack/Training Food

24–30 ounces of PowerBar Endurance sports drink, at least an equal amount of water, and 1 PowerBar or cereal bar

Post-Training Food

16 ounces of PowerBar Recovery drink

Dinner

Penne Pasta with Tomatoes and White Beans (page 285), 1½ cups of mixed vegetables, 2 cups of mixed-greens salad with 2 tablespoons of non-fat dressing, and 2 dinner rolls

Evening Snack

3 chocolate-chip cookies (approximately 3-inch diameter) and 1 cup of soy milk

THURSDAY

TOTAL CALORIES: 4,054   CPF RATIO: 70-12-18

Breakfast

Whole-grain bagel with 2 tablespoons of cream cheese, 16 ounces of berry-banana-peach smoothie, and 1½ cups of orange juice

Morning Snack

1 piece of fresh fruit

Lunch

Veggie burger on whole-wheat bun with tomato and provolone cheese slices; medium-sized baked potato or sweet potato, 1 piece of fresh fruit and 1 can of cola

Afternoon Snack
2–3 ounces of fig bar cookies

Dinner
Cashew Crusted Chicken (page 300) over 2 cups of long-grain wild rice; 2 cups of Tomato Florentine Recovery Soup (page 307) and 1 slice of garlic bread

Evening Snack
A handful of graham crackers (approximately 8) and 1 cup of chocolate-raspberry pudding (or flavor of your choice)

FRIDAY

TOTAL CALORIES: 3,764   CPF RATIO: 72-14-14

Breakfast
Seriously Filling Strawberry Oatmeal Breakfast Smoothie (page 311), 1 oat-bran muffin

Morning Snack
1 medium-sized bowl of low-fat yogurt with a handful each of raisins and low-fat granola; 1½ cups of fruit or vegetable juice

Lunch
Chicken-breast sandwich on a whole-wheat bun, 2 cups of pasta salad, 1 piece of fruit, and water

Afternoon Snack/Training Food
16 ounces of PowerBar Endurance sports drink, at least an equal amount of water, and possibly 1 energy gel

Post-Training Food

16 ounces of PowerBar Recovery drink, 1 cereal bar

Dinner

2 servings of Spinach and Black Bean Pasta (page 292), 2 slices of garlic bread, and 2 cups of mixed-greens salad with low-fat dressing

SATURDAY

TOTAL CALORIES: 3,964   CPF RATIO: 70-13-17

Breakfast

1 cinnamon-raisin bagel with 2 tablespoons of cream cheese, and a Bananerberry Smoothie (page 313)

Morning Snack/Training Food

30 ounces of PowerBar Endurance sports drink, at least an equal amount of water, and 1 energy gel

Post-Training Food

16 ounces of PowerBar Recovery drink, 1 cereal bar

Lunch

Smoked-turkey-breast sandwich on multigrain bread with provolone cheese, lettuce, and tomato; 1 cup grilled new potatoes, 1 piece of fresh fruit, and 1 can of cola

Afternoon Snack

2–3 ounces of fig bar cookies and 1½ cups of fruit or vegetable juice

Dinner

Grilled Atlantic salmon (4 ounces) over 2 cups of long-grain wild rice, lightly sautéed spinach and toasted almonds; 2 slices of garlic bread

Evening Snack
A handful of graham crackers (approximately 8) and 1 cup of chocolate-raspberry pudding (or flavor of your choice)

SUNDAY
TOTAL CALORIES: 4,130   CPF RATIO: 67-13-20

Breakfast
1 cup of oatmeal with ½ cup each of raspberries and blueberries;
2 slices of whole-wheat toast, 2 teaspoons of fruit preserves

Morning Snack/Training Food
20 ounces of PowerBar Endurance sports drink, at least an equal amount of water, and 1 cereal bar

Lunch
Fajita burrito with chicken, black-bean salsa, 1 cup of brown rice,
2 handfuls of tortilla chips, and 2 cups of fruit juice

Afternoon Snack/Training Food
20–24 ounces of PowerBar Endurance sports drink, at least an equal amount of water, and 1 energy gel

Post-Training Food
16 ounces of PowerBar Recovery drink, 1 cereal bar

Dinner
Pasta with Yogurt Sauce (page 286), 2 cups of mixed vegetables, and
2 whole-grain dinner rolls

Evening Snack
3 chocolate-chip cookies (approximately 3-inch diameter) and 1 cup of soy milk

Sample Meal Plan #8

Athlete: 195-pound triathlete

Training Period: Foundation

Training load: 9–10 hours/week

Recommended grams/pound body weight:
CARBOHYDRATE: 2.5–3.0 g/lb
PROTEIN: 0.5–0.6 g/lb

	Monday	Tuesday	Wednesday
Sample Training	Rest day	Endurance swim 45 min	Endurance running 1hr
		Endurance cycling 80 min w/8 x 10 sec Stomps™ (These workouts can be done separately)	Recovery cycling 1 hr (These workouts can be done separately)
% CPF	63-14-23	65-13-22	61-13-26
Calories	3,192	3,251	3,503
Carbohydrate (g)	525	550	548
Protein (g)	116	108	118
Fat (g)	84	81	102
Saturated Fat (g)	20	21	32
Fiber (g)	49	49	42

Average Daily CPF Ratio: 63-13-24

Energy (kcal)	3,313
Carbohydrate (g)	542
% Calories from Carbohydrate	63
Protein (g)	108
% Calories from Protein	13
Total Fat (g)	91
% Calories from Fat	24
Saturated Fat (g)	24
Cholesterol (mg)	117
Fiber (g)	47

Thursday	Friday	Saturday	Sunday
Rest day	Endurance swim 60 min	Endurance cycling 2 hrs w/4 × 5 min FastPedal™	Endurance swim 60 min
		Endurance run 45 min w/drills (These workouts should be done back to back)	
63-13-24	64-11-24	64-11-25	62-13-24
3,184	3,251	3,354	3,491
516	538	555	560
104	96	100	113
86	91	96	96
20	14	27	31
46	55	35	47

MONDAY

TOTAL CALORIES: 3,192   CPF RATIO: 63-14-23

Breakfast
2 cups whole-grain cereal with 1 banana and 1 cup of skim milk;
1 English muffin with 2 tablespoons of fruit preserves, 1½ cups orange
juice

Morning Snack
16 ounces of fruit smoothie

Lunch
Pasta with sautéed vegetables, 1 cup of Tomato Orzo Soup (page 305), 1
whole-grain roll, and 1 piece of fruit

Afternoon Snack
2 handfuls of mixed nuts and 1½ cups of vegetable juice

Dinner
Mediterranean Lemon Chicken (page 298), 1 small baked potato or
sweet potato, 2 cups of Greek salad (greens, olives, feta cheese, oil-and-
vinegar dressing), 2 cups of mixed vegetables, 1 cup of low-fat milk
(1% milkfat)

Evening Snack
1 small-to-moderate-sized slice of apple pie (⅛ or less of the whole pie)

TUESDAY

TOTAL CALORIES: 3,251   CPF RATIO: 65-13-22

Breakfast
1 cup of oatmeal (regular or instant) with ½ cup of raspberries and
blueberries; 1 slice of whole-wheat toast

Morning Snack/Training Food

1 banana with 2 tablespoons of chunky peanut butter; 20 ounces of PowerBar Endurance sports drink, water

Lunch

Fajita burrito with chicken, black-bean salsa, 2 handfuls of tortilla chips, and 2 cups of fruit juice

Afternoon Snack/Training Food

16–20 ounces of sports drink, at least an equal amount of water, and 1 PowerBar or cereal bar

Post-Training Food

16 ounces of PowerBar Recovery drink

Dinner

Pasta with Yogurt Sauce (page 286) with 2 cups of steamed mixed vegetables and 1 dinner roll

Evening Snack

2 chocolate-chip cookies (approximately 3-inch diameter) and 1 cup of soy milk

WEDNESDAY

TOTAL CALORIES: 3,503   CPF RATIO: 61-13-26

Breakfast

1 fruit-and-oat-bran muffin with 2 tablespoons of fruit preserves; 1 4-ounce container of low-fat yogurt (any flavor), 1½ cups orange juice

Morning Snack

1 fruit-and-oat-bran muffin and 1 cup of fruit or vegetable juice

Lunch

Peanut-butter-and-jelly (2 tablespoons each) sandwich on whole-grain bread, 2 fig bars, and 1 piece of fruit

Afternoon Snack/Training Food

16 ounces of PowerBar Endurance sports drink (more like 24–30 ounces if you're doing the workouts back-to-back), at least an equal amount of water, 1 energy bar

Post-Training Food

16 ounces of PowerBar Recovery drink

Dinner

Spinach and Salmon Fettuccini (page 289), 1 cup of mixed-greens salad with non-fat Caesar dressing, and 1 slice of garlic bread

Evening Snack

½ cup of premium ice cream with ½ cup of fresh fruit

THURSDAY

TOTAL CALORIES: 3,184   CPF RATIO: 63-13-24

Breakfast

2 slices of whole-grain toast with 2 tablespoons of peanut butter, 1 banana and 1½ cups orange juice

Morning Snack

1 medium-sized slice of carrot bread with 1 teaspoon of butter and 1½ cups of fruit or vegetable juice

Lunch

Butter-bean burger (page 319) on whole-wheat bun with spinach and tomato, 1 cup of Tomato Florentine Recovery Soup (page 307) with a handful of crackers, 1 small bag of barbecue potato chips, water.

Afternoon Snack
Bananerberry Smoothie (page 313)

Dinner
Spinach and Black Bean Pasta (page 292) with 2 cups of steamed broccoli, 1 cup of mixed-greens salad with 2 tablespoons of non-fat Caesar dressing and 2 dinner rolls

Evening Snack
1 medium-sized slice of carrot bread

FRIDAY

TOTAL CALORIES: 3,251   CPF RATIO: 64-11-24

Breakfast
2 muffins and 1 Seriously Filling Strawberry Oatmeal Breakfast Smoothie (page 311)

Morning Snack/Training Food
20–24 ounces of sports drink, an equal amount of water

Post-Training Food
16 ounces of PowerBar Recovery drink, 1 cereal bar

Lunch
Black-Bean Hummus (page 317) in a pita pocket with cucumber, romaine lettuce, tomato slices, and carrot slices; 1 cup of fruit salad and 1½ cups orange juice

Afternoon Snack
2 handfuls of trail mix (mixed nuts, dried fruit, M&M's, etc.)

Dinner
Speedy Gnocchi (page 295) with marinara sauce, tossed with sautéed spinach and almonds, 1 slice of garlic bread

Evening Snack
1 fruit popsicle

SATURDAY
TOTAL CALORIES: 3,354   CPF RATIO: 64-11-25

Breakfast
1 cup of oat-bran cereal, 1 cup of skim milk (or soy milk), 1 piece of fresh fruit, and 1½ cups of fruit or vegetable juice

Morning Snack
1 muffin with honey spread and 20 ounces of sports drink

Lunch
1½ cups of cheese ravioli with marinara sauce, 1 whole-grain roll, and 2 cups of garden salad with low-fat dressing

Afternoon Snack/Training Food
About 24–36 ounces of PowerBar Endurance sports drink, at least an equal amount of water; 2 energy gels and 1 energy bar, OR, 1 energy bar and either 1 piece of fruit or 1 cereal bar

Post-Training Food
16 ounces of PowerBar Recovery drink, ½ turkey sandwich

Dinner
Grilled beef tenderloin (4 ounces) with broccoli-and-tofu gratin, grilled new potatoes, and 1 dinner roll

Evening Snack
A handful of graham crackers (approximately 8) and 1 tablespoon of peanut butter

SUNDAY

TOTAL CALORIES: 3,491   CPF RATIO: 62-13-24

Breakfast
1 cup of oatmeal (regular or instant) with ½ cup each of raspberries and blueberries; 1½ cups orange juice, and 1 serving of Quick Start Breakfast Drink (page 312)

Morning Snack/Training Food
About 20 ounces of PowerBar Endurance sports drink, at least an equal amount of water, and maybe 1 energy gel

Post-Training Food
16 ounces of PowerBar Recovery drink, a handful of graham crackers (approximately 8) with peanut butter

Lunch
¼-pound hamburger on a whole-wheat bun, topped with avocado slices, lettuce, and tomato; 1 cup of Black Bean and Rice Salad (page 318), 1 piece of fruit, and 1 can of cola

Afternoon Snack
2 cups of sports drink, fruit juice, or soy milk, and 2 big handfuls of pretzels

Dinner
Artichoke and Sun-Dried Tomato Pasta (page 280), 1 slice of garlic bread, and 1 cup of low-fat Caesar salad

APPENDIX: THE CTS FIELD TESTS

The CTS Cycling Field Test

The CTS Cycling Field Test consists of two short time trials, preferably over the same course. This can be the complete workout for most athletes, especially when you include warm-up, recovery between efforts, and then a cool-down. Depending on your circumstances (weather or terrain), these can be time-based efforts (8 minutes in duration) or distance-based (3 miles). I recommend a field test every 6 to 8 weeks throughout the year.

When performing the CTS Field Test, collect the following data:
Time of each effort (mm:ss)
Average heart rate for each effort
Average power (if available) for each effort
Average cadence for each effort
Weather conditions (warm vs. cold, windy vs. calm, etc.)
Course conditions (indoors vs. outdoors, flat vs. hilly, point-to-point vs. out and back, etc.)
Rate of Perceived Exertion (RPE) (how hard you felt you were working) for each effort

You are going to repeat this field test several times throughout the year, and the data you gather needs to be comparable between tests. Repeated field tests establish baseline data that you can use to evaluate training progress. The more consistent you keep your field test location and conditions, the more accurately you can judge your progress over time. Try to reduce the number of variables between tests by using the same course under similar conditions (temperature, wind) every time. The following are instructions for the CTS Field Test:

Step #1: Find/Create a Test Course
Locate and measure, to the best of your ability, a flat, 3-mile course. Ideally, try to select roads that aren't busy, and remember that traffic has the right of way.
Step #2: Fuel Your Body Properly
If possible, don't eat any solid foods for the two hours immediately prior to the test. This helps eliminate stomach upset during the test and heart rate variations due to the foods themselves. However, in the 45 minutes or so immediately prior to effort #1, consume about 16 ounces of a high-carbohydrate sports drink that you are comfortable with. Make sure you record your food intake prior to the field test, so you can duplicate this for future tests.
Step #3: Warm-up
The warm-up should last 10–20 minutes at a minimum, and it should include 2 or 3 high-intensity efforts. These should be 1–2 minutes in length, with at least 2–4 minutes of recovery after each effort. By the end of the effort, you should be physically warm, sweating, and prepared for effort #1. You want about 10 minutes between the completion of the warm-up and the start of effort #1.
Step #4: Begin Effort #1
The effort begins with a standing start. Your gear selection should allow a fast, stable start; not so small that you spin the gear out before you are able to sit down, and not so large that you can barely get it moving. As you gain speed, gradually move to a sitting position and shift into a higher gear.

Step #5: Find Your Ideal Gear
Once you are up to speed, your gearing should allow you to maintain a cadence between 90 and 95 rpm on flat terrain and between 80 and 85 rpm if climbing. Avoid the impulse to "mash," or push a big gear at low rpm. This leads to premature fatigue, which ultimately means a slower time.
Step #6: Achieve Maximum Sustainable Intensity
When you reach a speed that you feel you can barely maintain for the entire time of the effort, settle into a steady breathing rhythm. From this point forward, the effort is going to be challenging. Force the pace all the way to the end of the effort.
Step #7: Collect the Data
Complete the effort, and immediately collect the data listed above. It is also good to record subjective observations that may prove insightful, including your RPE, how hard you started, and how comfortable you felt with the cadence.
Step #8: Recover Between Efforts
Allow 10 minutes of active recovery between the first and second efforts. During this time, ride at low intensity, but high cadence, in an easy gear. Active recovery leads to quicker recovery than complete rest and helps keep your legs warm for effort #2.
Step #9: Effort #2
(Repeat Steps #4 through #7)
Step #10: Cool-down
Once you complete effort #2, the field test is over. Instead of 10 minutes of active recovery, conclude the ride with 15–30 minutes of active recovery. Once you return home, record any additional data, such as course and weather conditions. Good job!

Moving the CTS Cycling Field Test Indoors

Using Your Own Bicycle:

Sometimes, it's not possible to perform a field test outdoors due to inclement weather, lack of a suitable and safe course, or lack of daylight or time. When performing the field test using your bicycle on an indoor trainer, you can perform time-based efforts (two 8-minute efforts) instead. Although you won't be able to use "time" of efforts to determine improvement, you can still at least observe any changes to your average heart rate for each effort. If you have a power meter, then you can still determine if your average watts has improved.

Using a Bicycle in the Gym:

If you're doing the CTS Cycling Field Test in your local gym, you can perform it on a "spinning" bike, like those used in stationary-bike classes. The big difference from using a regular bicycle is the absence of gears. This can make it more difficult to judge the resistance you're pedaling against, especially when you try to repeat the field test at a later date.

Resistance on a "spinning" bike is usually adjusted by turning a knob that increases or decreases the pressure that brake pads are applying to a large, heavy flywheel. You want to set the resistance so you can maintain a cadence of 90 to 100 rpm for the entire 8-minute effort of the field test. In order to accurately repeat the test at a later date, it is important to be able to set the bike up in the same manner. To do this, loosen the resistance knob until there is no resistance against the flywheel. Begin tightening the resistance knob, counting the number of times you completely turn it clockwise.

When performing the CTS Cycling Field Test, collect the following data:
Time of the effort (mm:ss)
Distance covered
Average heart rate
Weather conditions (warm vs. cold, windy vs. calm, etc.)
Outdoors or Indoors
Rate of Perceived Exertion (RPE) (how hard you felt you were working) for each effort

The CTS Running Field Test

The CTS Running Field Test is designed to get an accurate and reproducible gauge of fitness. In a nutshell, it's eight minutes of all-out running. This can be the complete workout for most athletes, especially when you include warm-up, recovery between efforts, and a cool-down.

The following are instructions for the CTS Running Field Test:

Step #1: Find a track
Find a track in your area. If you cannot find a track, pick a stretch of flat road at least two miles long.

Step #2: Warm up
Jog easy for 15 minutes, get a good stretch, and do a few FastStrides™. Make sure your muscles are loose and your lungs are ready (you'll need them).

Step #3: Hammer down
When you reach a pace that you feel you can barely maintain for the entire effort, settle into a steady rhythm. From this point forward, the effort is going to be challenging. Force the pace all the way to the end of the effort. Grind out the eight minutes and go as far as you can. Be sure not to go out too fast and fizzle at the end.

Step #4: Cool-down
Finish with 15 minutes of easy jogging to clear the lactic acid, and then do some more stretching. Record your average heart rate as well as the distance you covered.

Step #5: Collect the Data
Complete the effort, and immediately collect the data listed above. Record the time of the effort to the nearest second. It is also good to record subjective observations that may prove insightful, including your RPE, how hard you started, and how you felt in the last two minutes.

Moving the CTS Running Field Test Indoors

The CTS Running Field Test can easily be moved indoors onto a treadmill. Following a good warm-up, be sure to reset the distance to zero so that you get an accurate measurement for how far you run during the eight-minute test. If you plan on training primarily outdoors, incline the treadmill to simulate a 1-to-2% grade. I've found that doing this leads to results that are more comparable to outdoor field tests. If you're going to be primarily training on a treadmill, it's okay to set the treadmill up flat for the field test. You're going to record the same information as you would from the outdoor field test, and be sure to record the incline setting so you can duplicate the same conditions in later tests.

Using Your Field-Test Data

Estimating the Fuels You're Burning

As I mentioned in Chapter 2, your heart rate can give you a good idea of what fuels you're burning as your exercise intensity changes. Simply take your average heart rate from the CTS Running Field Test, or the higher of the two average heart rates you observed during the CTS Cycling Field Test, and apply that number to the table on page 29.

Calculating Training Heart Rates

When I was working with Lance Armstrong during his comeback from cancer, I wanted to increase the precision of his heart-rate training. Lance could only handle a limited workload, and I wanted to make sure he was using his time effectively. One of my major departures from conventional training methodology was to move away from using widely accepted "heart rate zones." Instead, I began using "ranges" that are much narrower (3 to 6 beats) as opposed to "zones" which I found to be excessively wide (20 beats) for critical workouts.

For example, using a zone system based on maximum heart rate, if an athlete's peak (or "max") heart rate during a field test was 195 beats per minute, and his target training zone was 75 to 85% of max HR, then this would create a training zone between 146 and 166 beats per minute—a 20-beat difference. My experience is that for most individuals, even if the max HR is valid, this "zone" is still much too wide. With a zone that wide, the relative contributions from various energy systems change considerably from one end of the zone to the other. If your goal is to develop aerobic endurance, exercising at the low end of the zone may be too easy, and exercising at the high end of the zone may be too hard.

At CTS, we use average heart rates from your field test to determine heart-rate ranges for interval workouts and heart-rate ceilings for endurance and recovery workouts. From the cycling field test, we use the higher of the average heart rates from the two efforts. Since there's only one effort in the running field test, there's only one average heart rate to use. Below are just a few of the percentages we, and you, can use to establish heart-rate intensities for training. First, take the appropriate heart-rate number from your field test and multiply it by the given percentage to establish the low number of the range. Next, add 2 to 4 beats to determine the high number of the range. For even more information and assistance in applying heart-rate information to training, I encourage you to start working with a CTS coach.

	Adult (<35 years)	Master (≥35 years)
EnduranceMiles™ (cycling)	≤91%	≤88%
EnduranceRun™ (running)	≤97%	≤96%
Tempo™ (cycling)	88% (low) +2–4 beats (high)	87% (low) +2–4 beats (high)
RecoveryMiles™ (cycling)	50–70%	50–70%
RecoveryRun™ (running)	50–85%	50–85%

For example, take an adult whose average heart rates during the CTS Cycling Field Test were 183 (effort #1) and 185 (effort #2). The lower limit of her heart-rate range for a Tempo interval workout would be: 185 × 0.88 = 163 bpm. To generate the heart-rate range for Tempo workouts, add 2 to 4 bpm to 163 (we will add 4). The Tempo heart-rate range for this adult athlete becomes 163 to 167.

I recommend using "heart rate ceilings" during endurance workouts (longer, moderate-paced runs and rides) and recovery workouts (shorter, active-recovery runs and rides) instead of prescribing small heart-rate ranges. These heart-rate ceilings are useful because they provide a specific marker that you should stay under in order to facilitate development of the aerobic energy system. By only providing a ceiling, you have a great deal of freedom during endurance and group-training sessions.

Your goal should be to spend at least 95 percent of the endurance training time below your heart-rate ceiling. For example, if the total run or ride time is 90 minutes, then you should spend at least 85 minutes below the ceiling. It's okay for your heart rate to go above the ceiling sometimes, like during short, steep climbs, etc., as long as these efforts are short (ideally less than 30 seconds), and there aren't too many of them. If you ignore the heart-rate ceiling often, you will hinder the development of your aerobic energy system during the Foundation and Preparation Periods, and that will decrease your performance potential later in the season.

SELECTED REFERENCES AND RECOMMENDED READING

Ball, T., Headley, S., Vanderburgh, P., and Smith J. Periodic carbohydrate replacement during 50 min of high intensity cycling improves subsequent sprint performance, *Int. J. Sport Nutr.*, 5, 151, 1995.

Bland, J. B., et al. *Clinical Nutrition: A Functional Approach,* Gig Harbor, WA: The Institute for Functional Medicine, 1999.

Borer, K. T. *Exercise Endocrinology,* Champaign, IL: Human Kinetics, 2002.

Brooks, G. A., Fahey, T. D., and White, T. P. *Exercise Physiology: Human Bioenergetics and Its Applications.* Mountain View, CA: Mayfield Publishing Company, 1996.

Bucci, L. *Nutrients As Ergogenic Aids for Sport and Exercise.* Boca Raton, FL: CRC Press, 1993.

Burke, E. R. *Optimal Muscle Performance and Recovery,* New York: Avery Publishing Group, 2003.

Burke, E. R. *Serious Cycling.* Champaign, IL: Human Kinetics, 2002.

Coggan, A. R., and Coyle, E. F. Carbohydrate ingestion during prolonged exercise: effects on metabolism and performance, *Exerc. Sport Sci. Rev.*, 19, 1, 1991.

Coyle, E. F. Fuels for sport performance, in *Perspectives in Exercise and Sports Medicine: Optimizing Sport Performance*, Lamb, D. R. and Murray, R., editors, Carmel, IN: Cooper Publishing Group, 1999.

Coyle, E. F., Coggan, A. R., Hemmert, M. K., and Ivy, J. L. Muscle glycogen utilization during prolonged strenuous exercise when fed carbohydrate, *J. Appl. Physiol.*, 61, 165, 1986.

Drinkwater, B. L., Nilson, K., Chestnut III, C. H., Bremmer, W. J., Shainholtz, S., and Southworth, M. B. Bone mineral content of amenorrheic and eumenorrheic athletes. *NEJM.* 311: 277–81, 1984.

Drinkwater, B. L., Nilson, K., Ott, S., and Chestnut III, C. H. Bone mineral density after resumption of menses in amenorrheic athletes. *JAMA* 256: 380–2, 1986.

Duyff, R. L. *American Dietetic Association Complete Food and Nutrition Guide*, 2nd edition. Hoboken, NJ: John Wiley & Sons Publishing, Inc., 2002.

Engall, D., and Hirsch, E., Environmental and sensory modulation of fluid intake in humans. In Ramsay, D. J. and Booth, D. A., editors, *Thirst: Physiological and Psychological Aspects.* London: Springer-Verlag, 382–90, 1991.

Fielding, R. A., and Parkington, J. What are the dietary protein requirements of physically active individuals? New evidence on the effects of exercise on protein utilization during post-exercise recovery. *Nutr. Clin. Care* 5(4): 191–6. Review, 2002.

Fletcher, R. H., and Fairfield, K. M., Vitamins for Chronic Disease Prevention in Adults, Clinical Applications, *JAMA* 287, no. 23, 2002.

Gastelu, D., and Hatfield, F. *Dynamic Nutrition for Maximal Performance*, Garden City Park, NY: Avery Publishing Group, 1997.

Greenleaf, J. E. Environmental issues that influence intake of replacement beverages. In: *Fluid Replacement and Heat Stress.* Washington, D.C.: National Academy Press: XV: 1–30, 1991.

Hoffman, J. *Physiological Aspects of Sport Training and Performance*, Champaign, IL: Human Kinetics, 2002.

Jeukendrup, A. E., editor, *High Performance Cycling*, Champaign, IL: Human Kinetics, 2002.

Koutsari, C., and Sidossis, L. S. Effect of isoenergetic low- and high-carbohydrate diets on substrate kinetics and oxidation in healthy men. *Br. J. Nutr.* 90(2): 413–18, 2003.

Lall, S. B., et al. *Indian Jour. of Exp. Biol.:* vol 37, Feb 1999: 109–16 ref article.

Lin, P. T., et al. *Xenobiotica,* 21 (1991), p. 205.

Martin, W. H. III, Effects of acute and chronic exercise on fat metabolism, *Exerc. Sport Sci. Rev.,* 24, 203, 1996.

Maughan, R. J., and Murray, R. *Sports Drinks: Basic Science and Practical Aspects,* Boca Raton, FL: CRC Press, 2001.

Montain, S. J., and Coyle, E. F., Influence of graded dehydration on hyperthermia and cardiovascular drift during exercise, *J. Appl. Physiol.,* 73, 1340–50, 1992.

National Research Council. *Recommended Dietary Allowances,* 10th edition. Washington, D.C.: National Academy of Sciences, 1989.

Nielson, B., Kubica, R., Bonnesen, A., Rasmussen, I. B., Stoklosa, J., and Wilk, B. Physical work capacity after dehydration and hyperthermia. *Scand. J. Sports Sci.,* 3, 2–10, 1981.

Perron, M. and Endres, J. Knowledge, attitudes and dietary practices of female athletes. *J. Am. Diet. Assoc.* 85: 573–6, 1985.

Physician's Desk Reference: PDR for Nutritional Supplements, 1st edition, Montvale, NJ: Thompson Healthcare, 2001.

Ridker, P. M., Rifai, N., Rose, L., Buring, J. E., and Cook, N. R. Comparison of C-Reactive Protein and Low-Density Lipoprotein Cholesterol Levels in the Prediction of First Cardiovascular Events. *NEJM* 347: 1557–65, 2002.

Romijn, J. A., Coyle, E. F., Sidossis, L. S., Gastaldelli, A., Horowitz, J. F., Endert, E., and Wolfe, R. R. Regulation of endogenous fat and carbohydrate metabolism in relation to exercise intensity and duration, *Am. J. Physiol.,* 265, E380, 1993.

Saltin, B., Costill, D. L. Fluid and electrolyte balance during prolonged exercise. In Horton, E. S., Terjung, R. L., editors, *Exercise, Nutrition, and Metabolism.* New York: Macmillan, 150–8, 1988.

Schmalz, K. I. Nutritional beliefs and practices of adolescent athletes. *J. School Nursing.* 9:18–22, 1993.

Spriet, L. L., and Watt, M. J. Regulatory mechanisms in the interaction between carbohydrate and lipid oxidation during exercise. *Acta Physiol. Scand.* 178(4): 443–52, 2003.

Wardlaw, G. M. *Perspectives In Nutrition,* 4th edition. New York: WCB/McGraw-Hill Companies, 1999.

Wilber, R. L. and Moffatt, R. J., Influence of carbohydrate ingestion on blood glucose and performance in runners, *Int. J. Sport Nutr.,* 2, 317, 1992.

Wildman, R. E. C., and Miller, B. S. *Sports and Fitness Nutrition,* Belmont, CA: Wadsworth Publishing, 2004.

Wolinsky, I. *Nutrition in Exercise and Sport,* 3rd edition. Boca Raton, FL: CRC Press, 1997.

Wolinsky, I., and Driskell, J. A. *Nutritional Applications in Exercise and Sport.* Boca Raton, FL: CRC Press, 2000.

Wolinsky, I., Driskell, J. A. *Energy-Yielding Macronutrients and Energy Metabolism in Sports Nutrition.* Boca Raton, FL: CRC Press, 2000.

Zawadzki, K. M., Yaspelkis III, B. B., Ivy, J. L., Carbohydrate-protein complex increases the rate of muscle glycogen storage after exercise, *J. Appl. Physiol.,* 72, 1854–9, 1992.

Ziegler, E. E., Filer, L. J., Jr. *Present Knowledge in Nutrition,* 7th edition. Washington, D.C.: International Life Sciences Institute, 1996.

ACKNOWLEDGMENTS

Chris Carmichael

To the love of my life, my wife, Paige, how we continue to grow, build, and create new and wonderful opportunities for each other. I am consumed by our love; I love you forever.

To my children: Anna and Connor, you both are wonderful, sparkling balls of life for Paige and me.

I would like to thank all the people who make up Carmichael Training Systems for their dedication to making my vision a reality. Many of the CTS coaches, especially Kathy Zawadzki and the talented coach and chef, Greg Brown, played integral roles in putting this book together. You all are the best.

To Tanya, Stephanie, and all the folks at PowerBar, it was a blast working together; what's next?

Of course, this section would be incomplete without thanking Lance Armstrong and all the athletes I have had the pleasure of coaching over the many years. I cannot imagine a career more fulfilling than this one.

To my mother and father, who were my first and always my best coaches, you have my eternal gratitude. The same is true for my brother and sister, who have always been there for me.

Thank you to Susan Petersen Kennedy, Brian Tart, and Anna Cowles at Penguin Group for supporting this project from beginning to end.

And finally, a very special thank you to Jim Rutberg, my friend and colleague. How you do what you do; I have no idea, but thank God you do! Love ya.

Jim Rutberg

I'd like to thank Chris Carmichael for helping me reach my athletic and career goals, and Kathy Zawadzki for her expertise in, and passion for, sports nutrition. I would also like to thank the incredible group of coaches I have had the pleasure to learn from and work with: Jim Lehman, Craig Griffin, Dean Golich, James Herrera, Mike Niederpreum, Jason Koop, Bryan Bergman, Renee Eastman, Ashley Kipp, and Kate Gracheck. Thank you for helping ensure we didn't forget anything.

A special thank you to Greg Brown for his dedication to creating great recipes for this book. Above all, I thank Leslie Pearlman for her love, patience, and editing skills; and my family for always supporting my dreams.

Thank you to Brian Tart and Anna Cowles at Penguin Group, whose skilled and thoughtful editing was an essential and much appreciated part of bringing this book to print.

Kathy Zawadzki

I am grateful that I was given the opportunity to explore the dynamic relationship between nutrition and athletic performance while a graduate student at the University of Texas. That introduction sparked my career in coaching and sports nutrition. Thanks to Jay T. Kearney, Ph.D., and

Randy Wilber Ph.D., from the U.S. Olympic Training Center, for guiding me in the process of applying scientific knowledge to real-world athletes. And thanks to Chris Carmichael and his team of coaches for providing me the opportunity to share this with athletes.

Special thanks goes to my father, John T. Zawadzki, for providing a life-long example of healthy eating and staying physically active, even before it was in vogue. Above all, I would like to thank my husband, Jon, and daughter, Madeline, for their patience and ongoing support during the long hours involved in the writing process.

INDEX

ABOUT THE AUTHORS

Chris Carmichael is an endurance coach and advisor to Olympic athletes and teams around the world. He is Lance Armstrong's personal coach. In 1999, Carmichael was named the U.S. Olympic Committee's Coach of the Year. That same year, while guiding Lance Armstrong to his first Tour de France victory, he founded Carmichael Training Systems (CTS) to bring quality coaching to elite athletes and other active people. Carmichael lives in Colorado Springs with his wife, Paige, and their children, Anna and Connor.

Jim Rutberg graduated cum laude from Wake Forest University with a BS in health and exercise science. A former elite-level cyclist coached by Chris Carmichael, Rutberg has worked with Carmichael and CTS since 1999. In 2003, Rutberg coauthored *The Ultimate Ride* with Chris Carmichael. Rutberg lives in Colorado Springs with his wife, Leslie.

Kathy Zawadzki is a certified sports nutritionist and a licensed cycling coach working at CTS. Kathy's interest in sports nutrition started while in graduate school, where she did one of the first studies looking at the effect of carbohydrate and protein supplementation on athlete recovery. She has spent the last fifteen years working as a coach and nutritionist to help athletes maximize their training. As the mother of a two-year-old, Kathy also enjoys training and competing as a masters' athlete. Zawadzki lives in Littleton, Colorado, with her husband, Jon, and daughter, Madeline.

Learn more about a limited-time offer of ONE FREE* MONTH
of CTS Fitness and Nutritional Coaching
by going to

www.foodforfitness.net

Just enter the special promotion code:
foodforfitness and that's it!
It's that easy. Start your coaching today!

Questions about this offer:

E-mail your questions to: **askcts@trainright.com**

*A one-time registration fee of $4.95 applies to this offer